WESTERN MATERNITY AND MEDICINE, 1880–1990

W0234865

Studies for the Society for the Social History of Medicine

Series Editors: David Cantor
Keir Waddington

Titles in this Series

1 Meat, Medicine and Human Health in the Twentieth Century
David Cantor, Christian Bonah and Matthias Dörries (eds)

2 Locating Health: Historical and Anthropological Investigations of
Place and Health
Erika Dyck and Christopher Fletcher (eds)

3 Medicine in the Remote and Rural North, 1800–2000
J. T. H. Connor and Stephan Curtis (eds)

4 A Modern History of the Stomach: Gastric Illness, Medicine and
British Society, 1800–1950
Ian Miller

5 War and the Militarization of British Army Medicine, 1793–1830
Catherine Kelly

6 Nervous Disease in Late Eighteenth-Century Britain: The Reality of a
Fashionable Disorder
Heather R. Beatty

7 Desperate Housewives, Neuroses and the Domestic Environment,
1945–1970
Ali Haggett

8 Disabled Children: Contested Caring, 1850–1979
Anne Borsay and Pamela Dale (eds)

9 Toxicants, Health and Regulation since 1945
Soraya Boudia and Nathalie Jas (eds)

10 A Medical History of Skin: Scratching the Surface
Jonathan Reinarz and Kevin Siena (eds)

11 The Care of Older People: England and Japan, A Comparative Study
Mayumi Hayashi

12 Child Guidance in Britain, 1918–1955: The Dangerous Age of Childhood
John Stewart

13 Modern German Midwifery, 1885–1960
Lynne Fallwell

Forthcoming Titles

Human Heredity in the Twentieth Century
Bernd Gausemeier, Staffan Müller-Wille and Edmund Ramsden (eds)

Biologics, A History of Agents Made From Living Organisms
in the Twentieth Century
Alexander von Schwerin, Heiko Stoff and Bettina Wahrig (eds)

Bacteria in Britain, 1880–1939
Rosemary Wall

Health and Citizenship: Political Cultures of Health in Modern Europe
Frank Huisman and Harry Oosterhuis (eds)

Institutionalizing the Insane in Nineteenth-Century England
Anna Shepherd

The Politics of Hospital Provision in Early Twentieth-Century Britain
Barry M. Doyle

Psychiatry and Chinese History
Howard Chiang (ed.)

Stress in Post-War Britain
Mark Jackson (ed.)

WESTERN MATERNITY AND MEDICINE, 1880–1990

EDITED BY

Janet Greenlees and Linda Bryder

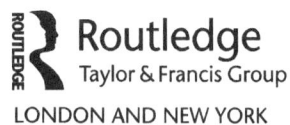

Routledge
Taylor & Francis Group

LONDON AND NEW YORK

First published 2013 by Pickering & Chatto (Publishers) Limited

Published 2016 by Routledge
2 Park Square, Milton Park, Abingdon, Oxfordshire OX14 4RN
711 Third Avenue, New York, NY 10017, USA

First issued in paperback 2015

Routledge is an imprint of the Taylor & Francis Group, an informa business

© Taylor & Francis 2013
© Janet Greenlees and Linda Bryder 2013

BRITISH LIBRARY CATALOGUING IN PUBLICATION DATA

Western maternity and medicine, 1880–1990. – (Studies for the Society for the
Social History of Medicine)
1. Maternal health services – Western countries – History – 19th century. 2.
Maternal health services – Western countries – History – 20th century. 3. Pregnant women – Western countries – Attitudes.
I. Series II. Bryder, Linda editor of compilation. III. Greenlees, Janet, 1966– editor of compilation.
362.1'982'0091821-dc23

ISBN-13: 978-1-138-66300-8 (pbk)
ISBN-13: 978-1-8489-3434-4 (hbk)
Typeset by Pickering & Chatto (Publishers) Limited

CONTENTS

Acknowledgements   ix
List of Contributors   xi
List of Tables   xiii

Western Maternity and Medicine: An Introduction – *Linda Bryder and*
   Janet Greenlees   1
1 Safely Delivered? Insights into Late Nineteenth-Century Australian
   Maternity Care from Coronial Investigations into Maternal Deaths
   – *Madonna Grehan*   13
2 Pregnancy, Pathology and Public Morals: Making Antenatal Care in
   Edinburgh around 1900 – *Salim Al-Gailani*   31
3 'The Peculiar and Complex Female Problem': The Church of Scotland
   and Health Care for Unwed Mothers, 1900–1948 – *Janet Greenlees*   47
4 Taking 'Advantage of the Facilities and Comforts ... Offered': Women's
   Choice of Hospital Delivery in Interwar Edinburgh – *Alison Nuttall* 65
5 'What Women Want': Childbirth Services and Women's Activism in
   New Zealand, 1900–1960 – *Linda Bryder*   81
6 'Twixt God and Geography: The Development of Maternity Services
   in Twentieth-Century Ireland – *Lindsey Earner-Byrne*   99
7 Test Tubes and Turpitude: Medical Responses to the Infertile Patient
   in Mid-Twentieth-Century Scotland – *Gayle Davis*   113
8 Women's Experiences of the Maternity Services in Berkshire and
   Oxfordshire, *c.* 1970–1990 – *Angela Davis*   129
9 From *Muller* to *Johnson Controls*: Mothers and Workplace Health in
   the US, from Protective Labour Legislation to Fetal Protection
   Policies – *Allison L. Hepler*   147

Notes   163
Index   209

ACKNOWLEDGEMENTS

We are grateful to many people who have helped bring this project to fruition. The idea grew out of a workshop held at the Centre for the Social History of Health and Healthcare (CSHHH) at Glasgow Caledonian University, Scotland in April 2010. The initial idea for the workshop arose from a number of conversations and a desire to assess new directions and possibilities for research in the history of maternal health care. That workshop, 'Perspectives on Modern Maternal Health and Healthcare, c. 1850–2000', brought together a diverse range of scholars from a number of countries. It was financially supported by both the Wellcome Trust and the Economic History Society, and we are grateful to them for their support. Despite travel disruptions from the volcanic ash in Iceland, most participants managed to attend at least part of the workshop. Those grounded by the ash ensured their papers could be presented through other formats. The workshop not only highlighted new directions for future research in many areas of maternal health and health-care provision, but many papers posed significant challenges to previous arguments about the development of maternal health care in many countries. Consequently, at the end of the workshop, participants agreed the benefits of collecting papers into an innovative edited volume of studies that challenged current historical understandings of the development of maternal health care. A careful selection of studies from the workshop was supplemented by inviting additional contributions to ensure a coherent volume that covered a range of Western countries. This allowed us to highlight similarities between women's growing expectations of maternity care in Western countries and the many stakeholders who contributed to women's experiences of maternity since the nineteenth century. We are grateful to the workshop participants and the authors in this volume. We would also like to thank David Cantor for both his advice and practical support in putting this collection together.

JANET GREENLEES AND LINDA BRYDER

LIST OF CONTRIBUTORS

Salim Al-Gailani is a Research Associate at the Department of History and Philosophy of Science, University of Cambridge, funded by a Wellcome strategic award in the history of medicine. He completed a PhD at Cambridge in 2010 on J. W. Ballantyne and the early history of antenatal care in Edinburgh. He is currently developing his doctoral research into a monograph.

Linda Bryder (DPhil Oxon) is a Professor of History at the University of Auckland. She teaches the history of health and medicine, and has published widely in that area. Specific interests include the history of tuberculosis, infant health, maternity and women's health in the twentieth century. She is currently working on a history of New Zealand's National Women's Hospital.

Angela Davis is a British Academy Postdoctoral Fellow, Department of History, University of Warwick. She is currently researching the provision and experience of pre-school childcare in Britain during the years 1939–79. Her wider research focuses on motherhood in post-war Britain and Israel.

Gayle Davis is a Senior Lecturer in the History of Medicine at the University of Edinburgh. Her current research examines the social, medical and political response to infertility in later twentieth-century Scotland. Her published work includes *'The Cruel Madness of Love': Sex, Syphilis and Psychiatry in Scotland, 1880–1930* (Amsterdam and New York: Rodopi, 2008) and (jointly authored with Roger Davidson) *The Sexual State: Sexuality and Scottish Governance, 1950–80* (Edinburgh: Edinburgh University Press, 2012).

Lindsey Earner-Byrne lectures in Modern Irish History in the School of History and Archives, University College Dublin, Ireland. She has published on the history of welfare, gender and medicine. Her publications include *Mother and Child: Maternity and Child Welfare in Dublin 1920s–1960s* (Manchester: Manchester University Press, 2007) and several articles and book chapters, including 'Moral Prescription: The Irish Medical Profession, the Roman Catholic Church and the Prohibition of Birth Control in Twentieth-Century Ireland', in C. Cox and M. Luddy (eds), *Cultures of Care in Irish Medical History, 1750–1950* (London: Palgrave, 2010), pp. 207–28, and 'Child Sexual Abuse: History and the Pursuit of Blame in Modern Ireland', in K. Holmes and S. Ward (eds), *Exhuming Passions: The Pressure of the Past in Ireland and Australia* (Dublin: Irish Academic Press, 2011), pp. 51–70.

Janet Greenlees is an Assistant Professor of History at Glasgow Caledonian University, Scotland. Her research interests include American and British employers' provision of health care, environmental health, maternal health care and women's history. Her publications include *Female Labour Power: Women Workers' Influence on Business Practices in the British and American Cotton Industries, 1780–1860* (Aldershot: Ashgate, 2007), as well as articles in journals and edited collections.

Madonna Grehan is an Honorary Fellow in Nursing at the University of Melbourne's School of Health Sciences. She is examining aspects of health care history in nineteenth- and early twentieth-century Australia, focusing on the provision of maternity care. Madonna is the Hon. Director of the Australian Nursing and Midwifery History Project, a web-based resource aimed at raising the profile of nursing and midwifery history.

Allison L. Hepler, a Professor of History at the University of Maine at Farmington, obtained her PhD from Temple University in Philadelphia. In addition to her work on women and workplace health, she has studied labour activism on behalf of worker health and, more recently, the impact of McCarthyism on small-town America. She is also deeply involved in local history where she lives, in Woolwich, Maine.

Alison Nuttall is an Honorary Fellow and former Wellcome Research Fellow in the School of History Classics and Archaeology, University of Edinburgh. Her recent publications include (edited, with Rosemary Mander) *James Young Simpson: Lad o Pairts* (Erskine: Scottish History Press, 2011), and 'Maternity Charities, the Edinburgh Maternity Scheme and the Medicalisation of Childbirth, 1900–1925', *Social History of Medicine*, 24:2 (August 2011), pp. 370–88. She has also contributed the nineteenth-century midwifery sections to A. Borsay and B. Hunter (eds), *Nursing and Midwifery in Britain Since 1700* (Basingstoke: Palgrave Macmillan, 2012) and a report on professional self-regulation for the Nursing and Midwifery Council.

LIST OF TABLES

Table 3.1: Occupations of the women admitted to the Church of
Scotland's home for unwed mothers, 1915–17   53

WESTERN MATERNITY AND MEDICINE:
AN INTRODUCTION

Linda Bryder and Janet Greenlees

The period 1880–1990 saw dramatic transformations in women's experiences of pregnancy and childbirth in the Western world. The most prominent was the change of location of childbirth, from the home to the hospital. This era also saw the establishment and public acceptance of scientific medicine in Western society, including infertility, antenatal and childbirth services. In the twentieth century the health of mothers as well as their newborn babies became the subject of much political and public concern and attention. From the 1930s, there was a steep and constant decline in maternal mortality and later in perinatal mortality. The relationship between all these changes has been the subject of immense historical analysis, with authors adopting very different perspectives, and the ways in which the narrative has been told has altered markedly in line with the wider social and cultural changes of the late twentieth century. Much of the writing from the 1970s came from a feminist political perspective. The vast expansion of the discipline of the history of medicine over subsequent decades has seen others enter the field from a less ideological perspective. The authors of this volume fall into the latter category. Whilst drawing on that earlier literature (outlined below), these essays offer fresh perspectives, contributing to a broader, more nuanced understanding of the cultural, social and political history of pregnancy and childbirth in the modern Western world. They do not seek to cover all Western countries or all periods, but focus on particular aspects of the story, through a case study approach, to pose questions about women's experiences at this important time in their lives and the factors which influenced those experiences. The subjects of the volume are the various stakeholders in childbirth services – women, midwives, physicians, governments and the voluntary sector – as well as the broader ideological and religious concerns that underlay the services provided, and how these stakeholders and concerns have shaped women's experiences of childbirth.

Feminism and Women's Agency

In 1960 Sir Dugald Baird, Regius Professor of Midwifery and Gynaecology, University of Aberdeen, delivered a lecture on 'The Evolution of Modern Obstetrics'. He began by explaining that in Glasgow forty years earlier, when he was a medical student, 'childbirth was a dangerous and wasteful process'. He proceeded to explain the 'advances' since then, noting that 'in many areas the maternal death-rate has now almost reached an irreducible minimum'. Those advances included sulphonamides and penicillin for puerperal sepsis, once the major cause of death in childbirth, blood-transfusion services for haemorrhage, and improved ante-natal care for eclamptic toxaemia. In his view, high death rates had not only been due to inadequate treatment methods, but also 'the lack of a well-organized maternity service staffed by well-trained doctors and midwives'.[1] The trajectory for him was one of scientific progress, professionalization and social reform.

Two decades later, medical sociologist Ann Oakley presented a very different account of the history of obstetrics. Calling her 1984 book *The Captured Womb*, she sought to explain the evolution of antenatal care and obstetrical intervention as a 'strategy for the social control of women'.[2] Whilst she acknowledged that 'in the battle to prevent every fatality that is conceivably preventable, medical antenatal care must be counted as an essential ally',[3] she nevertheless labelled obstetricians and the State as 'misogynist', and explained how 'womanhood and motherhood have become a battlefield for not only patriarchal but professional supremacy'.[4]

Oakley's book was both part of and a contribution to a new approach to the history of Western medicine more broadly. The move away from a celebratory approach to medical history occurred with the introduction of social history or what was called 'history from below' into university history departments from the 1970s and with it a new interest in women's history. In the introduction to her groundbreaking 1986 history of childbirth, *Brought to Bed: Childbearing in America 1750–1950*, Judith Walzer Leavitt explained, 'This book focuses on the phenomenon of birth precisely because of its centrality to women's lives. By understanding childbirth we can understand significant parts of the female experience'.[5]

Leavitt's study included an analysis of diaries, letters and autobiographies, from which she concluded that women were active agents of change in American childbirth history until childbirth moved to the hospital in the twentieth century. Then, women lost control over the birthing experience to the medical profession, 'and began their quest, continuing today, to recover some of that control'.[6] This statement indicates how her interpretation, like that of Ann Oakley, was rooted in the modern social and political movement of feminism. The new women's health movement had been heralded by the Boston Women's Health Collective's handbook, *Our Bodies, Ourselves*, which from its first edition in 1971 urged women to assume greater control over all aspects of their bodies and lives, including pregnancy and birth. The dominant feminist view of childbirth in the 1970s was summarized by American feminist academic Sheryl Ruzek who claimed in 1978 that,

> obstetrician-gynecologists fight to keep delivery their exclusive domain, even if it requires transforming what might be otherwise normal births into surgical events. In the hospital – particularly in the delivery room – the obstetrician can become the star of the obstetrical drama. Deferred to and waited on by nurses and other lower-status personnel, physicians enjoy their status and omnipotence.[7]

The new women's health movement, particularly prominent in America, quickly spread around the Western world.[8]

New histories of childbirth were also influenced by sociological studies of professions and professionalization, and concepts of power and social control as expounded by Michel Foucault. Significantly Oakley, who drew heavily on Foucault, was herself a sociologist rather than an historian, as was William Ray Arney, a much-cited contemporary writer on the rise of the profession of obstetrics in America.[9] Jane Lewis was another sociologist who turned her attention to history to explain 'the politics of motherhood', the title of her formative 1980 monograph.[10] But, whereas Oakley demonized the medicalization of childbirth, Lewis had a more nuanced account that gave women more agency.

The point can be made by looking at the conclusion of Lewis's chapter on the hospitalization of childbirth in Britain where she referred to the tendency among 'some present-day sociologists and feminists ... [to] dismiss all aspects of hospitalised childbirth as bad'. She cautioned that, 'Looking at the inter-war period, when the trend towards hospitalisation accelerated so rapidly, it is not so easy to reach such a clear-cut conclusion'. Doctors working in midwifery

> saw the chance to make the changes they honestly believed necessary ... Besides, the clinical causes of maternal death did need investigation and sepsis in particular did require more stringent aseptic and antiseptic procedures. Women themselves recognised this and supported more medicalised management of childbirth.[11]

Ten years later, she went further and argued after surveying records of the early twentieth-century Women's Cooperative Guild:

> What is clear is that women of all social classes in the early twentieth century expressed fear of childbirth in terms of both the pain and the considerable chance of subsequent health problems. Their fears were real and arose directly from the conditions of maternity they experienced. When these are understood, their demand for hospital births becomes readily comprehensible.[12]

Despite this recognition of women's agency, she still argued, however, that, 'The move to hospital births was dictated more by professional developments and the changing status of obstetrics as a specialty than by women's campaigns, although the latter were invoked to legitimize the change'.[13] Significantly she declared, 'Ann Oakley is probably correct when she argues that the wombs of women are containers to be captured by ideologies'.[14]

Oakley's imagery of the captured womb proved to be a powerful and enduring one. In the case of America, anthropologist E. Davis-Floyd explained in 1992 that she had journeyed through American feminist writings on birth and the women's health movement, including studies by Suzanne Arms, Gena Corea, Barbara Ehrenreich and Deirdre English, Michelle Harrison, Emily Martin, Adrienne Rich, Diana Scully, Nancy Stoller Shaw and Barbara Katz Rothman.[15] She believed these writers 'explosively and consistently exposed the intense patriarchal bias in the American Way of Birth and in the medical treatment of women and their bodies'. Yet, she continued,

> the more I immersed myself in these works and their point of view, the more I was forced to notice the dissonance between this feminist critique of birth and the beliefs, desires, reactions, and behaviors of the women I was interviewing ... I have therefore tried in this book to move beyond the perspective that sees women's choices for birth technology as 'false consciousness' waiting for the feminist conversion.[16]

Yet, as Wendy Mitchinson later pointed out in her 2002 history of childbirth in Canada, while Davis-Floyd did not blame women for making the choices they did, she still suggested a 'cultural determinism that lessens recognition of women's agency'.[17] In her 2009 history of anaesthesia in America, Jacqueline Wolf provides much evidence from the lay press and women's magazines of women making choices relating to childbirth procedures over time, but still lectures them that 'Ultimately, the normalization of obstetric anesthesia has taught women to view themselves as helpless victims of a bodily process rather than as the most important participants in that process'.[18]

In her 1995 'critical history of maternity care' in Britain, Marjorie Tew did not even consider the possibility of women's agency. She argued that women were indoctrinated by doctors to go to the hospital to give birth rather than stay home: 'In the sphere of maternity care the obstetricians' objective was to make their profession the sole repository of confidence. To achieve this objective required an unremitting campaign of propaganda'.[19] Further, she claimed of the obstetrician,

> He reasserts his superiority most emphatically when he cuts open the womb and extracts the baby without any co-operation from the mother, an intervention apparently so deeply satisfying to the operator that, now that its danger to life is relatively small, is imposed on ever slighter pretexts.[20]

Building on this interpretation in her 1998 study of the history of childbirth in Ireland, Jo Murphy-Lawless also explored the motives of the male obstetrical profession, explaining how 'what the practitioners fear is losing control over childbirth and part of their response is to try to frighten women by raising the possibility of death'.[21] She believed that 'Over the last 250 years, the desire to administer and control life has been embedded in obstetric medicine', and she referred to the 'problem of male power over the body, our female bodies, and of the corresponding diminution of our sense of autonomy and control, of what can be termed our personal agency'.[22] Explaining the historiography since the 1970s, she wrote,

> writers have converged around the convincing thesis that male medical control of childbirth has disempowered women as mothers and as care-givers, principally through its argument that childbirth is full of risks and danger, that it is pathological and thus requires the medical expert to oversee the event.[23]

This historiography extended around the Western world, including New Zealand where two late twentieth-century histories certainly embraced this thesis.[24]

Thus the dominant understanding of the history of childbirth, emerging from the social history and feminist movements of the 1970s, was one of progressive male domination and oppression or disempowerment of women. In her 2003 overview of childbirth and maternity in the twentieth century Hilary Marland noted that 'The Twilight Sleep phenomenon is interesting because it shows that demand for intervention did not necessarily come from doctors, but could result from the vigorous campaigns of women's groups'. Why does Marland find this 'interesting'? She does not say, but presumably because it upsets the paradigm, the conventional (feminist) wisdom of doctors forcing interventions on women. This shows how pervasive the literature has been.[25]

Yet Marland and others have attempted to uncover agency among childbearing women. In their 1992 edited volume, Valerie Fildes, Lara Marks and Hilary Marland explained in the introduction that the essays investigated the 'many actors who were involved in conceiving and implementing programmes [relating to maternal and infant welfare]: women's organisations, local voluntary associations, doctors, midwives, health visitors and public health administrators, local and national governments'.[26] In her 1996 study of London's 'metropolitan maternity', Marks came to her subject matter from this angle. As she explained in her introduction, she focused on initiatives from local voluntary groups, political pressure groups and labour organizations, as well as the efforts of individual women themselves. She found the 'voices and demands [of users] had a profound influence on the facilities provided, a factor which is all too often overlooked by historians'.[27] Around the same time, Susan Williams investigated the part played by the National Birthday Trust Fund in reforming childbirth services in Britain from 1928 to 1993,[28] and in Australia Kerreen Reiger studied the influence of voluntary women's organizations on childbirth reform from the 1950s to the 1990s.[29]

Such attempts to address mothers' agency in a meaningful way and move away from victimization theories have been further developed in this volume. Indeed, in this volume we are tackling the old victimization theories head-on, in part because, as we have indicated, they persist in historical scholarship despite efforts to challenge them. In her chapter on interwar Edinburgh, Alison Nuttall utilizes hospital case books from a range of Edinburgh's voluntary maternity hospitals in the 1920s and 1930s to examine the move to hospital birth, and concludes that far from being forced into hospital by male doctors, women made rational choices when they opted for hospitalized birth, based on experience of care and rest offered in the institutions.[30] Like Lara Marks in London, Linda Bryder considers the lobbying by women's groups in New Zealand and shows how they persuaded the government to provide free hospitalized childbirth there in 1938, and also how women's groups kept up the pressure to influence hospital policy in their interests once hospital childbirth became the norm in the 1950s. Discussing the move to hospital births in Ireland, Lindsey Earner-Byrne stresses the role of health visitors as advocates for improved maternal care, and argues, 'The motivation for this advice was largely practical: poor mothers might get better food in hospital and some much needed rest'.

Angela Davis also brings women's voices to the fore in her chapter in this volume. Drawing on seventy oral history interviews with women from Berkshire and Oxfordshire, she focuses on women's accounts of their childbirth experiences, and in particular their views of the modern obstetrical interventions of the 1970s, including ultrasound scans, episiotomy, induction, epidural anaesthesia and caesarean section. She found a great diversity of views amongst the mothers she interviewed, and concludes that it was not medical interventions *per se* that formed the basis of most of their complaints, but rather hospital routines and insensitive staff, whose number included nurses and midwives as well as doctors.[31] She makes the important point that historical accounts of maternity care which have focused simply on what was being done to women miss the importance of subjective factors such as their knowing and liking the person who was doing it. One of the topics she investigated was women's attitudes to home birth. She found her interviewees expressed very different attitudes from those in the contemporary literature from the activist voluntary organization, the National Childbirth Trust, with the oral history material less supportive of home birth and more critical of ideas about natural childbirth more generally. Very few women recalled wanting home births but being prevented by doctors, or that the fear of medical complications stopped them choosing a home birth.

Midwifery Marginalized

Another strand in writing the history of childbirth since the 1970s, apart from the narratives of oppression of women by male obstetricians, has been that of the undermining of midwives. This thesis also emerged from gender studies and the

1970s feminist movement. American writers Barbara Ehrenreich and Deirdre English, in *Witches, Nurses and Midwives* (1973), portrayed American obstetricians as 'self-serving individuals who "had no real commitment to improved obstetrical care", and who systematically sought to outlaw midwifery in order to gain a monopoly over this potentially lucrative field of practice'.[32]

In her 1977 history of the 'struggle for the control of childbirth', as she described it, Jean Donnison plotted the undermining of the traditional English midwife from the eighteenth century, which culminated in the 1902 Midwives Act, placing them in a 'uniquely disadvantaged position among the professions',[33] totally disempowered by the 'obstetrical Establishment'.[34] Donnison urged the 'restoration and development of the midwife as an independent practitioner in her own right, acting truly as the "with-women" to the mother, rather than as a machine-minder to the obstetrical engineer'.[35]

Tew explained the policy of hospitalization of childbirth thus:

> The policy of the increasing hospitalisation of birth advocated by doctors, allegedly to improve the welfare of mothers and babies, was in fact a very effective means of gaining competitive advantage by reducing the power and status of midwives and confirming the doctors' ascendancy over their professional rivals [and as a] promising gateway to assuring their [doctors'] social importance.[36]

Some historians have attempted to contextualize the changes, rather than frame the demise of midwives as a result of male domination. For instance, Charlotte Borst wrote in her 1995 history of childbirth in Wisconsin that midwives there 'were not pushed out of practice by elitist or misogynist obstetricians. Instead, their traditional, artisanal skills ceased to be valued by a society that had come to embrace the model of disinterested, professionalized science'.[37] Women, like men, embraced science as modern and progressive, and Borst clearly felt the need to stress that the situation was more complex, or less conspiratorial, than some historical accounts might suggest.

In the understanding of the historical contest between the doctor and the midwife, the latter found a surprising ally in retired British general practitioner-turned-historian, Irvine Loudon. Loudon later explained that when he undertook the research for his 1992 history *Death in Childbirth*, covering the period 1800 to 1950, 'I found that I arrived at a conclusion I had not expected'. Just as Professor Thomas McKeown had challenged the 'role of medicine' in bringing about the major improvements in life expectancy in Britain during the nineteenth and twentieth centuries, by carrying out a major historical epidemiological study,[38] Loudon performed the same conceptual transformation for the history of childbirth. Loudon found that the professionalization of obstetrics from the late nineteenth century to the mid-twentieth century did not correlate with an improvement in the chances of survival for women in childbirth. He found in the early twentieth century it was safer for women to be attended by midwives in childbirth than by doctors, as the former were less likely to intervene. Yet, significantly, as he later explained, this was not necessarily the traditional midwife, the demise of which was lamented by some feminist and other historians. He explained,

> Between 1850 and World War II, the lowest rates of maternal mortality were found in those countries, regions or areas in which maternity services were based largely or wholly on *trained* midwives. I found no exceptions, but it was also clear that the success of midwives was dependent not only on effective training, but also on being accepted and respected as professionals by the communities they served, and preferably by the medical profession as well. It was also important that where possible the midwife should be able to obtain skilled obstetric assistance rapidly when complications arose. But the unexpected finding was that even where such help was unavailable or available only with great difficulty ... it was still possible for trained midwives to provide a maternity service with a very low rate of mortality compared with national rates before World War II.[39]

Thus he found that midwives were effective health practitioners but he also considered it important to stress that he meant *trained* midwives. Mitchinson has argued that there has been a tendency in much of the literature to romanticize traditional home birth.[40] When Leavitt explained women's preference for the 'modern practices in the birthing rooms of medical science', she added that women also wanted to incorporate into that regime the 'psychologically comforting practices of their traditional birthing rooms'.[41] This was an imagined past.

In this volume, using Melbourne, Australia, as a case study, Madonna Grehan explores the reality of home birth before the twentieth century. In doing so, she builds on her 2009 PhD thesis in which she argued that midwives themselves embraced the changes to their regulation and education in the early twentieth century, rather than viewing them as a subordination process to the medical profession. Through their professional training they purposely distanced themselves from the image of the traditional untrained midwife with her domestic work status.[42] In her chapter in this volume, Grehan utilizes coronial inquests into maternal deaths in an age of truly 'natural' childbirth, i.e. before the advent of modern technologies of care. These inquests show how many of the attendants were ill-equipped to deal with the exigencies of labour, where things could go wrong very quickly. In this context, it was perhaps unsurprising that women welcomed the introduction of trained birth attendants and the shift of childbirth to the hospital.

Just as Loudon highlighted the importance of trained midwives and their acceptance as legitimate practitioners in their communities, so too does Janet Greenlees. Greenlees discovers that the key to success of the maternity home in Glasgow which she studied was the presence of the midwifery-trained matron, who was highly respected by medical practitioners and patients alike. Lindsey Earner-Byrne also cites Loudon that it was 'not the site of delivery but the morale and the standard of co-operation and integration between all concerned in maternal care' that was crucial to maternal mortality in twentieth-century Ireland,[43] and notes in that respect that rural Irish women were distinctly disadvantaged. As she puts it: 'Women outside of Dublin who could not (or did not wish to) pay for private care depended on a haphazard and poorly funded system that varied significantly from county to county'.

The Return of the Physician

At the same time, in the history of women's experiences of childbirth we cannot ignore the efforts, motivations and opinions of the health practitioners who care for them while pregnant, during, and after birth. Turning her attention to physicians, Wendy Mitchinson cautioned in her 2002 history that, 'Just as women exhibited agency, physicians experienced constraints in their practice, although feminist scholars have not been quite as willing to detail them'.[44] Mitchinson is one modern feminist historian who argued that women had agency, that childbirth services were negotiated rather than imposed.[45] But her major contribution was to introduce the study of physicians as legitimate subjects of inquiry for social historians of childbirth, without condemning them or characterizing them as motivated only by money and/or power. Focusing on the medical profession is not to be an apologist for doctors, nor is it a return to the old celebratory histories. Rather it is, as she explained, a serious attempt to understand 'how doctors worked in their world'.[46] In this way, Mitchinson also reflects the modern trends in social history which are represented in this book. In her chapter, Bryder shows how sometimes women could form alliances with doctors in their quest for improved maternity services. The latter were not necessarily dismissed as the 'enemy' as some historical accounts have intimated.

Salim Al-Gailani makes no apologies, and nor should he, for focusing his attention on the 'career and the professional, scientific, evangelical and political influences' on the early twentieth-century Scottish medical professional, John William Ballantyne. Al-Gailani examines the environment in which Ballantyne worked, comparing the 'pre-maternity' practices of Edinburgh's Royal Maternity Hospital (RMH) where Ballantyne was based, and the Lauriston Home for unmarried mothers. The latter served a social function, whereas the former became a site for 'systematic investigation of antenatal morbid states' under Ballantyne, whose patients became experimental subjects.[47] Yet, Al-Gailani does not portray this in a negative light of male domination of these pregnant women; rather he proceeds to show how they influenced the development of broader antenatal services at a regional and national level.

In contrast to Al-Gailani, Gayle Davis presents a darker side of medical attitudes towards maternity in her account of how doctors in mid-twentieth-century Scotland characterized and treated infertile patients. Such was the concern engendered by this subject that a Departmental Committee was appointed in 1958 to investigate infertility and its treatment through artificial insemination. Davis analyses medical testimony to that committee, as well as clinical records from the Royal Infirmary of Edinburgh out-patient infertility clinic, to gain insight into medical thinking and practices relating to infertility. Crucially, she argues that not only did physicians regard women who sought artificial insemination as somehow exhibiting a pathological version of the maternal drive, they were equally critical of sperm donors and husbands who 'allowed' their partners to seek treatment. Davis reminds us that if women's experience of maternity could be pathologized by physicians, so too could men's experiences. She also hints at another stakeholder group that helped to shape women's experiences of maternity and childbirth – men, as husbands, partners, and in this case sperm donors. This book is unable to more fully explore these issues, nor to look more at other family members – children, mothers and other relatives – who also shaped experiences of maternity.[48]

Religion and Rights

So far we have suggested that women's experiences of maternity and childbirth were shaped by a variety of stakeholders – including women, midwives and physicians – and that the story is more complicated than some early feminists and others have suggested. However, if we want to explore how women's experiences were shaped by stakeholders, we also want to explore how stakeholder's views were shaped by broader social, political and cultural concerns, notably those concerning religion and rights. In her chapter, Gayle Davis shows that doctors' views on the subject of infertility were shaped as much by their social, moral and religious views, as by their medical training. Al-Gailani also highlights the evangelical influences on Ballantyne's career and work. And in Ireland, Earner-Byrne explains how the religious landscape was an important determining factor in pregnancy outcomes. So too does Janet Greenlees in her chapter on Scotland. Social and religious values form an important backdrop for her discussion of the provision of maternity services for unmarried mothers in early twentieth-century Glasgow. She discusses the role of the Church of Scotland in filling a gap in the social services provided by the government, but in a way that ensured religious values were upheld. As noted, key to its success was the matron, who was both church member and qualified midwife. Greenlees also shows how the church's institution was relatively unusual in helping the unmarried mother to keep her child rather than adopt it out. Central to this policy was the religious belief in the sanctity of the family. Her chapter reveals how important it is to look beyond the interaction between women and their health professionals and incorporate institutional providers of health care in order to understand the shape of maternity services.

Discussion of fetal rights – or the rights of the fetus versus the rights of the mother – was another area of academic study to emerge from the 1960s, in the context of the campaigns to reform abortion laws in particular.[49] In her chapter in this volume, Allison Hepler analyses how modern concerns about fetal rights and a narrowing of the definition of motherhood changed practices in the workplace in America over the twentieth century. She identifies the new women's movement as bringing significant advances for women in the workplace from the 1970s, while noting that those advances which decreed equal treatment could also make women more vulnerable in their role as potential mothers; it was a double-edged sword.

The case studies presented in this volume have been organized chronologically. We begin with Madonna Grehan's case study of births in late nineteenth-century Melbourne and Salim Al-Gailani's analysis of the development of prenatal care in Edinburgh at the turn of the twentieth century. Janet Greenlees's chapter on the provision of childbirth services for unmarried mothers in early twentieth-century Glasgow, Scotland follows. Alison Nuttall's chapter takes us into interwar Edinburgh and women's choices of where to give birth, while Linda Bryder discusses women's activism relating to birth facilities in New Zealand in the period 1900–1960. Lindsey Earner-Byrne's essay spans the twentieth century more generally in Ireland, taking her discussion up to the 1990s in her analysis of the 'curious mix of religion and geography' in the development of maternity services in Ireland. Gayle Davis concentrates on the mid-twentieth century in her discussion of fertility services in Scotland, and Angela Davis focuses on women's experiences of childbirth in the 1970s and 1980s. Allison Hepler takes a longer view, ranging from the turn of the twentieth century to the 1990s, when she looks at changes relating to 'fetal rights' and fetal protection laws in the United States. Through this chronological ordering of our case studies, we aim to explore and elucidate the historical experience of women as mothers and potential mothers over time and place, and how this experience was shaped by a variety of stakeholders and concerns.

The literature on the history of childbirth which emerged following Dugald Baird's 1960 analysis provides an essential foundation for the discussions here. While recognizing the important contributions of the literature on the history of childbirth that came out of the feminist and social history movements of the 1970s, a central theme of this book is that women were not victims of a dominant male medical profession, but were rational beings who made the best choices they could for themselves and their children, either individually or collectively, under the circumstances in which they lived. This does not mean women were free agents; they were also subject to wider cultural influences.

For instance, like men of the early twentieth century, they were persuaded by the benefits of science, and later they were influenced by modern consumer and feminist movements. In neither case, however, did they absorb these cultural trends passively, but rather weighed up the information available to reach their own decisions. They were also subject to other influences and constraints, such as those imposed by churches, or by governments through their social policies, or by the cultural values of particular social and ethnic groups (the last a subject beyond the scope of this book).[50] Within the narratives developed here, the medical profession is not portrayed as simply intent on exploiting women's bodies for power or financial gain, as has so often been suggested. At the same time, neither is our story one of medical progress. While the advances Baird highlighted were undeniable, they do not tell the whole story. Health professionals, like the women they served, were subject to social, cultural and political constraints. Indeed, the essays in this book highlight how the full social context in which childbirth, or any other medical event occurs, has to be considered to understand its history. The value of this volume to the historiography of motherhood and childbirth is that all our authors bring the historian's craft to bear on the subject matter, drawing from a vast array of primary sources to throw new light on various episodes, influences and developments within the history of maternity and childbirth during an important period of change, from the late nineteenth to the late twentieth century.

1 SAFELY DELIVERED? INSIGHTS INTO LATE NINETEENTH-CENTURY AUSTRALIAN MATERNITY CARE FROM CORONIAL INVESTIGATIONS INTO MATERNAL DEATHS

Madonna Grehan

According to histories of maternity care written throughout the twentieth century, having a baby in nineteenth-century Australia and throughout the British Empire was a very risky business, largely because maternity cases were attended by women without any education or training.[1] Such histories celebrated the removal of uneducated women from midwifery practice as a health reform welcomed by women, and emphasized medicine's and trained nursing's superior scientific knowledge as pivotal in transforming maternity care. More recently, this long-standing perspective has been questioned by some within the profession of midwifery, and by midwifery advocates in Australia and elsewhere. This follows a worldwide professionalizing movement aimed at uncoupling midwifery from its association with nursing and installing midwifery as a separate and distinct profession. In part, this professionalizing stance has been justified on a revisionist interpretation of maternity care history.[2] As the argument goes, midwifery in the nineteenth century was an ancient lore practised by autonomous women who had childbearing women's best interests at heart. This perspective contends that doctors, aided by the nascent profession of nursing, hoodwinked women into biomedical care based in hospitals by declaring home births unsafe and by denigrating women who attended them. Revisionists argue that medicine simply wanted to control maternity because it was a lucrative area of practice.

Given the polarization of these perspectives, it is hard to know if either reflects the reality of birth for women in the nineteenth century. This chapter focuses on the colony of Victoria in Australia with a view to examining that reality. Uncovering maternity care history in this period has its challenges, the main one being a lack of primary sources on which to draw. The deficit stems from confluent factors, particularly the haphazard way in which colonial Victoria was settled and developed.[3] Victoria covers almost 227,000 square kilometres, around the same area as mainland Britain.4 When gold was discovered around Victoria during the second half of the nineteenth century, the colony's population rose rapidly: up from 98,000 people in 1851 to 1.160 million in 1891. A similar proportional increase occurred in registered births: up from 3,000 in 1851 to 38,500 in 1891. More than half of the colony's births occurred in rural and semi-rural areas, often in remote and sparsely settled parts of the colony.[5] For most women, birth happened at home or in small lying-in hospitals, the latter increasing markedly in number throughout the colony over the last quarter of the century.[6] In this domain of private attendance, neither practitioners nor their activities were regulated, unless that practitioner was a doctor.[7] The corollary is very few documentary sources describing the care that women may have received. Women and sometimes their husbands wrote about birth and its aftermath in diaries and correspondence, but references to reproductive episodes tend to be euphemistic and sparse,[8] such as an acknowledgement that the mother's life was spared.[9]

The lack of evidence about domiciliary birth contrasts markedly with ample and detailed records of the care provided to women in institutions in the same period, such as the Women's Hospital in Melbourne, Victoria's capital city, seen in the work of historian Janet McCalman.[10] The Women's Hospital opened in 1856 and rapidly developed a reputation nationwide for leading research and practice in maternity and gynaecological care. That care was carefully documented, but those who received it constituted a small sector of the colony's nineteenth-century childbearing population. Of Victoria's 26,148 registered births in 1880, only 590 (2.25 per cent) occurred at The Women's; of the 33,000 births registered in 1887, The Women's accounted for 479 (1.45 per cent).[11] The immense value of these institutional patient records is not disputed, but there remains a gap in our knowledge of how women fared when they had their babies at home, outside the regulated environment of a hospital.

The research presented here offers a window into that private realm, drawing on an alternative source for evidence of care in the community: extant case records and newspaper reports of coronial investigations into maternal deaths between 1880 and 1900. A statistical analysis of maternal deaths is not the intention of this paper. Rather, it paints a credible and nuanced picture of nineteenth-century birth and birth care, enabling us to test the veracity of existing accounts of maternity care history. The chapter begins by introducing the coronial investigation process and explaining how this research proceeded. The limitations of coronial investigations as primary sources are then discussed for two reasons: they impact on how the cases can be analysed and are likely to apply in other colonial jurisdictions. Using case reports, the chapter draws out the nature of birth care in this era: who was attending at maternity bedsides and what sort of circumstances and pregnancy complications those attendants faced.

It then considers a complex aspect of these cases: statements made to coronial courts about the use of violence in labour. Lastly, the outcomes of coronial investigations are discussed.

Maternal Death Records as Primary Sources

Having inherited conventions of the British legal system, Victoria's legislation concerning coronial investigations remained largely unchanged in the nineteenth century and was consolidated under the Coroners Act 1890.[12] Coronial investigations applied to 'sudden and unexplained deaths not certifiable by a medical practitioner'.[13] Their purpose was to examine 'when, where, how, and by what means' the deceased came by death.[14] Every investigation had a legislated chain of command, involving the male occupations of medicine, policing and the judiciary.[15] Most investigations were prompted when a medical practitioner declined to issue a death certificate for burial. A doctor, so inclined, notified the local police who, in turn, notified the district coroner who determined if an inquest was indicated. The district coroner was a 'police magistrate, barrister, solicitor or doctor', although a Justice of the Peace could preside over what was termed a 'Magisterial Inquiry'.[16] Magisterial inquiries tended to be held in geographically isolated regions. Coronial inquests were held before a jury of between five and twelve men.[17] It was the jury's role to determine if anyone should be held accountable for the death and recommended to criminal trial.

Ascertaining nineteenth-century childbirth-associated deaths is not as straightforward as one might expect using Victoria's resources. Newspaper reports of investigations can be found by published indexes and by searching digitized copies available online.[18] The database of Victorian inquests, *Knight's Index*,[19] has limitations, in part, related to the system of death reporting. First, no specific taxonomy for pregnancy-related death existed in the nineteenth century. Causes of deaths in pregnant women therefore were recorded variously and with compound terms such as 'exhaustion childbirth' or 'flooding [haemorrhage] childbirth'.[20] Second, the index contains many gaps such as basic demographic categories (sex and age of the deceased) not being recorded. Third, transcription errors have produced anomalies.[21] Fourth, some inquests reported upon in newspapers are not listed in *Knight's Index*. Other limitations manifest in the records of cases themselves. Case records are held at the state's repository for government records, Public Record Office Victoria, but some files are not extant, some are designated 'missing', while other case files do not correspond with the index entry. The volume of evidence in each file varies greatly.

The research reported here comes from nineteen cases of maternal death in the years 1880 to 1900. Fifteen cases of likely maternal death were located in newspapers, some of which were contained in *Knight's Index*. From *Knight's*

Index itself, seventy childbirth-associated death cases were identified. Causes of death recorded in this twenty-year period include: birth, childbirth, exhaustion, haemorrhage, ruptured uterus, flooding, complicated labour, protracted labour, preterm labour, peritonitis, sepsis and pyaemia.[22] A random selection was made of twenty-five possible cases listed in *Knight's Index* from metropolitan and rural areas. Of these twenty-five cases, two concerned men, two files were missing, one investigated the suicide of a 50-year-old woman and six of the cases were abortion-related. The abortion cases were set aside because the research reported here was focused on deaths in childbirth.[23] Despite what are considerable deficits in terms of rigorous epidemiological analysis,[24] these records offer a unique view on the private world of nineteenth-century birth.

Attendants at the Maternity Bedside

In 1881, Dr James Jamieson, a lecturer in Obstetrics and Gynaecology at the University of Melbourne, and later Health Officer for the City of Melbourne, complained that uneducated women were responsible for 'Excessive Mortality among Lying-in Women' in the colony of Victoria.[25] By Jamieson's reckoning, around half of Victoria's registered births were attended by women, and in greater numbers in rural areas of the colony. Jamieson's assessment accords with the more recent work of historians Strachan, Pensabene and Swain and Howe,[26] and was borne out in the coronial cases examined. In each case, at least one female was present at the bedside at some point during labour. In the investigation records, these female attendants described themselves, or were referred to by others, as: mother, mother-in-law, daughter, sister, sister-in-law, friend, neighbour, nurse, midwife, ladies nurse or monthly nurse.

Some women were said to prefer relatives to attend at confinements. For example, Mrs Rebecca Dukes, aged twenty-nine, who died from haemorrhage after her placenta was retained, reportedly had wanted no attendant at birth other than her mother-in-law.[27] Mrs Mary Kirby, who died in 1882 aged thirty-two, had only her daughter present.[28] Miss Kirby's age was not recorded, but is likely to have been no more than sixteen. Other women, even when close to death, declined to have a nurse, midwife or doctor present as did Elizabeth Welsh, a mother of eight, whose husband told the investigation into his wife's death that 'I wished to go for the doctor earlier in the evening [but] the deceased did not wish it'.[29] Similarly, the husband of Ann Hayes went in search of a doctor to aid his wife in labour in February 1890. Mrs Hayes initially was attended by her sister and a sister-in-law. A second sister-in-law arrived to help just after the baby was born, at which time Mrs Hayes felt all right and insisted that her sister and two sisters-in-law should 'send after the doctor and prevent him from coming'.[30] That women dismissed professional help seems surprising, but it is possible that they were conscious of cost. If a midwife *and* doctor both attended and each expected to be paid for that attendance, the cost may have been significant, and in retrospect, if all went well such an expense may have seemed wasteful. These examples also suggest that women, despite feeling very unwell, were accustomed to making the best of their circumstances.

As well as establishing who was involved in maternity cases, coroners' investigations sought to ascertain in what capacity attendants were present at the bedside, that is, as a neighbourly gesture or in a professional capacity. The cases examined show that some attendants had considerable experience, others had some education/training, while others had no experience whatsoever. As one investigation heard, on a stormy night in 1886, Mary O'Connor, a mother of thirteen, called a heavily pregnant neighbour for help. Mrs O'Connor's neighbour, a mother of seven, told the investigation that 'I have never attended a confinement case' and as far as the deceased's husband was concerned, their neighbour had 'acted kindly as a Christian woman'.[31] Mrs Margaret Jones had been attended by two women, with one a nurse. The deceased's husband explained that his wife

> had the doctor in attendance at two previous confinements but in the other cases only a nurse. I [Mr Jones, husband of the deceased] had every confidence in Mrs Edgar and also in Mrs Campbell [the nurse] the latter of whom had previously attended her in three of the confinements.[32]

Coronial investigations appear to have drawn a distinction between acting simply in a neighbourly way and attending cases as a nurse or midwife, the latter inferring payment for services rendered and possibly claims to qualifications such as a midwifery diploma or certificate. In 1892, Mrs Harriet Walton told a maternal death investigation that 'I went to her [the deceased's] house to attend her during childbirth. I having been in the habit of doing so at times but this was the first occasion on which I attended Mrs Richardson.'[33] A deceased's husband in an 1881 case said of his wife's attendant:

> Mrs McClelland came to my wife merely as a neighbour, not as a nurse. As Mrs McClelland objected to attend as midwife in my wife's case knowing that on a previous occasion my wife had been very ill in her labour.

The neighbour, Mrs McClelland, concurred, saying 'I am not a midwife. I came as a neighbour only'.[34]

Several of the cases examined made reference to the certification of midwives. At a lengthy inquest leading to a criminal trial in early 1892, Mrs Hannah Goldstein told the court 'I am a certificated midwife', having obtained the certificate 'In Poland'.[35] In the case of Mrs Margaret Pitt Martin, no witness could say if Mrs Ramsay, the woman's nurse, was 'certificated as a midwife'. The doctor who attended had known Mrs Ramsay for six years and did consider her 'capable of acting as nurse in cases of ordinary labour'. John Martin, husband of the deceased woman declared 'I did not pay Mrs Ramsay as midwife. I understand she was to be paid. I believe my wife engaged her. She was recommended but I did not inquire whether she was a certificated midwife'.[36]

Certification implies that the holder was educated in maternity care, but without regulatory oversight, there was no way to judge the bona fides of an individual and their certificate. Training in maternity care was available locally in Victoria, but it is difficult to judge how many women availed themselves of it. In the city of Melbourne, as early as 1859 doctors ran courses privately along the lines of Scottish models, giving lectures and issuing signed certificates to attendees.[37] The Women's Hospital in Melbourne ran a course for pupil nurses in the care of women, successful candidates of which earned a certificate as a 'Ladies Monthly Nurse and Sick Nurse'.[38] In the 1860s, the course consisted of three months of practical tuition and lectures, combining maternity (midwifery) and gynaecological care of women. The course enjoyed little prominence and after the Women's Hospital's monthly nurses were criticized in 1869, amid a coronial investigation, they were defended in writing by the hospital's resident medical officer. He declared them skilled practitioners able to undertake cases of natural labour and educated well enough to know when to seek help for complications.[39] For nurses who trained up to the 1880s, that education was provided according to the principles of miasmatic theory. After training, there were no professional fora where that foundational knowledge could be updated and by the 1880s that education was out of date, given the emergence of germ theory. This contrasted with parts of Europe where midwives and nurses were educated, practice regulated, professional fora existed and where maternal death rates in the late nineteenth and early twentieth centuries were substantially reduced.[40]

Women all over the colony appear to have accepted whatever attendance was available locally. In several of the cases examined, the birth attendant marked her sworn deposition with an 'X' in lieu of a signature. The fact that a woman was illiterate does not appear to have been an impediment to private engagements as the case of Annie Bibby shows. Bibby was a midwife whose deposition was marked with an X. She told a maternal death inquiry in 1886 that 'I have been engaged as a midwife for upwards of nineteen years in all, during fourteen of which I have resided at Harrietville' – a Victorian rural settlement.[41] These cases emphasize the enormous variation in those providing maternity care: women with certificates, women with experience, women with no experience and women who were unable to read and write.

Practices and Practicalities

Aside from illuminating who was attending at the maternity bedside, coronial records offer insights into what those attendants were doing: the ordinary, everyday practices performed. Most women appear to have given birth in bed after being taken 'ill' with labour pains, while several walked about for as long as possible. Mrs Alice Rochford's baby, however, was born on the floor of the house, on a sheepskin mat.[42] Her attendant, Ann Coutts, whose deposition was signed with an X, told the inquest that Mrs Rochford returned to bed after the birth, but that:

> She fainted in bed. I was trying to remove the afterbirth. [The] Haemorrhage from the birth of the child unto her death was not more than usual. I did not consider she was a long time in labour. I put her on a [chamber] pot of hot water to try to get the afterbirth away she was very cold. I have done the same thing once or twice before and it was successful. I do not hold a certificate or diploma.[43]

Some of the practices that individuals employed were frowned upon. The doctor testifying at Alice Rochford's inquest concluded that the midwife's action in sitting Mrs Rochford on the chamber pot probably hastened the deceased's demise. Even so, the inquest did not apportion blame to anyone.[44] At the investigation into the death of Mrs Margaret Pitt Martin in 1889, the doctor deposed: 'I examined the deceased. She had a bandage on it [the abdomen] ... It is usual but improper in my opinion to bandage the abdomen after delivery'.[45] Mr Martin thought that the midwife in attendance, Nurse Ramsay, 'appeared very assiduous' in her care, being careful to remove the large volume of blood-soaked linen from the lying-in room, discreetly, to avoid alerting the Martins' children to the awful situation.[46] Nurse Ramsay recommended to Mr Martin that he should burn the placenta in the fire; when he did not do it, she buried it in the back yard. In this case, the deceased's body had been exhumed two weeks after burial because of 'certain rumours that had gained currency that the death was not altogether due to natural causes'.[47] The inquest heard the attending doctor intended to inform the police when Mrs Martin died but that Mr Martin was 'a little put out' at not receiving a death certificate and so, reluctantly, the doctor provided one. It is possible to read this as an attempt by Mrs Ramsay, the nurse, to destroy evidence, but this seems unlikely. Disposing of the placenta by fire was recommended practice in an 1888 treatise on *Antiseptic Midwifery* authored by Dr Walter Balls-Headley of the University of Melbourne and the Women's Hospital.[48]

Evidence of other practices, including the provision of pain relief and sustenance, can be found in coronial investigations. For example, brandy was requested by Mary Ann Kilmartin to relieve her labour pain.[49] It was given as a stimulant after birth to Margaret Pitt Martin, Alice Richardson and Mary O'Connor,[50] and given during labour as sustenance for the ailing Agnes Harley whose labour was obstructed. Miss Harley's midwife, Mrs Hannah Goldstein, had called in a doctor for help. Diagnosing the patient's imminent collapse, the doctor instructed Mrs Goldstein to administer 'restorative medicine, to feed her for every half-hour on brandy and egg – a spoonful at a time – and to keep her strictly quiet'. The doctor later attempted to deliver the baby using obstetric instruments, but was unsuccessful. In her deposition to the inquest, Mrs Goldstein stated that 'Ether was not administered to the woman [Agnes Harley] in my house', indicating that delivery was attempted without any anaesthetic.[51] Agnes Harley's inquest was the only one of those examined in which the use of an anaesthetic was raised. In fact, chloroform was generally the anaesthetic agent of choice for births, with ether used only as a secondary option if the chloroform was ineffective or could not be tolerated.[52] Establishing the extent of use of anaesthetics in the private domain will require further examination.

Coronial records also shed light on the practicalities of providing care in late nineteenth-century Australia, highlighting the enormous effort that families and communities expended when women went into labour. Usually several people were involved at births: attending at the bedside, sending messages or travelling to get help. Evidence from coronial investigations underscores how hard obtaining skilled assistance could be and it shows that, on occasion, doctors declined to respond to desperate calls for help. For example, Mrs Mary O'Connor lived 2 km/1.5 miles out of the town of Sandhurst in rural Victoria. When she went into labour suddenly one evening in 1886 at midnight, her husband went to town and rang the doctor. The doctor was ill and could not come. Mr O'Connor then visited two other doctors in the town, but both declined to attend Mrs O'Connor because they had not been pre-engaged for the case. Mr O'Connor returned home at 3 am to find a neighbour, who had no knowledge of midwifery, at the bedside. The baby was born subsequently, but haemorrhage ensued. In the daylight, Mr O'Connor returned to town and eventually secured the services of another doctor who arrived at O'Connor's home at 4.30 pm. By that time Mrs O'Connor had died.[53] A local newspaper took a rather dismal view of the three doctors who would not attend, expressing concern that the inquest did not question them. The newspaper reported, however, that 'The coroner was particularly careful to exonerate from blame the neighbour's wife who kindly attended the deceased woman'.[54]

The difficulty in obtaining help was not confined to rural areas. In 1881 Mrs Jane Pollovineo, the 29-year-old wife of a Melbourne street grocer, died from inversion of the uterus and ensuing haemorrhage. Her nurse Mary Daley had sent for a doctor just before the baby was born, but the doctor declined to attend. Dr Charles S. Ryan, formerly a surgeon with the Turkish army in 1876–8 and honorary surgeon to the Melbourne Hospital, arrived eventually, but Mrs Pollovineo died shortly after.[55] Similarly, in 1883, Mary Thompson's husband ran for help at the attending midwife's behest when Mrs Thompson suffered a sudden, severe haemorrhage, but the doctor declined to come because he had not been engaged for the case in advance.[56] These are not isolated cases of a lack of professional support of female attendants. The reasons for it are complex, but there are two explanations of which there is evidence. First, doctors would not attend women if they suspected the family could not pay. Second, doctors did not want to attend 'hopeless' cases, particularly if a midwife or other attendant was involved, because of a perception that the doctor would be blamed for an adverse outcome when his help had been sought too late to make a positive difference to the outcome.[57]

Pregnancy Complications

Given Dr James Jamieson's claims that uneducated female practitioners were responsible for an excessive maternal death rate, and in the light of the more recent debates about biomedicine's unwelcome intrusion into what was a domain of woman-led birth, it is useful to examine what attendants did or did not do when a complication manifested. In the majority of cases examined, the primary cause of death was haemorrhage, arising from a combination of uterine and placental status (rupture or atony of the uterus, a delivered/partially delivered/retained placenta or placenta praevia/accreta).[58] Substantial blood loss happened to seemingly healthy but, in all likelihood, anaemic women, often without any warning and quickly. In fact the speed with which haemorrhage afflicted women proved an insurmountable force, particularly in geographically isolated places where medical or other help was distant and necessitated travel on foot or by horse. Whether by day or night, these journeys took time and, as the cases examined have demonstrated, help was not always forthcoming.[59] The inquests and inquiries examined confirm that those by the bedside were ill-prepared to deal with the complication of post-partum haemorrhage.

At the inquiry into the death of Mrs Elizabeth Welsh in 1892, the midwife attending explained that Mrs Welsh became delirious not long after the birth and lost a 'great deal' of blood. Mrs Welsh died two hours later, while her husband was away seeking a doctor.[60] Similarly, Mrs Elizabeth Cook haemorrhaged at her home in the tiny hamlet of Annandale in the far north-east of Victoria. She had been in good health when her husband left for work at 7.30 that morning. Labour ensued during the day and after six hours she gave birth to a healthy girl in the company of female neighbours. But within half an hour, her colour had changed. She haemorrhaged for the next three hours and died at 6 pm. Witnesses told the investigation into her death that 'There was no means of sending for doctor before death'. The nearest doctor was a round trip of some 32 km/20 miles away, and only when one of the women's spouses returned at nightfall was there someone available with a horse to make the hazardous journey to get help.[61]

A 40-year-old mother of fifteen, Mrs Margaret Jones, died just before Christmas in 1886, following rupture of her uterus. Her labour had commenced at around 4 pm. The contractions became so violent that her neighbour in attendance, Mrs Edgar, sent for Mrs Campbell, a nurse, to help but the situation worsened at 9 pm. At that point, Mr Jones, a carpenter, sent his son by horse to a town 8 km/5 miles distant, so that a telegram could be sent to the nearest doctor, but the hour of 10.30 pm was too late for the telegram to be transmitted. The young man rode a further round trip of 40 km/25 miles to fetch the doctor himself. In the meantime, at around 3 am Mrs Jones's labour pains stopped. She sank and died eventually at 9.30 am. The post mortem revealed that the 'enormous' fetus had entered the abdominal cavity when the uterus ruptured.[62]

Mrs Mary Ann Kilmartin went into labour at dusk in mid-winter in a small central Victorian rural settlement. Mrs Kilmartin, a 34-year-old, had the usual 'show' when the bloody mucous plug dislodged from the cervix, but she did not immediately have violent labour pains. Her husband told the inquest that when the pains did become worse at 7 pm, he 'did not send for any nurse as my wife did not consider she was at her full-time', instead his wife asked for a neighbour to come.[63] At 9 pm, his wife asked for brandy to relieve her distress. Mr Kilmartin ran 8 km/5 miles to the nearest public house and back, for the brandy. The baby was born at 10 pm and the mother immediately became weak. Her husband wanted to fetch the local midwife, but Mrs Kilmartin begged him to stay, insisting that she would be all right in time. Mr Kilmartin sent a neighbour by buggy to collect the midwife, who lived 9 km/6.5 miles away, while another went on horseback to get help from a town 21 km/13 miles away, in case the midwife was not at home. By the time the midwife did arrive, Mrs Kilmartin had expired. These grim scenarios demonstrate that when haemorrhage struck, death could follow very soon after confinement or hours after birth. Even when professional help was obtained, it was sometimes too late to save the mother.

What to do about deaths in childbirth and how to improve the safety of women had been the subject of discussion in medical society publications since the 1850s. Newspapers took up the cause in the 1860s, reporting regularly on coronial investigations with much criticism directed at those who interfered in the natural process of labour. At the inaugural obstetrics course at the University of Melbourne in 1865, Dr Richard Tracy emphasized to his students that nature was the safest midwife for most women, and that interference was the mark of an ignorant birth attendant.[64] Interference included activities such as forcibly stretching the cervix after each contraction, tearing the perineum well in advance of the birth, or pulling at the fetal parts to hasten the birth and in the process scoring fragile mucous membranes with sharp fingernails. Pulling on the umbilical cord, and therefore the placenta before it had separated from the uterine wall, was another form of interference.[65] Pushing on the uterus via the abdomen also was considered interference, as was asserted in the case of Eliza Elliot in her care of Mary Belle Seymour, whose uterus ruptured.[66] In the mid-nineteenth century, these actions were understood to lead to haemorrhage but by the 1880s, and the emergence of germ theory, unnecessary interference in labour was more directly associated with the mortal danger of puerperal sepsis. These insights came with the understanding of human beings as vectors of infection.[67] Thus, Dr James Jamieson's analysis of puerperal fever and erysipelas in Australia pointed the finger squarely at female attendants who reportedly did not understand the danger of infection or the modern antiseptic precautions necessary in maternity cases to guard against it, including personal cleanliness and frequent washing of hands.[68] The condition of the deceased's body was often the most useful witness to any interference having been employed.

Statements about Violence

Husbands and other witnesses, police officers in charge of deceased persons and doctors who performed autopsies made statements in their depositions about violence, or evidence of violence, having been inflicted on the deceased. Individuals could describe what attendants did, but signs of violence were the most important. These manifested as bruising, breakages of the skin or bones or as torn tissues, internally and/or externally.[69] In the case of Mrs Ann Hayes, the doctor found 'no external marks of violence ... [the] Umbilical cord was hanging from the vagina and had been properly attended to'.[70] Similarly, Constable O'Brien said of the body of Mrs Jane Renton who died from haemorrhage: 'There were no marks of violence visible'.[71]

At his post-mortem of Miss Nannie William Thomas in 1880, Dr Hugh Boyd observed that the 'body was ... free from external marks of violence. There was no evidence of any other irritant'.[72] Thomas was a 24-year-old woman who had concealed the pregnancy from her mother, delivering her baby of nine months' gestation in the family's backyard fowl house one evening. When Miss Thomas returned inside after an absence she was noticed to be very pale, but immediately retired to bed. Two hours later, she declared herself to be dying and confessed to the birth. Dr Boyd attended, finding the placenta still adhered to the uterus; he gave Miss Thomas stimulants, but she died from haemorrhage around seven hours after the birth. The baby was discovered dead in the fowl house, also from haemorrhage because the umbilical cord had not been tied. The fact that the effects of 'violence' were not evident indicated that labour had not been induced.

With suspicions about how Mrs Margaret Pitt Martin died resulting in exhumation of her body two weeks after death in 1889, the findings at post-mortem were critical. The woman's inverted uterus and half of the placenta were found in the coffin, but the examining doctor stated that extrusion of the womb had occurred after death because there were no signs of violence to indicate otherwise.[73] In the case of Mrs Mary O'Connor, the 41-year-old mother of thirteen, her attendant Ann Weiland told an inquiry:

> I am the mother of seven children. I never before attended a confinement case. I did
> not succeed in removing the afterbirth. I tried, but the deceased was too weak to assist
> or help in anyway. I am not a nurse. I used no violence.[74]

At an inquest into the death of Miss Agnes Harley, reports of which featured
in newspapers over January and February 1892, a midwife and at least six doctors were scrutinized about their practices. Miss Harley, a servant, was pregnant
for the second time and residing at the house of a midwife, Mrs Hannah Goldstein. When Miss Harley laboured at the midwife's house for some time without
progress, delivery of the baby was attempted with instruments applied by a Dr
Fenwick and his colleague. Dr Fenwick had a prior engagement interstate and
after several hours handed Miss Harley's case to his colleague. After review by
another doctor, Miss Harley was removed by taxi-cab to the nearby Women's
Hospital with her baby partly delivered but wedged in the pelvis. The lengthy and
difficult extraction of the dead fetus was achieved by doctors using instruments
at The Women's. Miss Harley died twenty-four hours later. Post mortem revealed
'Two abrasions of a considerable size on her hip, bruises and breakages on other
parts of the body' of Miss Harley.[75] In the unborn baby, every bone was 'smashed',
destruction which was said to have taken place at the midwife's house.[76]

Miss Georgina Graham, a 23-year-old unmarried woman, died of erysipelas
two weeks after delivering a live baby boy. She had come to town from the country accompanied by her mother to give birth in a rented room and was attended
by an unnamed midwife. Reportedly, a doctor was called in because of 'a bad
labour and [it] required instruments'.[77] Miss Graham, ill almost immediately
after confinement, was subsequently admitted to Melbourne's General Hospital
where she died. Post mortem revealed a rent in the vaginal wall, a suppurating
mass in the pelvis, as well as severely lacerated tissue in the cervix, vagina and
uterus. Aside from stating that the birth occurred 'outside' the hospital, the limited inquest record makes no comment on what inflicted this extensive damage
to Miss Graham's reproductive tract. It may have been caused by the instruments
themselves, or by human hands with sharp nails attempting to pull the baby out.
No criminal charges appear to have been laid against any person.

Statements made about violence are a complex element of the coronial investigation to unravel. The precise questions asked by coroners were not recorded,
making it tempting to read intentions into questions where they may not exist.
However, this line of questioning did try to pinpoint whether behaviours of
attendants were appropriate. What can be said is that the application of violence was not unique to any category of attendant. Most of the cases, read now,
display some element of violence about them, no matter who was involved. At a
time when caesarean section or obstetric forceps were not widely available, there
was no alternative other than to extract a baby with brute force. In the absence

of modern understandings of the physiological separation of the placenta, it is not surprising that attendants may have applied force to extract an adherent placenta. Procedures performed by some medical practitioners, such as those at the Women's Hospital in the case of Agnes Harley, were accepted as a measure to save life 'in the interests of humanity'.[78] Those undertaken by other doctors, such as Dr Fenwick, or performed by women, appear to have been less acceptable. How the courts determined what was an appropriate application of violence and what was inappropriate is a complexity beyond the scope of this chapter, but worthy of further research. What can be said is that the way the Victorian coronial courts assessed attendants' actions towards those in their care inevitably impacted on conclusions to coronial investigations: arriving at an outcome.

Outcomes from Inquests

Coronial investigations sought to understand the entire circumstances leading to death, from which conclusions could be drawn. Thus, they could elicit a range of outcomes. A death could be recognized as one unforeseen and one that no-one, reasonably, could have prevented. For example, the coroner determined that Mrs Alice Rochford came to her death in 1895 'from the afterbirth adhering to the womb, thereby causing haemorrhage resulting in her death and that under the exceptional circumstances of the case no blame is attachable to any person'.[79] Equally, the coroner presiding at the Agnes Harley inquest in January 1892 concluded that the midwife, Hannah Goldstein, could not be charged with delay in sending for medical assistance.[80] In the case of Elizabeth Welsh, the doctor called in to help reported that:

> I found on examining the deceased that the nurse had paid the usual attention as thorough as she was able, but, that the deceased had lost a large quantity of blood by flooding, which was the cause of death. The deceased was liable to flooding at her confinement. I was called to her six years ago when she had an attack of the same kind from which she nearly died.[81]

Dr Sweetnam, who examined the body of Margaret Jones, told the court that her death was a result of 'shock caused by rupture of [the] uterus ... which could not have been averted by medical attention unless very early in the confinement. This case was beyond the skill of any nurse.'[82] Sweetnam's assessment was accurate. Delivery of the baby by fetal destruction, as occurred in the Harley case, was the only option to save the mother. Going by the inquest notes and newspaper reports, the nurse attending in this case, Mrs Mary Campbell, was not questioned,[83] which infers that she was not blamed.

Juries sitting at coronial inquests could censure women publicly. After an hour of deliberation, the jury in the case of Mrs Martin determined that her nurse, Mrs Ramsay, had not exercised due care, but that the want of care did not amount to criminal neglect.[84] Where negligence was found by an inquest jury, the case could be sent to a sitting of the Criminal Court. In 1885, the jury hearing the inquest into the death of Mrs Mary Ann Stones found certificated Ladies Nurse and midwife, Susannah Thompson, guilty of manslaughter. Thompson had 'ignorantly and recklessly' overdosed Mrs Stones through failing to follow the written instructions on a bottle of laudanum.[85] In this case, the jury added a rider acknowledging that the laudanum was given medicinally but ignorantly, and sent Thompson to trial. One month later she appeared in the Supreme Court where the jury returned a verdict of 'not guilty at the same time recommending the prisoner to be more careful in future'.[86]

Similarly, Eliza Elliot, the 'nurse or midwife' was found guilty of accelerating the death of Mrs Mary Belle Seymour by her undue interference. When sending her to trial, the inquest jury recommended her to mercy.[87] Eliza Elliot subsequently was found not guilty.[88] In the Agnes Harley case, the midwife, Mrs Hannah Goldstein, was called to answer that she had delayed in sending for medical assistance, but exonerated.[89] At criminal trial Dr Fenwick was found guilty of negligence for leaving Miss Harley when she was so ill, but he was not found guilty of manslaughter.[90]

Inquests presented an opportunity for some critics of maternity care to declare what should be done about childbirth deaths. With more than half of the colony's births attended by women, much critique centred on installing training and regulation for female attendants. Dr James Neild, a vocal critic of women as attendants, performed the post-mortem of Mrs Margaret Pitt Martin after exhumation. Although the midwife was not blamed for the woman's death, Neild told the inquest that:

> The person who delivered the deceased ought to have known that the afterbirth had not been entirely removed. It is not a difficult matter to ascertain whether the whole of the afterbirth has come away when in its natural state. It is the duty of every midwife to ascertain if there is any unusual bleeding. With ordinary care and skill in my opinion deceased should have recovered after delivery.[91]

Similarly, the doctor who was called in the case of Alice Rochford implied at the inquest that the midwife was not fit for the task. His assessment reads:

> I have been called in cases where Mrs Coutts has acted as midwife. I have not had sufficient experience of Mrs Coutts to say whether she's experienced or not ... If a certified or registered midwife had had the case she would have sent for a doctor instead of attempting to remove the afterbirth. By registered midwife I mean a person that has had a training and holds a diploma from some medical hospital that the person is a fit person to practise as midwife.[92]

The outcomes of the cases examined in this chapter give the impression that the courts exercised a degree of leniency towards the birth attendants concerned. Further research will establish if that impression is justified. In practice, the courts had few avenues under criminal statutes for sentencing those seen to be negligent in their maternity attendance. No licensing system prescribed what the work was and who could practise it, making coronial investigations the only mechanism in the nineteenth century by which midwives and others could be held to account for their actions. The cases examined here convey a sense that maternal death continued to be accepted in this period as an event that befell women, regardless of the qualities of those who attended them. Leniency may simply have reflected the broader public opinion, represented in the juries of men who made judgements on inquest cases.

Within medical circles, of course, maternal death was viewed as a serious problem that could be, and should be, prevented with better training. Dr James Jamieson continued to argue for compulsory training for midwifery attendants and a system of registration under the governance of a board.[93] While there was some impetus in Victoria to impose regulations on midwifery work in the 1890s to control who attended at maternity bedsides, the government was disinclined.[94] Australian historian Patricia Grimshaw notes that concern about maternal health grew in Australia in the late 1890s as the colonies moved towards a federation of states under a new constitution and a new flag; women in this context were seen as the 'mothers or potential mothers' of the embryonic nation and deserving of the protection of the state.[95] By the turn of the twentieth century, most Western countries were moving to protect the lives of mothers and babies by regulating midwifery practice, and Australia was to follow in the first quarter of the twentieth century.[96]

Although reform of maternity care was driven by medicine and actively supported by the emerging profession of trained nursing, it was sanctioned by women too, as evidenced in the aspirations of the Country Women's Association, an apolitical organization for rural women launched in Victoria in 1928. Among the foundational aims of the organization were the provision of 'proper maternity facilities' equipped with trained staff, and telephones at a cost within reach of all small householders.[97] Rural women no longer wanted to run the gauntlet of birth as their grandmothers had done throughout the nineteenth century.

Conclusion

The research presented here confirms that records and reports of coronial inquests into maternal deaths can make a valuable contribution to understanding how maternity care was practised in communities during the nineteenth century. The inquest records offer credible and nuanced insights into the practicalities and perils faced by women and their attendants in an age of truly 'natural' childbirth: who was providing care, how they were prepared for it, everyday practices and how long it took to obtain professional help. In light of this evidence, what can be said about received and revisionist perspectives of Australia's maternity care history?

A central tenet of received histories is that birth in the nineteenth century was a risky business, a risk aggravated by the ignorance of female attendants. The inquest cases examined here confirms that birth was indeed hazardous for some. Before the advent of modern technologies of care (antenatal surveillance, caesarean section, blood transfusion and so on), women could lose their lives when common complications manifested unexpectedly. A caveat applies here: coronial inquiries represent the worst of all possible outcomes, and do not account for the myriad women without complications in pregnancy and birth. That said, for any woman whose pregnancy and/or labour was not straightforward, the outcome was unpredictable and contingent.

The blame for maternal mortality prevalence, according to received histories, lay squarely at the feet of women attendants, but precisely how much mortality can be attributed to the 'ignorance' of women is a moot point, requiring further investigation. There is no doubt that a plurality of women attended at maternity bedsides just as Dr James Jamieson had claimed was the case in 1881. Inquest records show that many of those attendants were ill-equipped to deal with the exigencies of labour. The fact that some women were performing neighbourly duties, and doing all that could be reasonably expected of them, was recognized by the coronial courts. Without doubt, some female attendants were entirely unaware when birth complications manifested. It is reasonable to conclude that these women lacked knowledge of the state of maternity. Labelling them as 'ignorant' may seem harsh, but is a valid description, given the context.

Other women attendants had limited knowledge and were capable of recognizing something amiss, but either did not know what to do about complications (for example in cases of haemorrhage) or were unable to do anything (in cases of obstructed labour for which surgery was the solution). Thus, putting all of these women in the same category of 'ignorant' *is* harsh because, in some cases, these same attendants actually understood their practice limitations and sought the help of medical doctors, who then declined to assist. This means that the label 'ignorant' is unhelpful. It applies a broad brush to all female attendants, without sufficient context to justify it.

Revisionist histories apply their own broad generalizations no less frequently. Justifying a connection between present and past midwifery practice has been a foundation of midwifery's professionalizing movement in Australia, as was noted in the introduction to this chapter. Historical links, such as maternity being midwifery's natural 'turf', and the idea of midwives sharing a unique and ancient lore, are used as justification for midwifery's separation from nursing in the professionalizing process. But the inquest cases reported here do not support the idea of a lore 'shared' between female attendants, because the primary feature of the maternity landscape in nineteenth-century Australia was its plurality of practitioners, coupled with vastly different preparation for maternity attendance, confirming earlier reports.[98] That plurality does not mean that all women attendants were uneducated or 'ignorant', it merely underscores diversity, a lack of uniformity. But of the female attendants who claimed education, certification and/or experience, some employed questionable practices, earning the censure of Victoria's coroners for unnecessarily interfering in labour when watchful waiting was recommended as the safest practice. The proclivity of some women in interfering in labour without justification appears to have been mostly strongly associated with the derogatory descriptors of 'ignorant' and 'incompetent'.

The inquest cases described here amply demonstrate the grim reality of natural birth for those unfortunate enough to deviate from a straightforward labour. This is a brutal truth of maternity care history in the nineteenth century and critical to understanding the changes that scientific medicine brought to bear with a focus on the safety of women and babies. However, revisionist histories prefer to position medicine's foray into maternity care as an unjustified takeover of professional turf. In this way, revisionist histories ignore the awful circumstances faced by some women during natural labour, thus contributing to a nostalgic, romantic and imagined history of midwifery and birth. On the cases discussed here, it is difficult to support the argument that women somehow were hoodwinked into hospital birth, or that they did not embrace educated trained personnel in maternity care.

There are lessons for contemporary practitioners in understanding and accepting their history, warts and all. The safety of women and babies still guides the regulatory arrangements governing midwifery practice in Australia. With the enormous emphasis now placed on pregnancy and birth as healthy episodes in the reproductive cycle, and with a trend away from births in hospital, it is timely for midwives to acknowledge that, historically, birth has presented insurmountable difficulties for women and for practitioners. That is not likely to change. Pregnancy and labour may be normal physiological processes in the reproductive cycle, but they are unpredictable and when a perfectly natural and uncomplicated labour deviates from that normal status, the consequences for all can be devastating and irreparable, just as they were in the nineteenth century.

2 PREGNANCY, PATHOLOGY AND PUBLIC MORALS: MAKING ANTENATAL CARE IN EDINBURGH AROUND 1900

Salim Al-Gailani

In the decade or so before the outbreak of World War II, welfare reformers in Britain declared the systematic provision of care to mothers and young children by the state 'one of the most successful developments of public health work': infant mortality had more than halved between 1900 and 1925.[1] Leaders of the maternal and child welfare movement credited this new 'hope for baby' to the realization around 1900 that infant mortality was preventable and were optimistic that the medical supervision of pregnancy would further reduce the 'still disgraceful death-toll' of mothers and neonates.[2] What came to be described as 'antenatal care' around the time of World War I was one of several new health and welfare programmes – the regulation of midwives, the expansion of health visiting, infant feeding centres and baby clinics – usually taken to mark the origins of a welfare state which prioritized mothers and infants.[3] Much historical writing has analysed the contested 'politics of motherhood' these initiatives responded to and continued to shape.[4]

While we have many general accounts of the introduction of antenatal care as part of a package of state-sponsored maternal and infant welfare reforms in Britain and elsewhere, we know less about its early history, especially at a local level prior to legislation.[5] Those reformers arguing for the expansion of medical supervision of 'expectant mothers' draw on the perceived success of initiatives in several countries, but most histories recognize Edinburgh as pioneering.[6] The obstetrician John William Ballantyne (1861–1923) oversaw the world's first dedicated 'pre-maternity' ward at the Edinburgh Royal Maternity Hospital from 1901 and, in a widely discussed series of articles, set out the rationale for the medical supervision of pregnancy. At the suggestion of James Haig Ferguson (1862–1934), the hospital began to offer the first outpatient antenatal clinics in Britain. Ferguson combined maternity hospital practice with directorship of an institution known as the Lauriston Pre-Maternity Home. Founded in 1905, the home provided board and medical supervision for unmarried pregnant women.[7] The local authorities formally linked these institutions through the council-run Maternity and Child Welfare Scheme in 1917, making the availability of antenatal clinics to all poor expectant mothers a central objective of municipal public health.[8]

While this much is known, the development and realization of these initiatives remains little studied. Early histories were written by obstetricians interested in promoting Edinburgh as the 'birthplace' of a progressive medical innovation.[9] Revisionist accounts, shaped by late twentieth-century concerns over the medicalization of pregnancy and childbirth, regarded antenatal care as subjecting women to medical and social control.[10] These perspectives have tended to focus on questions of individual, institutional and national priority for the 'idea' of antenatal care. Yet antenatal care should be seen neither as purely a triumph for preventative medicine, nor as an instrument of social control. This chapter revisits Edinburgh around 1900, not merely to reinterpret the standard origin stories, but to explore the complex social and intellectual context in which antenatal care was conceived and debated, as well as the large network of people, institutions and skills that contributed to its development.

The chapter begins by focusing on Ballantyne's career and the professional, scientific, evangelical and political influences on his work. It explains how his understanding of pregnancy came out of an interest in the causes of congenital malformations, but was increasingly shaped by wider concerns that many contemporaries grouped together as problems of 'public morals': the declining birth rate, degeneration and population health. The second section draws on previously unused archives to compare and contrast the different forms of 'pre-maternity' practice offered by Royal Maternity Hospital and the Lauriston Home in the two decades before the establishment of the municipal welfare scheme. The final section argues that these institutions were increasingly promoted as serving complementary goals. To appreciate how and why antenatal supervision became an established part of maternity care, we need to examine how its leading advocates communicated to and were understood by different, but often overlapping audiences in Edinburgh and beyond: philanthropists, evangelicals, medical colleagues, public health reformers and, above all, pregnant women.

'A Gospel of Hope': John William Ballantyne and Antenatal Hygiene

Before the turn of the twentieth century, antenatal care was more the responsibility of the expectant parents than the medical practitioner, with whom few women would have had any formal contact before confinement. Consulting an accoucheur during pregnancy nonetheless became more common among wealthy women in mid-Victorian Britain.[11] A burgeoning nineteenth-century genre offering specific advice on pregnancy and lying-in to middle-class women suggested readers 'engage [their] future medical attendant early'.[12] Some European and American maternity clinics informally admitted patients days or weeks in advance of labour and in the late nineteenth century began informally to offer health instruction to pregnant women. Yet at whatever stage women recognized they were pregnant, early twentieth-century oral testimony in Scotland indicates that the doctor or midwife was rarely called until childbirth was imminent.[13] Serious medical interest in the supervision of expectant mothers appears to have begun only around 1900. Although early initiatives in antenatal care developed in quite different contexts in France, Britain, the United States, Australia and New Zealand, they were strongly informed by one another. By World War I, antenatal care reformers internationally recognized John William Ballantyne as the movement's 'great apostle'.[14]

Ballantyne was part of a group of elite Edinburgh obstetricians who began their careers assisting Alexander Russell Simpson, nephew of the anaesthetic pioneer James Young Simpson.[15] A. R. Simpson inherited the university chair of midwifery from his uncle in 1870 and thereafter 'dominated Edinburgh obstetrics and gynaecology' through appointments to the gynaecological pavilion of the Royal Infirmary and the Royal Maternity Hospital.[16] Bound together by scientific and professional interests, family connections, philanthropic activities and a deep commitment to the United Free Church of Scotland, Simpson's circle was close-knit.[17] Simpson's assistants followed him not only into senior hospital appointments, but also into positions of leadership of the evangelical movement in Edinburgh. From the late 1870s until the 1920s, their intimate involvement with revival meetings, temperance campaigns and missionary work reinforced the strong connection between obstetrics and evangelicalism in the Scottish capital.

Ballantyne converted as a student and climbed the ranks of the city's evangelical community to become president of both the Edinburgh Medical Missionary Society and the Pleasant Sunday Afternoon Brotherhood, founded to encourage working-class religious worship. By the second decade of the twentieth century, he spoke regularly at United Free Church Congresses, temperance demonstrations and meetings of the Scottish chapters of the Alliance of Honour and the National Council for Public Morals on the importance of making an 'effort to lead a simple, self-controlled life'.[18] For Ballantyne and other members of Simpson's circle, alcohol and syphilis were chiefly responsible for a range of social problems: moral and physical degeneration, disease, crime and poverty.[19] As obstetricians, they thought themselves especially well qualified to appreciate the effects of intemperance and deviant sexuality on account of their 'unparalleled acquaintance with family secrets'.[20] It was as 'public moralists' that they were best able to establish a presence as members of Edinburgh's 'distinguished citizenry' and civic leadership.[21]

This group participated not only in evangelical communities, but also in the scientific community by cultivating identities as anatomical experts. As a mentor and patron, Simpson directed the work of his assistants by giving them privileged access to anatomical resources and extensive supply networks cultivated through the Edinburgh Obstetrical Society, founded in 1840. In the 1880s and 1890s, the 'Edinburgh school' produced influential work on the anatomy of the female pelvis and pregnant uterus. Ballantyne participated, but distinguished himself from his colleagues by focusing on the fetus and newborn infant. He used this anatomical work to launch an academic career as a lecturer in obstetrics and the emerging speciality of paediatrics. Because Edinburgh was a small city with a limited supply of wealthy private patients, practitioners relied upon teaching and publication far more heavily than their London counterparts. This gave Edinburgh medicine its characteristically academic culture and meant many practitioners devoted a significant part of their time to research.[22] It was in this context that Ballantyne established an international reputation as the preeminent British teratologist, or expert on what were then termed 'monsters'.[23] He rode a wave of renewed scientific interest in the field in the late nineteenth century as museums of anatomy and pathology sought to expand and catalogue their collections of specimens and experimental physiologists manipulated animal embryos to create monsters in the laboratory. Anthropologists and alienists (psychiatrists) also increasingly adopted teratological concepts by making congenital malformations morphological signs of a spectrum of conditions associated with degeneracy, including insanity, alcoholism and criminality.[24]

Ballantyne spent the 1890s 'engrossed in teratology'. This included founding a short-lived journal, collecting, dissecting, drawing and classifying rare forms of fetal abnormality and experimenting with hen's eggs to produce monstrous chicks.[25] His lectures and publications culminated in the leading English-language manual of teratology in 1904.[26] Ballantyne justified this work in an internationally anatomist-dominated field by highlighting the obstetrician's advantage, that only he could compare the health of the mother during pregnancy with that of her fetus or child. He claimed that the obstetrician's familiarity with his patient, her family and her social circumstances enabled him to construct a pathological genealogy for any given case. While obstetricians had long dissected fetal anomalies, preserved them for anatomical museums and reported them in journals, Ballantyne insisted that the systematic collection of case histories by obstetricians would make teratology clinically relevant. By framing clinical histories as a crucial component of the investigation of fetal anomalies, he promoted a new discipline: 'antenatal pathology'.[27]

Positioned between obstetrics and teratology, Ballantyne initially struggled to find an audience for what even he conceded was 'extraordinarily dry and marvellously unpractical work'.[28] Advice from colleagues, journal editors and book publishers to write on a subject that was more obviously marketable to clinicians encouraged a reorientation from pathology towards the hygiene of pregnancy and public health. Beginning in the late 1890s, Ballantyne promoted 'antenatal hygiene' by harnessing his project to broader concerns about the 'future of the race'. Blending together teratological science with temperance reform, antenatal hygiene helped promote an understanding of pregnancy that laid particular emphasis on the environment. Against the dominant view that the mother's placenta and womb offered protection from toxins and injuries, Ballantyne proposed that the fetus 'is not beyond the influences of her environment, nay, her body is his immediate environment, and he is profoundly affected by it for good or evil, for health or disease'.[29] He insisted that every child had 'the right to be engendered by self-respecting individuals, to be conceived in soberness, and to be developed under healthy conditions of intrauterine life'. What Ballantyne termed the 'antenatal death roll', especially from the 'morbid influences' of alcohol and syphilis, became a recurrent theme of his polemics as the declining birth-rate and infant mortality was made nationally central after 1900.[30]

Such rhetoric was increasingly commonly deployed in a national discourse on depopulation, physical degradation and social and moral decadence. The distinctiveness of antenatal hygiene was Ballantyne's insistence upon the necessity of carrying 'to the infant yet unborn some of the benefits of modern medicine and hygiene'.[31] This meant enabling qualified medical practitioners to provide 'scientific' health advice to pregnant women about diet, exercise, clothing and mental and sexual hygiene and, above all, educating the medical profession and the wider public in the 'value of antenatal life'. Articulated within the context of renewed concern over the practice of criminal and increasingly also medical abortion, Ballantyne sought to establish obstetricians as natural advocates of the unborn child. The systematic use of obstetric anaesthesia and antisepsis led to growing medical unease about such operations as craniotomy 'which either kill the foetus or subject it to a grave risk in order to improve the maternal prognosis'.[32] These arguments had a direct impact on intertwined debates over abortion, the declining birth rate and midwives' registration. Amid fears that unsupervised and unlicensed practitioners would increase the business of criminal abortion, obstetricians could claim a moral imperative to protect antenatal life, and so reinforce their status over midwives.[33]

Newly charged debates about heredity, syphilis, alcoholism and infant mortality provided opportunities to bring antenatal hygiene to even wider audiences. Ballantyne helped promote the work of French advocates of 'intrauterine puériculture' – the general principle that medical, charitable and governmental assistance to pregnant women would improve the quality of both individuals and the population as a whole – within Anglo-American medicine. Like 'puériculture', antenatal hygiene was underpinned by the widely held 'neo-Lamarckian' belief in the possibility of offsetting the worst results of heredity by manipulating the environment, before and after birth. As William Schneider has noted, such arguments were attractive to the French medical and educational establishment because they were both optimistic in their prospects for change and supportive of work in health and social reform.[34] Antenatal hygiene similarly appealed to those groups in Britain seeking to promote the goals and values of both preventive medicine and temperance reform against the challenge of negative eugenics.

Addressing a national audience increasingly preoccupied with the degeneration of the British population, Ballantyne argued that by 'clean living' and 'antenatal hygiene', individuals could guarantee their own and their progeny's redemption from sin and physical degradation.[35] He opposed those eugenicists who he believed placed too great an emphasis on irreversible morbid heredity at the expense of medical and moral improvement. Favouring the temperance language of 'dereliction' that could be ameliorated through social intervention, he insisted that it was 'better to try to turn the weeds into flowers rather than to suppress them'.[36] These arguments became especially valuable tools against eugenicists who accused the medical practitioner of 'busying himself in preserving weedy lives and in counteracting the benefit of the survival only of the fittest'. For reformers opposed to the perceived 'fatalism' of negative eugenics, antenatal hygiene could be framed as a 'gospel of hope'.[37]

Ballantyne's views on pregnancy, heredity and hygiene developed within the milieu of Edinburgh obstetrics, but also in an evangelical context that saw individual spiritual salvation as a means of social improvement. Both teratology and temperance reform offered him not only 'a glimpse of the true form of prevention which is set at work before birth' but also the authority to speak as an expert on this subject.[38] By aligning antenatal hygiene with public morals, a project originally focused on anatomy was transformed by discussion in new settings and assimilated into broader debates about public health and welfare. As the recognized pioneer of antenatal hygiene, Ballantyne joined a diverse coalition of intellectuals, social welfare campaigners, public health officials, medical practitioners and clerics who aimed to regenerate the nation's moral life by positive education.[39] These broad social and moral reform movements drove new understandings of expectant motherhood in the early twentieth century.

'Pre-Maternity' in Edinburgh: Institutions, Patients and Practices

Teratology, temperance and antenatal hygiene were pivotally important for providing a framework in which antenatal care could enter public discourse around World War I. Yet Ballantyne's 1901 appeal in the *British Medical Journal* for the establishment of a 'pre-maternity hospital' described the innovation for which he is best known. Reprinted in medical journals internationally, the article argued for dedicated institutions for women who were ill and pregnant, offering a means of 'scientifically investigating' 'prenatal diagnosis and treatment ... on a large scale and in a systematized fashion'.[40] To help understand how antenatal care emerged from Ballantyne's comparatively narrow vision for the hospital, this section explores the history of 'pre-maternity' practice and its various meanings at two Edinburgh institutions: the Royal Maternity Hospital (RMH) and the Lauriston Home for unmarried mothers. Focusing locally illuminates how these institutions sought legitimacy by accommodating the needs and expectations of a wider network of doctors, philanthropists and most importantly, the pregnant women for whom they cared.

Shortly after Ballantyne's 1901 plea, a 'pre-maternity bed' was endowed at the RMH, and named in honour of the university's first professor of midwifery, James Hamilton. The benefactor was officially anonymous, but later acknowledged to be the wealthy A. H. Freeland Barbour, A. R. Simpson's brother-in-law and, from 1907, professor of gynaecology. After Simpson donated a further bed himself in 1905, the Hamilton came to be known as the 'pre-maternity ward'. Though administrative changes in the RMH around 1870 formally excluded medical staff from the lay board of directors, Simpson and his allies were in fact increasingly dominant figures and among the largest individual donors to the hospital.[41] Ballantyne's connection with Simpson's circle and their influence within the RMH explains why the pre-maternity ward could be established there.

Founded in 1844, the RMH served the dual purpose of providing relief for the pregnant poor and training to fee-paying medical students and midwives. Until around 1900 it was the only provider of in-patient care in the city.[42] Like most maternity hospitals elsewhere in the nineteenth century, the RMH generally admitted only those patients who were already in labour. The Hamilton pre-maternity ended this practice by accepting women in any stage of pregnancy – some dated as early as two months – diagnosed with complications or abnormal obstetric histories. The Hamilton admitted around forty patients per year by 1909, some of which were documented in the single extant casebook and in published case records. Like existing lying-in institutions, the pre-maternity patients came almost entirely from Edinburgh's 'lower and middle working classes'.[43] But ill pregnant women came to the pre-maternity ward from as far afield as Cumberland; the wife of a Glasgow minister with a history of miscarrying, meanwhile, was sent by her doctor to stay in the ward for a month in 1911.[44] Though numbers were always too small to ascertain patterns of attendance and experience, such cases indicate the growing reputation of the Hamilton as a centre of medical expertise to which general practitioners could refer difficult cases.

While all senior physicians at the RMH attended patients in the Hamilton, Ballantyne oversaw and promoted its work. He insisted the criteria for admission were based strictly on medical need rather than on ability to pay a fee, or marital status. Ballantyne needed to respond in particular to suspicions that he was 'advocating a place for the reception of unmarried pregnant women, where they might get every attention, medical and hygienic; that I was thus making things easier for fallen women, and possibly even encouraging what everyone wished to hinder'.[45] He sought to secure a public role for the Hamilton ward by suppressing the moral assumptions that underpinned the work of the numerous charitable shelters for destitute, homeless and unwed pregnant women established across Europe and North America in the late nineteenth century. In Britain, the 'maternity home movement' was largely associated with the Salvation Army as part of their broader mission to 'rescue' 'fallen women'.[46]

Though the Salvation Army did similar work in Edinburgh by World War I, Edinburgh's first such institution was founded in 1899 as the St Luke's Home by John Halliday Croom, another RMH physician who succeeded Simpson as professor of midwifery in 1905. That year this institution was transferred to larger premises adjacent to the RMH where its charges were delivered, and was renamed the Lauriston Pre-Maternity Home, where James Haig Ferguson, formerly Croom's private assistant, took over as director.[47] Although neither Croom nor Ferguson were so obviously involved in Edinburgh's evangelical networks as Ballantyne or Simpson, local clergymen from various churches participated in managing and promoting the Lauriston's 'Christlike' work. The home was in fact explicitly nondenominational: each woman was 'put in touch with minsters and church-workers of her own persuasion'.[48] Supporters could justify the home's role with reference to Edinburgh's illegitimacy rate, among the highest in Britain: 8.5 in every 100 births compared to 7 in Glasgow and 4 in London in the period between 1905 and 1909.[49] The Lauriston remained the largest and highest profile maternity shelter in the city, accepting women from across Scotland, Ireland and the north of England until its closure in the 1970s. Annual reports, intended to publicize the home and encourage donations, survive from 1908; these help to recover the objectives and practices of directors and staff.

Maternity rescue work built on the assumption that offering shelter to women who had engaged in alleged sexual misconduct and become pregnant would protect them from being further corrupted, and slipping further into vice by becoming hardened prostitutes. Unmarried mothers were regarded as the most hopeful of all rescue cases and the Lauriston claimed high success in returning the women to family or friends or finding employment, usually in domestic service. The Lauriston was supported not only by prominent local clergymen and doctors, but also by members of the women's movement, who proclaimed sisterhood with women under their care. At the home's annual meeting in 1912 Lady Frances Balfour, a high-profile suffragette, proclaimed maternity rescue work 'emphatically a woman's question'.[50] Such work allowed women to contribute to a public discussion about the problems of sexuality, pregnancy and illegitimacy to a mixed audience.

The only prerequisite for admission to the Lauriston was that women were in their first pregnancy, to protect the institution from the charge of encouraging vice. But the directors favoured charges who came from 'honest work' and could return to it after their confinements, and could pay their own board. The home had room for about fourteen cases at a time, usually between sixty and eighty per year.[51] The standard narrative in annual reports and occasional publicity in the local press was that unmarried mothers were vulnerable women 'drawn from respectable surroundings', 'more sinned against than sinning', 'terrorised victims' of male lust and seduction. Reports were filled with tales of 'selfish' rogues and 'heartless scoundrels' and sought to 'draw the special attention of Christian workers to the *extreme* youth' of their charges.[52] These stories echoed fictional narratives in the contemporary penny press and were designed to appeal to the sympathies of potential donors.

The Lauriston's first concern was to restore unmarried mothers to moral life and economic self-sufficiency. But the philosophy of maternity rescue work was that 'fallen women' would find redemption by 'awakening the sanctity of motherhood'. It relied on the mother's 'overwhelming passion for maternity' to effect reformation, rather than a lengthy period of penance and discipline, as in rescue homes for prostitutes.[53] Nurturing the maternal bond was seen as an effective method of ensuring unmarried mothers would avoid moral relapse. In 1912 the directors opened a mother and baby home where women could live with their newborns for two months before the child was boarded out. Of the babies born between 1908 and 1919, a third returned home with their mothers, roughly a quarter of who found employment in domestic service. This was favoured because rescue workers reckoned adoption removed the burden of the child's support, which was meant to serve as a constant reminder of the consequences of the woman's sin. For one benefactor of the Lauriston, 'if these women are to be saved they are to be saved through the child ... it is the idea of motherhood that will help them ... what was a curse may become a salvation'.[54] The blueprint for the redemptive environment of the home was therefore a 'period of valuable discipline' that combined 'softening influence, kindness, sympathy' and 'wholesome shelter' with a steady diet of religious and domestic training.[55] Moral education was supplemented with training for domestic service so that inmates would be able to support themselves after they left the institution, in order to provide for their infants. 'Salvation' therefore implied the conversion of fallen young women to middle-class standards of female propriety.

In contrast to the Lauriston, the language of *care* did not feature at all in the early public rhetoric of the Hamilton pre-maternity ward at the RMH. With publicity directed primarily towards medical audiences, Ballantyne stressed that the ward was a site for 'systematic investigation' of what he termed antenatal morbid states. It was an opportunity to collect empirical data to elaborate the relationship between mother and fetus, and its pathology.[56] More broadly, he aimed to test the efficacy of dietary regimens, obstetrical interventions, including induced labour, and therapeutics, such as calcium chloride, which 'did a great many strange things, which were not yet fully understood'.[57] Many of the poorer women who typically attended maternity hospitals had suffered from childhood rickets, which left them vulnerable to significant danger in childbirth.[58] Patients at the Hamilton diagnosed with contracted pelvises from rickets were put on a 'proteid diet' pioneered by the Hamburg obstetrician, Ludwig Protchownick. Protchownick experimented with nutrition in pregnancy hoping 'to keep the size of the child small and so facilitate labour', which it was thought might be induced 'about the seventh month and a half'. Protchownick's theory could only be adequately ascertained in such an institution 'as the ... pre-maternity hospital may yet turn out to be'.[59] Articles promoting the pre-maternity prophesied an obstetric future in which new scientific knowledge and medical technology would enable the physician to deliver every fetus live and healthy. Such rhetoric was essential for asserting the novelty of the Hamilton.

In reality, observation, management, treatment and intervention were all speculative: the pre-maternity was effectively Ballantyne's laboratory, and in this medical view, the expectant mother was an experimental subject. Despite initial concerns about the purpose of the Hamilton within the RMH hierarchy, by 1909, the directors considered pre-maternity work to have brought the 'spirit of research' to the hospital as a whole.[60] As early as 1908, Ballantyne was instrumental in reconfiguring the work of the RMH to facilitate physiological and pathological research. He persuaded the university to set aside an honorarium for a pathologist 'who could make use of the clinical material which the Hamilton Ward for pregnancy cases supplies us with' and in 1919 secured Medical Research Council funding for further research.[61] Ballantyne insisted that practical measures in antenatal hygiene, including advice to mothers and the medical management of pregnancy, must be underpinned by scientific research in 'antenatal anatomy, physiology, pharmacology and pathology'.[62]

Publicly, the RMH claimed to offer unrivalled obstetric care and its physicians increasingly saw it as their duty to encourage working-class women to make use of the maternity hospital. Yet directors recognized that it was 'not a popular Institution amongst the pregnant poor in Edinburgh'. Widespread rumours of infection, lack of privacy on the wards and unpalatable meals, rumours known to be rife among the city's pregnant poor, directly impaired the reputation of the pre-maternity ward.[63] That RMH directors were acutely sensitive to the perception that married women were not kept separately from the unmarried underlines the point that potential patients from the respectable working classes had to be convinced the Hamilton was entirely distinct from the Lauriston. Ballantyne conceded that it was often exceedingly difficult to convince women 'to submit themselves to hospital treatment', especially when 'they do not feel sufficiently ill, and their friends and relatives see no cause for their removal from home'.[64] Under early pressure by directors to justify pre-maternity work, Ballantyne made more active moves to advertise the Hamilton through ministers, missionaries, district visitors and 'others acquainted with the needs of poor women', and to encourage general practitioners to refer cases.[65] By 1908, he saw 'a rapidly increasing demand among medical men for some place – a hospital or nursing home – in which morbid pregnancies can be suitably treated; and there were indications that the patients themselves were beginning to share this feeling, some ... having entered the hospital on their own initiative'.[66]

While perceptions of both the Hamilton and the Lauriston were shaped by institutional practices, doctors, lay directors and philanthropists, their success more broadly therefore depended on the cooperation and approval of expectant mothers. Surviving records provide only a selective view of the activities of these institutions and the experiences of the pregnant women who sought their care. Those who applied to the Lauriston in desperate circumstances are likely to have treated the home as a place of refuge, a source of otherwise unavailable medical attention and the means to a 'self-respecting career'. While publicity invariably highlighted those women 'profoundly grateful for the shelter the Home affords', who were those who found God, married or returned to their families and employment, at least 7 per cent left or were dismissed from the home before their confinements.[67] Although reports do not elaborate what prompted women to leave, it is difficult not to interpret early departures as acts of resistance, perhaps in protest at the arduous work, or restrictions placed on them. The matron reported some women posed 'a difficult problem, requiring more restraint and time than the Home is designed to give'.[68]

Ballantyne fully recognized that pregnancy was a period of 'irksomeness, weariness, strain, inquietude' for all women, and in some cases extreme danger.[69] Many of the patients registered in the Hamilton casebooks had suffered traumatic experiences in past pregnancies, personal brushes with death during delivery, or slow and incomplete post-partum recoveries. Such experiences may have prompted women to seek medical attention where it was available, and to welcome the advice and reassurance provided by hospital staff. The casebooks suggest that childless women who had previously experienced miscarriages may have viewed the pre-maternity ward as a last resort. Campaigns for maternal and child welfare extolling the virtues of motherhood gained unprecedented importance in early twentieth-century public discourse, while testimonies of working-class women themselves represented childbearing as a long-desired 'life's work'.[70] For at least some of the Hamilton's patients, the intensive medical scrutiny may have represented hope for successful pregnancy and childbirth that had previously eluded them. For those women who already had families, the pre-maternity ward may have offered a place of extended rest from the tribulations of their daily lives.

The early history of the concept of 'pre-maternity' in Edinburgh shows that different medico-moral ideologies underpinned the care of the expectant mother in practice and rationale. For the clerics, doctors and philanthropists involved with the Lauriston, care was targeted at unmarried mothers; 'fallen women' who needed salvation through domestication. For Ballantyne, medical supervision within a maternity hospital offered an unprecedented opportunity for conducting research into the 'nature of pregnancy' and a blueprint for total medical control that prioritized the health of the fetus. Despite defining their purpose in different ways, the public roles of these institutions were constructed and evolved in continuing relation. Both the Lauriston and the Hamilton relied on similar networks of philanthropic support – Simpson's circle of obstetricians, for instance, were major donors to both institutions – and the acceptance of expectant mothers. Ballantyne and the RMH directors, moreover, had to convince doctors, philanthropists and the 'pregnant poor' that the pre-maternity ward was explicitly medical and therefore distinct from the forms of care offered by maternity shelters like the Lauriston.

From the 'Pre-Maternity System' to Antenatal Care

Despite the continuing moral association between institutional surveillance and illegitimate pregnancy, the Lauriston and the Hamilton were increasingly regarded as serving complementary roles. Physicians from the RMH had been involved with the Lauriston from the outset but, from around 1912, they emphasized the medical in addition to the moral benefits of rescue work. Every annual report after 1913 began with an extract from an article about the Lauriston in the *British Medical Journal* stating that because

> the young expectant mothers are under medical supervision whilst in the home … deviations from the normal healthy state of pregnancy can be at once detected and often cured; in more serious cases the woman can be transferred to the [Hamilton] pre-maternity ward.

Ferguson and his colleagues also insisted that broader obstetric lessons could be drawn from the experience of the Lauriston: 'rest before confinement, good food, healthy surroundings, and avoidance of excitement, seem to give the mother greater vitality, more perfect nutrition, full-term labours, and good recoveries'. For Ferguson, the 'condition of health which prevails unvaryingly among' the Lauriston's charges on confinement taught the 'enormous importance of prenatal care', which he argued should be available to all pregnant women.[71]

Meanwhile, RMH physicians sought to extend the hospital's pre-maternity provision. Starting in 1913, the Hamilton was coordinated with the work of the hospital's domiciliary staff. Arranging for home visiting by trained pre-maternity nurses who asked around for pregnant women not already under the care of a doctor or midwife helped to attract patients. To facilitate this work, Ballantyne provided nurses with printed cards to record consultations, thereby disciplining them to be sensitive to signs of impending danger; the nurse just had to put a cross next to 'danger signal'. The nurses were also trained to offer basic advice about hygiene, and indicate on the card that they had done so.[72] From June 1915, the RMH began to offer outpatient antenatal clinics on the premises in addition to home visiting.[73] Consultations were to identify potentially pathological cases, which would then be transferred to the Hamilton, offer expectant mothers basic health advice, and ask them 'to report themselves for further supervision'.[74] The physician-in-charge was assisted by two student medical officers and two nurses, seeing on average 8 or 9 women at each clinic in its first year, and 104 by December 1915. As physician-in-charge at the RMH during the summer quarter, Ferguson supervised the first outdoor clinics. Ballantyne took over in September 1915, and in subsequent publications referred to the clinics, the outdoor nurses, the Lauriston Home and the Hamilton as a single 'pre-maternity system', through which potentially pathological cases were identified for treatment or pre-term induction. By 1916, he routinely described this system as providing 'antenatal care of the babies'.[75]

The 'pre-maternity system' helped broaden the reach of the RMH to women who were not otherwise under medical surveillance. Yet it also aligned the previously distinct philosophies of the Lauriston and the Hamilton. As Ballantyne began to address new audiences in antenatal hygiene, the rhetoric he used to promote the pre-maternity system also became more explicitly moralistic. The redemptive story of an alcoholic woman kept from drink in the Hamilton and giving birth to a healthy baby tellingly became the symbolic narrative used to promote the Edinburgh system in such settings as the Society for the Study of Inebriety, the National Conference on Infant Mortality, the Sanitary Association and the United Free Church Congress.[76] Extending medical supervision to potentially all of the city's 'pregnant poor' was intended to cultivate awareness that good food, healthy surroundings, avoiding mental strain and abstaining from alcohol gave the mothers greater vitality, full-term labours and good recoveries. The pre-maternity system exhorted pregnant women to comply with various forms of health instruction, through clinics and advice literature, which physicians claimed could predict and prevent pathological pregnancies and deliveries. Though these first clinics only served a fraction of Edinburgh's expectant mothers, steadily increasing uptake suggests that many welcomed the availability of medical care.[77]

During World War I, the maternal and child welfare movement gathered momentum nationally and it was during these debates that the concept of 'ante-natal care' first emerged. Groups who took the Edinburgh system as a blueprint used antenatal care as a vehicle for advancing quite different political and professional concerns. Each patient who attended the Edinburgh antenatal clinics was given a pamphlet authored by Ballantyne and published by the Women's Cooperative Guild, 'Hints to Expectant Mothers'.[78] For the campaigning women of the guild, the expectant mother was in urgent need of state support,[79] and used Ballantyne's philosophy of antenatal hygiene to support this view. Ballantyne's mission to educate the public in the 'sacredness of human life before birth' was also useful to early twentieth-century women doctors and midwives seeking to legitimate their entry into the medical profession, who could claim special understanding and 'close contact with the problem of unnecessary suffering of mothers and unnecessary waste of infant life'.[80] For elite obstetricians in Edinburgh and beyond, antenatal supervision promised unprecedented opportunities to study the physiology and pathology of pregnancy, securing Medical Research Council funding from 1919.[81] Amand Routh, president of the Royal Society of Medicine's Obstetric and Gynaecological Section, credited antenatal pathology and hygiene with inspiring a 'new obstetric ideal' through prevention and research.[82] These new areas of expertise and public health roles invested the discipline with added prestige and authority.

Yet it was a new generation of politically influential public health reformers who would do most to advance the concept of antenatal care as 'state medicine'. Challenging the laissez faire ideology that had underpinned Victorian public health, reformers insisted that social welfare could and would enable the individual to overcome the structural contingencies of her environment. Women were singled out as the main target group under the assumption that they alone were the best and most natural trainers of their children. Increasingly prioritizing the medical scrutiny of the mother, including during pregnancy, the new public health was championed nationally by Arthur Newsholme and William Leslie Mackenzie, medical officers to the Local Government Boards of England and Scotland respectively, and George Newman, medical officer to the newly created Ministry of Health from 1919.[83] They invoked the Edinburgh pre-maternity system to argue that the scrutiny and care of the expectant mother was crucial to the health and welfare of the infant after birth. Mackenzie referred to 'ante-natal care' in a discussion on the 'duty of the State Towards the Early Environment of the Child' at the British Medical Association meeting in Aberdeen in 1914, the earliest apparent use of the term in the *British Medical Journal*.[84]

A series of reports on maternal and child health by the Local Government Board under the auspices of the Carnegie UK Trust in 1917, which stressed the importance of pre-maternity work and antenatal care, were part of broader campaign for legislative change.[85] Edinburgh's municipal maternal and child welfare scheme was introduced in 1917, taking advantage of central government's offer to fund half the costs of maternity and infant care in England, Wales and Scotland under the terms of the Notification of Births (Extension) Act, 1915. Designed to coordinate what were perceived to be fragmentary services offered by the city's voluntary agencies, the scheme established the RMH as the main centre of antenatal work in Edinburgh.[86] An annual grant from the Edinburgh Corporation (town council) required the hospital to hold twice-weekly clinics, provide a record of all cases to the public health department and stipulated that an antenatal physician should be available at 'any time for consultation as an expert in connection with Maternity Welfare'.[87]

This expansion of antenatal provision was accelerated nationally by the passing of the Maternity and Child Welfare Act of 1918. As a result of the Act, the Edinburgh Corporation established a Maternity and Child Welfare Department, a subsidiary of the public health committee, which was ultimately responsible for coordinating the broader municipal maternity and child welfare apparatus. This was by now a complex bureaucratic system that required the cooperation of a large network of individuals: doctors, midwives, health visitors; and institutions: hospitals, maternity centres, schools for mothers, pre-maternity homes, milk depots, schools, nurseries and children's shelters.[88] In line with national developments, the department emphasized that its chief aim was not 'to do things for mothers as to educate and to show them how to do things for themselves'.[89] Compared with elsewhere in the country, however, the Edinburgh scheme placed unusual emphasis on pre-maternity work.

The RMH credited the antenatal work with the increasing demand for hospital births: women attending the clinics could arrange in advance for admission to the labour wards.[90] Equally importantly, the incorporation of the antenatal work into the municipal scheme was a sign of both the Edinburgh Corporation's increasing stake in the management of the city's hospitals, and the transformation of the RMH into an instrument of the local authority's public health policy. This culminated in a 1919 agreement stipulating that the RMH provide treatment for VD cases under the terms of Venereal Diseases Act (Scotland) 1917 in return for a further annual grant. The VD clinic was coordinated with antenatal work, and both placed under Ballantyne's charge.[91] Public health officials perceived the moral surveillance and regeneration of patients as part of the functions of VD treatment clinics more broadly.[92] The maternal and child welfare schemes codified an important link between the medical supervision of pregnancy, moral hygiene and the control of venereal disease.

Conclusion

The municipal maternal and child welfare and VD schemes in Edinburgh marked the emergence of new institutional and political structures which made the systematic provision of antenatal clinics a key objective of a reformed public health. Their introduction allowed local and ultimately national authorities to define the scope of antenatal care and standardize its practice. The making of antenatal care as part of the new state medicine in Britain followed a broad political consensus that the medical supervision of pregnant women would improve the health of the population as a whole. Focusing on Edinburgh in the decades before the municipal scheme has helped to explain how this consensus was negotiated. This early history also suggests that antenatal care was not a static concept but was understood and practised in constantly evolving ways. Tracing its construction through Ballantyne's 'antenatal pathology and hygiene', the Hamilton Ward, the Lauriston Home and finally the pre-maternity system that would serve as a model for the municipal scheme shows how differently the objectives of medical and moral care could be promoted and perceived. Only by appreciating that these individuals and institutions secured roles in public health by appealing to and accommodating the interests of various groups – philanthropists, temperance reformers, medical practitioners and public health officials and, most importantly, expectant mothers – can we fully understand how antenatal care was made. Pregnant women's experiences of pre-maternity provision are difficult to recover, though their agency is essential to take into account. Ill pregnant women and unmarried mothers are likely to have perceived the Hamilton and the Lauriston in quite different ways from medical practitioners and from each other. Yet the success of both institutions, and antenatal care more generally, depended on their approval.

Acknowledgements

I am grateful to Linda Bryder, Janet Greenlees, Nick Hopwood, Malcolm Nicolson, Alison Nuttall and Jim Secord for comments on earlier versions of this chapter, the research for which was funded by Wellcome Trust (Grant 074298).

3 'THE PECULIAR AND COMPLEX FEMALE PROBLEM': THE CHURCH OF SCOTLAND AND HEALTH CARE FOR UNWED MOTHERS, 1900–1948

Janet Greenlees

In 1904 the Church of Scotland established a Committee on Social Work (CSW). With the broad aim of 'providing social services irrespective of class, creed or colour based on Christian gospel and carried out by committed Christian men and women', their network of health and social services gradually expanded so that by World War II, the Church was the largest single provider of social services in Scotland.[1] While some services targeted men, young single women living in cities were prioritized due to fears about rising immorality amongst young people and from the belief that women were the moral guardians of the family.[2] To address these anxieties and complement existing charitable provision, the Church of Scotland opened a network of hostels, 'preventive' homes for single, 'friendless' girls and boarding houses. And, in 1915, they opened a maternity home for unwed mothers in Glasgow to meet a 'very pressing need'.[3] Combined, these services sought to address the 'peculiar and complex female problem' present in Scotland's cities,[4] but it was the Church of Scotland's home for unwed Scottish mothers that secured the Church both medical and civic recognition for its high standards of maternal health and social care, while also meeting the Church's evangelical and political objectives.

The Church's entry into social work coincided with broader British anxieties about the health of the nation and a need for national efficiency. These were highlighted particularly well in the social enquiries of Charles Booth (1889) and B. S. Rowntree (1902), where improving maternal and infant welfare were core concerns and paralleled growing fears about population 'degeneration'.[5] At the turn of the twentieth century, the illegitimate birth rate was on average higher in Scotland than in England and most of Europe. Moreover, in Glasgow, death rates for illegitimate babies remained similar to that in 1873 at 286 deaths per 1,000 births – nearly double that for legitimate births, of 145 deaths per 1,000 births.[6] At the same time, the Scottish birth rate was falling steadily from a peak of 35.5 per 1,000 of population in 1876 to 25.5 in 1914.[7] These facts greatly concerned the Scottish government, Medical Officers of Health (MOH) and social reformers. As in many Western countries, Scotland's solution to reducing its high infant mortality rates centred on the mother.[8]

Histories of maternal and infant welfare reforms in Great Britain have emphasized the government's increasing role in reducing infant deaths.[9] While historians have noted wide variations in care, overall, the health reforms introduced by pre-World War I liberal governments and adapted postwar, led to improvements in maternal and child health in England and Wales.[10] These were not shared by Scotland.[11] Yet, as in England and Wales, in Scotland a series of legislation sought to lower infant death rates and improve maternal health. In 1903, The *Report of the Royal Commission on Physical Training (Scotland)* recommended dramatic improvements in the feeding and environment of children. Often seen as the Scottish equivalent to the Inter-Departmental Committee on Physical Deterioration, this legislation led to the establishment of milk depots to supervise the artificial feeding of infants. Glasgow's depot opened in 1904. In 1907, the Notification of Births Act required all births to be registered. Initially permissive, this was made compulsory in 1915. In 1908, the Children's Act tackled the neglect and abandonment of children, which Glasgow's MOH Dr A. K. Chalmers believed instrumental in reducing the death rate of illegitimate infants.[12] Chalmers's concerns about high infant mortality rates and national efficiency motivated him to help instigate the 1914 National Conference on Infant Mortality, where he argued the necessity of improved antenatal care.[13] Shortly thereafter, the 1915 Midwives (Scotland) Act sought to both improve and standardize midwifery training. Later, the 1937 Maternity Services (Scotland) Act addressed maternal mortality with broader maternity services. While slow to have a significant impact in Scotland, these Acts, and legislation more broadly, have fuelled debates about the increased medicalization of childbirth during the first half of the twentieth century.[14]

It was into this growing legislative environment of maternity that the Church of Scotland and other charities entered. While in England, local philanthropic services made a major contribution to maternal health within their area, we know little about the mixed economy of welfare and voluntary bodies in Scotland that provided many of the health-care services in the decades immediately after 1900.[15] Scotland relied on an array of charities to provide both health and social care, more so than England. Charity was also more of a Scottish tradition than an English one.[16] Charities were relied upon to fill Poor Law deficiencies, with local parishes remaining responsible for its members long after they left the parish and when they did not have the finances to do so. Moreover, the 1870s Scottish Poor Law reforms left mothers of illegitimate children ineligible for relief.[17] Well into the twentieth century, these women and their children were often dependent on charities for survival.

While the efforts of the Salvation Army, the Magdalene Homes, the Church of England and other charities towards unwed mothers are recognized, little is known about the Church of Scotland's provision for these women and their dependents.[18] This is partly due to the many rifts within Scottish Presbyterianism which meant there was little coordination of health and welfare initiatives until the early twentieth century. By then, despite the survival of many minor Presbyterian churches owing to the endemic divisiveness of Scottish Presbyterianism, there were two major denominations, the United Free Church (UFC) and the Established Church of Scotland.[19] When the UFC failed to grow, its social mission struggled. In contrast, from the early twentieth century, the Established Church of Scotland's social and political influence grew, with many church leaders gaining political posts. The centrality of the Church to Scottish life in the first half of the twentieth century meant that it was well placed to address health and welfare issues and to influence policymakers.

While all denominations provided welfare services, this article focuses on the Church of Scotland's maternal health and welfare initiatives for unmarried pregnant women. These were a continuation, expansion and formalization of previous informal and localized efforts. In addition to parish support for the poor, since at least the eighteenth century, the Church sought to provide and improve midwifery care in parts of Scotland. For example, in the mid-eighteenth century the Kirk Session of St Machar's Cathedral in Aberdeen was 'appalled by the ignorance of women practicing midwifery'. They recommended that all women wishing to practice midwifery undertake a series of lectures on related topics delivered by the local practitioner, Dr David Skene. If any woman could not afford the lecture fees, St Machar's Kirk Session followed the example of other Kirk Sessions and paid them.[20] By the nineteenth century, ministers were instrumental in recruiting midwives to the Scottish islands.[21] While such initiatives were dependent on the enterprise of individual ministers, broader medical evangelicalism formed part of the Church's foreign and home mission.[22]

By analysing the Church of Scotland's maternity provision for unwed mothers, this chapter highlights the complex intersections between morality, medicine, maternity and welfare. It proceeds by first examining the problem of illegitimacy in Scotland and the existing Glasgow health-care market for unmarried, pregnant women in the decades surrounding 1900, thereby highlighting the gap in the health and welfare market the Church of Scotland hoped to fill. It next considers the unique services the Church of Scotland's maternity home offered these mothers when it opened in 1915. The home's matron led and coordinated the Church's provision of practical services to enable the mother to keep her baby if she chose. This contrasted with many similar homes whose providers favoured the mothers' penitence and the child's future, often through adoption, but offered little practical help. It then traces the Church of Scotland's home during and after World War I, analysing the changes and continuities in their provision prior to the National Health Service (NHS), highlighting the pivotal role of the matron in ensuring the success of the home's health and social services. Lastly, it considers the impact of World War II and the NHS on the Church's maternity home. This chapter argues that the Church of Scotland made health and social care a connector between religion and the family. Both the matron's and the women's agency of choice helped build the home's reputation, while also helping secure its social mission. Yet, by targeting only a small section of its membership, while pursuing evangelical goals, this chapter also argues that the Church neglected the broader health and welfare needs of the majority of the poor in general, many of whom were also Church members.

Full details and case records from the Church of Scotland's health and welfare initiatives are missing. Indeed, much of the social information about the Church's mother and baby home was kept in the matrons' heads. There was no legal requirement to retain any records beyond their working life and, to ensure patient confidentiality, many were probably deliberately destroyed. Yet government and medical structures commended the Church's provision. Moreover, despite the missing patients' voice, existing records illustrate the changing provision, intent and reception of the Church's homes. They highlight the centrality of individual matrons to achieving the Church's aims and ambitions. The matron's success was evident in both the standards of care and the nonjudgmental empathy the home extended to unwed mothers in a society where these women brought scorn and shame to themselves and their families.

Illegitimacy and the Early Twentieth-Century Health-Care Market for Unwed Mothers in Glasgow

In the decades surrounding the turn of the twentieth century, community attitudes towards both the unwed mother and child differed in Scotland from that south of the border. Andrew Blaikie has shown how local culture was pivotal to the acceptance of an illegitimate child by their immediate and extended family and their community – including the local Kirk. Certain Scottish communities, such as those in the north-east, applied no stigma of shame to illegitimate children and their mothers. Their families were involved in the child's upbringing. Yet elsewhere in Scotland, the mother of an illegitimate child might be abandoned by family and friends and left unable to support herself and her child.[23] These regional variations in illegitimacy rates, marriage norms and any associated shame and stigma remained well into the twentieth century and much longer than in England. Even in the 1970s, hastily arranged marriages were common in parts of Scotland.[24]

Where women or their families were shamed by an out-of-wedlock pregnancy, they made use of 'mother and baby homes'. While policies varied widely, most British homes sought to adopt the babies out.[25] Arranging adoptions was difficult in Britain before the passing of the 1926 Adoption Act which allowed birth parents to transfer their parental rights to another couple. This legislation led to the establishment of adoption agencies, more mother and baby homes and greater monitoring of their activities. However, the Church of Scotland chose not to join the other religious and private agencies that entered adoption services, acknowledging that it lacked the skill and staff to do so.[26] Rather, the Church continued to prioritize preserving the Christian family. They encouraged mothers to keep their babies and arranged short-term fostering or extensive aftercare. This included accommodation for mothers and their babies, with childcare to enable the mother to work. Nevertheless, the Church recognized that adoption was sometimes the only solution. In these cases, the 'mother and baby' home worked with other agencies to secure adoption into a Christian home.[27]

The Church's social policy concerning unwed mothers differentiated it from that extant in Glasgow. By World War I, Glasgow had an established and varied health-care market for unmarried mothers. The first Lock Hospital for venereal diseases outside of London opened in Glasgow in 1805 and delivered some babies of presumably unmarried mothers. The Scottish Magdalene Homes for unwed mothers were among the first in Britain, with Glasgow's opening in 1815. From the mid-nineteenth century, the voluntary Glasgow Royal Maternity Hospital or Rottenrow accepted unwed mothers alongside married women, with some patients referred from private maternity homes.[28] In 1873, the Glasgow Home for Deserted Mothers opened to take pressure off the Magdalene Home. It served 'destitute and homeless (first time) mothers and their helpless infants'.[29] The following year, the YWCA opened a home for pregnant (unmarried) working-class women who had a certificate of character.[30] By 1913, the MOH Dr A. K. Chalmers noted that the number of private lying-in homes in the city had risen to about thirty, from only twelve two years earlier. Operated by charities or a few philanthropic individuals, these homes targeted unwed mothers and emphasized adoptions. Chalmers questioned whether these private homes should be registered and supervised by public health or Poor Law authorities. Yet it was 1927 before this became mandatory. Indeed, other than their existence, little is known about the private homes, such as who operated them, where they were located, whether they served specific client groups or provided medical attendance at birth.[31] However, they filled an important gap in Glasgow's medical market because the government had no consistent strategy or provision for unmarried mothers.

This ambiguity between health and morality lent itself to both paralysis and manipulation. This, in turn, enabled government to avoid responsibility and claim the issue too sensitive for its supervision. Nevertheless, the mere existence of an extensive variety of provision for unwed mothers in Glasgow and their inclusion in political and medical debates about maternal health care, highlights how the unwed mother did not belong to a 'class' by herself – namely, outside of any medical provision.[32] Rather, health care for the unwed mother was an integral part of charity health-care provision in Glasgow.

'The Keeping of Mother and Child Together is a Cardinal Point of Social Policy': The Early Years of the Church of Scotland's Home for Unwed Mothers

The mission of the Church of Scotland's maternity home was heavily influenced by the well-known Glasgow minister, social investigator and prolific author of innumerable articles and books on the 'social gospel', the Reverend David Watson. Watson was minister of St Clement's Parish Church, Glasgow between 1886 and 1938. Active on several social committees, he was vice-convener of the CSW when the home opened, becoming convener in 1927 and co-convenor with the Reverend John Mansie, formerly of the UFC, after the union in 1929.[33] Watson firmly believed in treating unmarried mothers as individual human persons. By actively seeking to keep mother and child together, Watson believed 'the child thrives better, and the presence of the child is an important factor in safeguarding, steadying, and strengthening the mother'.[34] Adoption and nursing out should only be used as a last resort. Watson also recognized the economic and social costs of pregnancy outside of wedlock. Consequently, the Church should help reunite the mother with her family or help the mother find work to support herself and her baby. Watson's long-term leadership of the CSW helped secure the welfare of mother and child as a core element of social policy and the careful selection of staff helped to secure this.

While the Church's rescue homes had accommodated the occasional unwed mother, the 1915 opening of a maternity home on Herbert Street, Glasgow formalized their provision for unwed pregnant women.[35] It was small with only six beds. The boundaries for admittance stated that only 'respectable' girls, who were pregnant for the first time, *and* who were either themselves or their families' members of the Church of Scotland, were to be admitted.[36] Implicit within 'respectable' was a certain amount of wealth. Unmarried, working-class women were deemed 'respectable' if they were in gainful employment. In the first two years of operation twenty-nine girls in paid employment entered the home (see Table 3.1).[37]

Table 3.1: Occupations of the women admitted to the Church of Scotland's home for
unwed mothers, 1915–17

Occupation	Number admitted
Domestic servants	18
Shop girls	4
Munitions workers	4
Clerkess	1
Saleswoman	1
Car driver	1

Source: W. L. Mackenzie, *Scottish Mothers and Children: Being a Report on the Physical
Welfare of Mothers and Children, Scotland* (East Port, Dunfermline: The Carnegie United
Kingdom Trust, 1917), p. 123.

These women were neither the unworthy poor nor prostitutes who received
most public scrutiny, despite some of these women also being Church members.
They had to be women of good character. Moreover, the Church of Scotland
sought to avoid stigmatizing the unwed mothers by treating them as individuals,
rather than as a faceless, collective group or as victims.[38] This philosophy characterized their reports and, to an extent, the services provided.

The health and social care offered by the Herbert Street maternity home was
at least as good as and probably better than unwed mothers would have received
in the other unregulated private nursing homes for illegitimate confinements
in Glasgow.[39] Miss Torrance, the matron of the Herbert Street home, managed
the home's finances and supervised a girl's care from when she entered the home
until she and her baby left. She was a qualified nurse, having passed the Local
Government Board Examination of Nurses at Eastern District Hospital in Glasgow in May 1907. By the time she was in charge of the Herbert Street Maternity
Home, she had also qualified in midwifery, probably under the 1915 Midwives
(Scotland) Act.[40] Hence, she would either possess a certificate from a hospital
approved by the Central Midwives Board for Scotland (CMBS) or she had been
in midwifery practice before 31 December 1914 and was of good character with
references to prove it – probably the former. Miss Torrance provided patients
with instruction on how to care for their baby, as well as some ante and postnatal
care, with time to spend with their baby and strengthen the mother–baby bond.
In addition, Dr Elizabeth Smith, physician to Glasgow's Lock Hospital, was the
honorary medical attendant. Not only did the provision of extensive health care
help build the Church of Scotland's reputation as a provider of quality health and
welfare services, it also highlights how the Church did not view unwed mothers
as marginal mothers, but as women deserving of excellent maternity care.

The Church's efforts did not go unnoticed. Social observers praised their
efforts at securing the health and well-being of both mother and child. In 1917,

the Local Government Boards, under the auspices of the Carnegie UK Trust, published a survey of maternal and child health throughout Britain. The Carnegie UK Trust *Report on the Physical Welfare of Mothers and Children ... Scotland* singled out the Church of Scotland's Glasgow home for favourable comment. Both its policy of keeping mother and baby together and the Matron's skills and empathy with the girls were commended.[41] Moreover, the Church also recognized that the matron was pivotal in helping reconcile an unwed mother with her family. In addition to providing the necessary and required medical and social services, Miss Torrance built a personal relationship with each girl. Her successes are measurable through her popularity with her clientele. Many former patients corresponded with her after leaving the home and visited with their babies.[42] Had the shame of unwed motherhood been pressed upon them, it is unlikely that they would have kept contact with the matron. Hence, both matron and patients exerted their agency of choice in terms of services and empathy provided and maternity care chosen, for mutual benefit. To that end, most women gave birth in the Maternity Hospital (Rottenrow) before returning to the home for postnatal care.[43] Thus, the maternity home reflected the Church's social theory and social reform agenda, core to which were the preservation of the biological family and the family of Christ. The Matron, Miss Torrance, was pivotal to the Church's success in achieving these goals.

The other Glasgow homes for unwed mothers adopted social policies that also emphasized the middle-class values of respectability but with a different methodology. The Home for Deserted Mothers sought to return the unwed mother to social respectability through vocation. Penitence could not be achieved while a woman cared for an illegitimate child. Therefore, as soon as possible after birth, the matron had the newborn placed under the 'care of proper and trustworthy nurses', implying that the mother was either not expected to or was believed unable to care for her own child. Instead, a mother's duty was to defray the costs of 'rearing and upbringing' her child, even through fostering until formal or informal adoptions were arranged.[44] While less is known about the matron(s) of this home, particularly her qualifications, she too was a pivotal figure in securing the home's goals. The other homes for unwed mothers, including the Magdalene's and the Lock Hospital, had comparable policies.[45] Both mother and baby would be better off if separated.

While the various Glasgow homes for unwed mothers served select and different client groups, they all involved small groups of social experts with narrow views of both the problem and the solution. All believed they were doing the best for both mother and infant and each matron was fundamental to the home achieving its goal. It was the means to this end that differed. The homes managed sexuality within the confines of the discourse of the time – in this case, the social welfare movement of the early twentieth century.[46] Helping indigent parents to help themselves was not a feature of most charity provision for unwed mothers.

The Interwar Years: 'The Effort to Render Practical Service in Christ's Name'

World War I and the Presbyterian Churches' perceived collective indifference to it weakened their moral authority and social influence in Scotland.[47] The Presbyterian Churches withdrew from broad social reform proclamations and associated political campaigns, which paralleled the post-war government's withdrawal from its pre-war social reform agenda. Instead, the Church of Scotland sustained Christianity in action by expanding its residential projects, including orphanages, boys' homes, homes for working girls, hostels, rescue and preventive homes for women, adding homes for unwanted babies and expanding their maternity home.[48] These homes were designed to fill both the practical needs of accommodation while also helping to remake post-war Scotland into a Christian country.[49] While their success depended on the staff, at the same time, prevailing social concerns influenced the homes' direction.

World War I increased public concerns about Scotland's persistently high infant mortality rates. The government responded with legislation designed to enable local authorities to raise money for maternity services, influence welfare provision and mandate reform. The 1918 Maternity and Child Welfare Act empowered local authorities to borrow money to fund schemes for maternal and child welfare. The Local Government Board for Scotland, replaced by the Scottish Board of Health in 1919, could now require local authorities to supply food and milk for pregnant women, nursing mothers and children under the age of five. Grants-in-aid were available to help set up maternity and child welfare centres.[50] However, these initiatives had little uptake. This, combined with the centres' prioritizing of educational and diagnostic advice over medical treatment, makes it probable that those women who needed the support most were unlikely to benefit from the schemes, namely single mothers – either unwed, abandoned or widowed. Therefore, considerable scope remained for charities to fill the gap in addressing broader maternal and child health and welfare needs. Instead of changing its focus to address these needs, the Church of Scotland turned inward, while also aggravating growing social tensions through both its calls for social reconstruction and its growing 'us' and 'them' attitude towards poverty and unemployment which saw middle-class congregations separating from working-class ones.[51]

The Church's new and existing health and social projects continued to reach only a minority of members and now targeted preserving their existing membership. The Church's Glasgow maternity home reflected this goal with the Matron,

Miss Torrance, remaining pivotal to its success. She provided the essential health care, empathy and welfare advice to women at a vulnerable time. Entwined within this was another goal, that of reconciliation. The Church sought to reconcile the woman with God and with her family. Despite the many potential difficulties surrounding these tasks, Miss Torrance achieved many successes. The expectant mothers spoke highly of the great kindness shown to them in the home, with many becoming 'greatly attached to the matron'.[52] Such attachments to the matron are unsurprising. She provided midwifery care and motherly empathy for girls isolated from their families during what was probably the most stressful and frightening period in their lives so far. Moreover, the girls 'often returned to her for advice after they have left the home'.[53] This close bond between the matron and former residents not only highlights how crucial an experienced and empathetic midwife was to the home's success, it also reinforced the Church's aim of trying to retain its members through regular opportunities for evangelism. The home's successes at reconciling and preserving families meant that when in 1923 the proprietors sought to resume possession of the building, rather than close, the committee purchased a larger house to broaden and continue its maternity services.[54] Miss Torrance agreed to stay on as matron of the new home and viewed the larger, improved facilities as an opportunity to expand the health and welfare services provided for expectant mothers.

In October 1924, the new 'mother and baby' home opened on 39 Lansdowne Crescent and civic and church leaders attended the opening. With forty beds, expectant mothers could now stay at the home for longer periods. They regularly came for about three months preceding the birth when pregnancy was most obvious, enabling the women or their families to hide any shame. Lengthier stays also allowed greater monitoring of the mothers' health and more time for Christian instruction. Women stayed at the home until they were about to give birth, when they were moved to a maternity hospital.[55] After giving birth the women returned to the home, where they remained for at least two months. During this time the matron provided instruction in mothercraft and the Bible, the women's health was monitored and they could 'find faith' and make arrangements for the future.[56] These additions were introduced shortly after the Scottish Board of Health made its short-lived commitment to fund hospital beds for expectant mothers in 1919–20.[57] They also marked the Church out as a rare provider of both antenatal and post-natal care in Glasgow.

Antenatal and post-natal care in interwar Scotland was becoming more common.[58] Since about 1900, antenatal care in Edinburgh had increased, largely due to the efforts of Drs John W. Ballantyne, James H. Ferguson and their teacher Alexander Russell Simpson.[59] Glasgow was not so fortunate. Dr A. K. Chalmers advocated antenatal care as important for lowering infant mortality rates. After

World War I, he opened antenatal clinics for both married and unmarried mothers in Glasgow, however, these were poorly attended and many closed.[60]

Concerns about poor antenatal care grew during the interwar period. In 1929, the Department of Health for Scotland commissioned an investigation into maternal deaths in Scotland. Between 1929 and 1933, over 2,500 maternal deaths were investigated. In 1935, the *Report on Maternal Morbidity and Mortality in Scotland*, also known as the Douglas and McKinlay Report, highlighted the need to improve all areas of maternity care, but particularly antenatal care.[61] Meanwhile, increasing numbers of medical professionals were critical of existing antenatal provision, including Dr Dugald Baird. After graduating from Glasgow University with a medical degree in 1922, Baird attended births in the Glasgow slums and worked as an obstetric surgeon at the Glasgow Royal Maternity Hospital. Between 1925 and 1934, while at the Royal, Baird conducted a study of 999 fatal maternity cases. He concluded that poor antenatal care was a significant contributor to Glasgow's high maternal mortality rates. He argued that 9 per cent of maternal deaths examined were of women where there had been a clear risk of a fatal outcome during pregnancy. He recommended increasing hospital accommodation for maternity cases, especially for antenatal assessment. Baird's calls for improved antenatal care were taken up more broadly in 1937 when the PEP *Report on the British Health Services* noted how only 35 per cent of expectant mothers in Scotland attended antenatal clinics, compared with 73 per cent in London and 63 per cent of women in the county boroughs.[62] Hence, the limited reach of the Church of Scotland's antenatal provision made little impact on broader maternal health in Glasgow.

Government concerns about maternal deaths also led to the increased regulation of maternity homes. The Church ensured its home met current legislative requirements by providing 'skilled nursing' and with a local doctor on call.[63] When in 1927, the Midwives and Maternity Homes (Scotland) Act mandated the registration and inspection of maternity homes, the Church of Scotland's home passed that and future inspections. In contrast, in 1929, the Glasgow MOH, Dr A. S. Macgregor, noted the varying quality of the facilities and record keeping at the private nursing and lying-in homes and the associated high rates of puerperal fever.[64] Hence, the Church of Scotland's maternity home not only fulfilled its own social and evangelical aims with its health and welfare services, it also met political and medical objectives and requirements.

The Church of Scotland's growing interest in health and social work was further stimulated by the 1929 union of the Established Church and the UFC. The establishment of a state church gave it the political strength to tackle social problems with larger, more coordinated and efficient services. Social provision was reorganized, while economic unity increased Church funds for publicity and modernizing the homes' facilities. For example, in 1931 electric lights

were installed in Lansdowne House and it was beautifully redecorated; however, births still took place at the maternity hospital.[65] The modernization and
publicity initiatives were rewarded with increased inquiries from ministers and
Church workers all over the country.[66]

At the same time, the Church acknowledged that modernization alone would
not have increased interest in the home. Rather, it was the skill, competence and
dedication of the long-serving Matron, Miss Torrance, her staff and the local doctor who was on call. Miss Torrance created an 'atmosphere of sympathy and love'
at the home, which was repeatedly acknowledged by the Church and the unwed
mothers.[67] Continuing testimony to Miss Torrance's influence was again found
in the numerous gifts and letters of gratitude she received from women who had
been under her care and from their return visits to the matron to tell her how
they were getting on.[68] Sadly, while their delivery is regularly noted in the Church
records, the actual letters have not survived. They would have provided great
insight into both the home's clients and the care provided. However, the mere fact
that these unwed mothers on the margins of broader social acceptability regularly
corresponded and visited with the matron suggests both high care standards and
that Miss Torrance was non-judgemental about the girls' plight.

Miss Torrance left Lansdowne House in 1938; shortly after the 1937
Maternity Services (Scotland) Act came into force. This Act targeted maternal
mortality and required that a midwife, doctor and obstetrician be available for
all women during pregnancy, with local authorities responsible for arranging
care.[69] Miss Torrance's successor, Miss Cecile Henderson, easily fulfilled her part
of this requirement. Miss Henderson, DCS, SRN, had extensive nurse training
and had previously worked as a missionary sister in charge of the Nurses' Training School at the Christian Medical College at Ludhiana in India. She then
worked in various other hospitals in India and Britain before coming to Glasgow.[70] Miss Henderson utilized her vast experience to maintain her predecessor's
high standards of cleanliness and health care at the maternity home. She was
aided in her mission by the staff and a local doctor who remained on call. Nevertheless, health care and social service were separate areas of provision. While the
former was pressured by the state between the wars, the latter was under strain
from changing social expectations.

The CSW remained committed to its health and social policies but its efforts
at keeping mother and baby together faltered. During the 1930s, the Church
increasingly fostered out babies or arranged adoptions. In 1939, nearly half the
babies born at Lansdowne House were adopted.[71] This figure corresponds with
studies of English and Welsh homes, where adoptions of illegitimate babies
increased significantly so that by World War II there was a presumption that these
babies would be placed for adoption.[72] Yet, explaining the change at the Church
of Scotland's home is more difficult because adoption was never a core point of

social policy. The rising adoption rate may simply relate to the women's individual circumstances. While the role of the matron in adoptions is unclear, the unwed mothers regarded Miss Henderson highly, leaving her gifts and holding her in great affection.[73] Hence, it is likely that rather than trying to persuade women to follow a certain path, she encouraged them to make their own decision. Indeed, it may have been the women's families who increased pressure on the unwed mothers for the babies to be adopted in order to hide the shame. From the mid-1930s, Lansdowne House reported how it had become 'a source of real comfort to *parents* into whose homes tragedy has come'.[74] Including the family in the service provision both aided and complicated evangelical aims.

As the Church of Scotland struggled to sustain its policy of keeping mother and baby together, the practicalities of hiding any shame became more difficult, while new legislation only increased women's options. The post-war introduction of health visitors made illegitimate babies increasingly difficult to hide.[75] Added to this, by the mid-1930s increasing shame and social blame was placed on unwed mothers, whom society often judged as incompetent. These women were blamed for poor child welfare and indeed women's own ill-health during pregnancy. The Douglas and McKinlay Report complained that many women refused to attend the antenatal clinics or to eat well during pregnancy.[76] Yet, unwed mothers would have been the least likely women to attend the clinics or to be able to afford to eat well. Lastly, the Adoption Act of 1926 made starting over easier for women than earlier. A woman could give up her baby and ensure that it would be well cared for. The Act also made it easier for voluntary providers to arrange adoptions. The Church of Scotland increasingly did so, preferring to work with other agencies rather than setting up their own. Hence, despite Scotland's growing disillusionment with evangelical Puritanism during the interwar years, the Church's commitment to social service provision and particularly for society's marginalized women – the unwed mothers – illustrates their sustained belief that evangelism through health and welfare services could heal the nation and preserve the Church. Yet the Church struggled with its priorities. They wavered between services for women, their parents and the babies, as well as associated social realities and social evangelicalism. Church leaders recognized the importance of individual matrons to achieving its medical, social and evangelical aims and in maintaining the 'excellent standard of work' at the Home.[77] Yet her role became more difficult as the Church wavered between its priorities. These dilemmas about the Home's mission continued into World War II and were compounded by a rapid turnover of matrons, while the war reinvigorated the Church's commitment to keeping mother and baby together.

World War II: 'The Effects of the War'

World War II brought yet another national resurgence of moral concern for women and children. Capitalizing on this, the Church sought to build a society in which motherhood would be welcomed and honoured. Lansdowne House formed part of the Church's efforts to aid the unfortunate.[78] This agenda placed new demands on the Church of Scotland's recently formed Committee for Christian Life and Social Work, a 1936 merger of the Committee on Social Work and the Committee of Life and Work. In 1941, the new Committee reorganized its social services and inaugurated a Moral Welfare Scheme. The Scheme sought to enable the Church to

> more efficiently ... exercise its social and redemptive ministry to Women, Girls, and Children in moral difficulty or danger and to make available for ministers of the Church and other Social Workers expert assistance in their work of moral welfare.[79]

It had three aims: prevention, treatment and aftercare. The 'mother and baby home' was to be a core feature of the treatment and aftercare.

Key to the success of the new Moral Welfare Scheme was the staff. While the Church recognized this, Lansdowne House experienced a fairly rapid staff turnover during the war. Miss Henderson resigned in 1941 due to illness. In 1942, she was replaced by Miss M. Craig, CMB, who had extensive experience in midwifery. She did not remain long at the home and an interim matron, a missionary nurse, replaced her, but returned to Nagpur Hospital in India in 1945. She was succeeded by Miss Dougall, who was also well qualified and had held posts of responsibility both in Scotland and abroad. Despite this rapid staff turnover, and the need for the home to be temporarily evacuated to Stirling, Lansdowne House retained its reputation for excellent care provision.

The home was well used during the war, including by women from HM Forces. By 1942, Lansdowne House was refusing applications for admission due to lack of accommodation.[80] The direct influence of the social and welfare workers on the mothers' decision-making is unclear, as is that of the staff and staff turnover, but the number of girls keeping their babies increased. This was despite the Adoption of Children (Regulations) Act 1943, which extended the options available to unwed mothers provided under the 1926 Act. Yet the Church still did not choose to register as an Adoption Society, preferring to sustain its commitment to the family and help each mother to make her own emotional decisions and to help her keep her child if she wanted to.[81] While the success of this decision is also difficult to measure, by 1944, no mothers at Lansdowne House chose to have their baby adopted and adoption rates remained low through 1948.[82] This contrasts with the adoption rates for illegitimate babies in England and Wales which rose during and immediately after the war. Indeed, there was a growing wartime presumption in England and Wales that illegitimate babies would be placed for adoption.[83] In Scotland, Lansdowne House provided important wartime resources when local authorities were struggling to supply adequate maternity services. Local authority initiatives at improving infant and maternal welfare were patchy, uneven or simply unable to tackle the size and scope of the problem.

Wartime demands meant the existing facilities at Lansdowne House could no longer meet patients' needs. In 1944, the Church purchased a larger property at 68 St Andrew's Drive in the wealthy Glasgow district of Pollockshields near the Victoria Infirmary and continued to call it Lansdowne House. Fitted in accordance with MOH guidelines, this building was better equipped than previous homes. It included birthing facilities which helped address the acute wartime shortage of maternity beds. Babies were delivered at the home into the 1950s when all confinements reverted to the hospital; this time the Victoria.[84] Continuing its recognition that the staff at the home was pivotal to its success, when Miss Dougall resigned her post as matron in 1948, the Committee appointed Miss Flora L. Davidson, SRN, SCM, as her successor. Miss Davidson had previously served the Church for twenty years as a missionary nurse. Such experience was desirable as she had spiritual gifts as well as nurse training. She also had a qualified nurse, Mrs Gordon, as an assistant.[85] Spiritual and medical expertise remained vital for enabling the Church to retain its independence as a provider of maternity care and for fulfilling its evangelical aims. Medical recognition of the home's health-care standards, combined with full maternity service provision, from antenatal care through delivery, postnatal care and social services also helped sustain demand. Indeed, the home continued to combine social and medical services long after both maternity and general hospitals had shifted away from social provision to a purely medical function.[86] The Church of Scotland provided a unique maternity service for its members in an increasingly sectionalized medical market.

During the war, the Church of Scotland's social services also faced challenges from the state. Most notably, the Beveridge Report of 1942 recommended the state provide more services, including health care for unwed mothers. In response, the Church reasserted its unique position in the health and welfare market as not merely financial, but touching the 'deeper needs of the soul'. To the Church, the war only highlighted the importance of keeping religion central to its projects. Moreover, while the law prevented discrimination in health care, it did not remove the social prejudices surrounding illegitimacy; nor did it address the economic realities faced by a lone mother. Once again, Lansdowne House found its social services complementing other provision. Its continued success remained partly due to its reputation as a provider of excellent health care by non-judgemental staff at a time when society continued to harshly judge the unwed mother.

Conclusion

The Church of Scotland's 'mother and baby' home provided only part of an extensive range of charity health and welfare provision available to unwed mothers in Glasgow. It filled a niche market by providing maternity care for unmarried Church members. During the first four decades of their home's existence, the Church remained committed to the belief that health was both an interconnector between religion and the family and a form of evangelism. While other 'mother and baby' homes also served particular markets, what distinguished the Church's home from the others was its consistent social policy of trying to keep mother and baby together. This commitment survived two world wars when illegitimacy rates were high, as were demands from childless parents to adopt. However, it was not simply the Church's social services or their social policy that helped secure the home's civic recognition. Rather, their success in achieving political and medical recognition related to their sustained high standards of health care provided by an experienced and empathetic midwife that filled a gap in municipal provision. The state had no policy on morality and health care, while both the state and society harshly judged the unwed mother.

The matron was crucial to the Church's success in gaining public recognition as a legitimate provider of maternity care and in fulfilling its social policy goals. Her freedom to run the home as she saw fit, her commitment to Christian values and her workload, all impacted on the mothers and the choices they made for their babies. Nevertheless, the matron's skill, commitment and empathy secured the girls' long-term affection.[87] The Home's first matron, the long-serving Miss Torrance, set high standards for her successors. Due probably to the range of health and welfare provision for unwed mothers in Glasgow, the matron was the fundamental person in establishing the excellent reputation of Lansdowne House. The fact that the home was regularly full is testament to both the matron's efforts and the unwed mother's or her family's choice for care in a religious setting. Yet these successes also aided the Church's political aims. Maintaining civic and medical recognition ensured the home independence from state control, while also securing the Church opportunities to influence policymakers on matters surrounding social care and illegitimacy.[88]

However, by prioritizing morality within its health and social service provision and emphasizing moral education, the Church ensured that its 'mother and baby' home excluded the poor in general, including married Church members. Many poor women would not meet the requirements of 'respectability', through appropriate employment or social standing, to be able to utilize the home's facilities. Yet poor women were less likely to seek antenatal and post-natal care or to have medical attendance at births. Consequently, they had correspondingly higher rates of maternal and infant mortality. Instead, Lansdowne House had become the State religion's official channel for approaching Scottish moral anxieties over the erosion of community and family values.

Acknowledgements

I am grateful to Linda Bryder, Derek Dow, Alison Nuttall and an anonymous reviewer for their comments on earlier versions of this chapter. The research for this was funded by the Wellcome Trust (Grant 095576).

4 TAKING 'ADVANTAGE OF THE FACILITIES AND COMFORTS ... OFFERED': WOMEN'S CHOICE OF HOSPITAL DELIVERY IN INTERWAR EDINBURGH

Alison Nuttall

Immediately before World War I, only a minority of Edinburgh parturients were confined in hospital. Home birth, typically attended by either the family doctor or pupil midwives from local training institutions, was the norm. However, by the outbreak of World War II, more than half chose to deliver in an institution, either a maternity hospital or a nursing home, electing to take 'advantage of the facilities and comforts ... offered by hospital treatment'.[1] This was both a rapid and a groundbreaking change for the city: in Britain as a whole, the tipping point of more than 50 per cent hospital births was only reached after World War II.[2] This chapter draws on contemporary institutional records of both inpatient and domiciliary deliveries to ask what caused such a major change in the behaviour of women in Edinburgh.

Implicit in much of the early historiography of the move to hospital birth is the belief that women were forced, by either direct medical pressure or the reduction of domiciliary services, to opt for inpatient care.[3] Less ideological examinations of the medicalization of childbirth have suggested that moving to hospital reduced women's fear of birth and were thus part of a gradual acceptance of the benefits of medical care.[4] More recent studies of contemporary behaviour, intended to increase understanding of the current choices made by women and thereby to reduce the very high percentage of hospital deliveries in Britain, have suggested a major role for 'social risk': the desire to conform to social norms, and to feel justified in the decision made.[5] Nonetheless, hospital records of the initial move to inpatient birth have not been examined in depth for the reasons to select such care, a deficiency which this chapter seeks to redress. The following section contextualizes the study by examining the interwar city, its maternity institutions and the sources they generated. The evidence for a move to hospital birth in Edinburgh is then explored, and the reasons for this analysed, focusing on the roles of deteriorating housing stock, increasing medical interest in maternal health, growing familiarity with the medical world and the immediate benefits of admission. The chapter concludes that although hospital records suggest that poor housing conditions played a major role in women's initial choice of hospital birth, the ensuing discovery of the care and rest offered to inpatients ensured institutional delivery increasingly became the social norm.

The City, its Maternity Institutions and their Records

Interwar Edinburgh is particularly well placed for such a study: although it was affected by the Depression, especially in its satellite villages, it was not a one-industry town and the effects were limited. In 1920, in the face of considerable opposition, the seaport, the independent burgh of Leith, was incorporated, coincidentally providing a contrast in public health management.[6] The city's long association with medicine, and particularly its medical schools and charitable facilities, ensured that all of its residents, in contrast to many in the interwar period, could make a genuine choice of place of confinement.[7] Equally, the need to provide the resulting large population of medical and midwifery students with domiciliary delivery experience ultimately deterred institutions from actively encouraging unnecessary admissions.[8] Finally, it was not only well provided with maternity institutions, but the records of many of those institutions survive and are available for research.

Two whole-year studies of the casebooks of a range of Edinburgh voluntary maternity institutions in 1924–5 and 1935 are examined here for evidence of reasons to choose hospital birth.[9] They are the Edinburgh Royal Maternity Hospital (ERMH), founded in 1844, based in the first custom-built maternity hospital in Scotland in Lauriston Place, and responsible for approximately 35–42 per cent of city births in the years studied; the Hospice (renamed the Elsie Inglis Memorial Maternity Hospital (EIMMH) after its move to Abbeyhill in 1925), an all-female provident hospital founded in 1904 in the High Street and responsible for 5–22 per cent of city births over the period; the Deaconess Hospital, established in 1894 in the Pleasance, which ran a mainly domiciliary service (inpatient care was provided for obstetric emergencies only) and cared for less than 2 per cent of city births; the Edinburgh Lying-In Institution (ELII), (1816–1933), also in Lauriston Place, of similar size to the Deaconess, and again providing mainly outpatient care; and the Western General Hospital maternity unit, opened by the city in 1932 as an adjunct to the Craiglockhart Poor Law Institution, and providing inpatient care only for approximately 3 per cent of city births in 1935.

The records themselves are of variable quality: those of the ERMH and Deaconess are both detailed and assiduously completed in comparison with the basic records of the Western General and Lying-In Institution; although the EIMMH intended to keep records of all its cases in considerable detail, these were rarely fully completed and not all have survived. It can be argued that the use of hospital casebooks implies an inpatient bias, but this is not the case. With the exception of the Western General, all the institutions studied provided both indoor and domiciliary care, allowing comparisons of behaviour to be made within individual institutions. Nonetheless, the women whose histories are recorded in such casebooks were not typical of the population as a whole but, even when able to make a small financial contribution to the costs of their care, came principally from the poorest levels of society. It is notable that, although its use as a regional centre for emergency cases widened slightly the social range of its patients (a trend already apparent in 1912),[10] there was a proportionate decline in attendance at the ERMH after the opening of the Western General, indicating that both hospitals admitted clients of similar social status, and that despite its efforts to increase its popularity, the ERMH cannot really be said to have broken away from its initial role as a maternity charity.[11]

The Move to Hospital

In 1912 approximately 10 per cent of births in Edinburgh took place within an institution. By 1938, 39 per cent of Edinburgh babies were delivered in voluntary or municipal institutions, with a further 12 per cent of confinements taking place in private nursing homes.[12] As the city's Medical Officer of Health (MOH) observed in 1938, '[t]he tendency of women to seek admission to institutions for their confinements [was] a progressive one'.[13]

Such an increase represented a major change in childbirth behaviour by Edinburgh mothers, and this is particularly apparent when the records of individual institutions are examined. However, the use of hospital records not only demonstrates a change in behaviour, but also fixes it chronologically. By 1925, when Edinburgh's MOH first began to publish detailed breakdowns of place of birth, institutional care was already dominant, with more than half of such deliveries taking place within voluntary hospitals.[14] Analysis of ERMH records shows that although it had provided almost certainly free inpatient care for the parturient poor from its inception until 1913, admission remained unpopular amongst its potential clients throughout the nineteenth century, and domiciliary births outnumbered indoor cases by two to one. Its Ladies Committee felt that this was the result of the presence on its wards of a large proportion of single girls, and campaigned for a separate Married Women's Pavilion.[15] However, although this was opened in 1895, married women continued to shun the ERMH, and to give birth in its care, but in their own homes. From 1916 this began to change, though the hospital initially ascribed this to the conscription of local doctors for war service. However, the newly acquired premises intended to house the war-time increase were never used, and by 1920 had been converted into additional nurses' accommodation.[16] Nonetheless, in 1921, for the first time, the percent-age of inpatient cases exceeded that of outpatient cases. Outdoor cases never regained their former dominance, and, by 1924, 58 per cent of patients delivered in the hospital, and only 42 per cent at home. By 1935 the proportions were 72 per cent and 28 per cent respectively.[17]

A similar process can be seen at the Hospice. In 1915, 80 per cent of its clients delivered at home, but, by 1921, inpatient births exceeded domiciliary. In 1924, as at the ERMH, 58 per cent delivered indoors, and 42 per cent at home. The move to a custom-built hospital in 1925 led to an immediate rapid expansion in inpatient numbers: recognizing the demand, even before the move the hospital management had already decided to complete the unfunded 'upper Hospital wing ... because the need for maternity beds is great, and because it would prove more economical in the end'.[18] One year later, 78 per cent of EIMMH patients delivered indoors, and 22 per cent at home, but thereafter the proportions fluc-tuated very little. In 1935, approximately 70 per cent were inpatients.[19] Such an instantaneous growth in inpatients in 1926 suggests that women were indeed keen to be cared for in hospital, rather than at home, and took prompt advantage of the new facilities. The decline in use at this time of the Deaconess Hospital, and the closure of the Lying-In Institution in 1933, both of which provided prin-cipally domiciliary care, also indicate enthusiasm for hospital confinement.[20]

Initially it was argued that this increase indicated a major change in the nature of the hospitals' population, particularly at the ERMH, the result of associating the expansion in inpatients with the growth in admission of married patients.[21] However, there was no essential change in the type of woman admitted. The fall in their average age and the increase in primiparity among admitted post-war married women combine to suggest that they resembled more closely the single and not the married ERMH inpatients of 1912, and that instead it was the tim-ing of the decision to marry that had changed.[22] The move to hospital was rather a change in behaviour in an already established client population. The increase in inpatient deliveries was not matched by an equivalent increase in share of city births at either hospital, as might be expected if the increase represented a widen-ing of their populations. Although at the ERMH this trend was partly obscured by the growth in the admission of women living outwith the city (the result of its use as a regional maternity centre for local maternity and child welfare schemes), nonetheless, while its indoor deliveries rose by 16 per cent between 1921 and 1930, the hospital's share of total city births only rose by 14 per cent, suggesting that what was happening was partly a re-organization of its usual clients, rather than expansion into a new market. This trend can be seen more clearly at the Hospice, whose share of city births remained relatively stable at approximately two per cent from 1919 to 1925, during which time inpatient deliveries increased from 40 to 58 per cent. The Hospice was not so much expanding its patient base, as changing the behaviour of its established clientele, a point made in its Annual Report for 1923: '[p]atients show a greater desire to come into Hospital for confinement and the proportion of booked cases is steadily increasing'.[23]

The combination of data drawn from hospital annual reports and those published by the Edinburgh Public Health Department have indicated that the move to hospital delivery in the city began towards the end of World War I and was in part the result of a change in behaviour by established users of domiciliary services. However, such data are much less forthcoming about the motives for such a change, a role better filled by detailed analysis of casebook content. The following sections examine the personal health records held by individual Edinburgh maternity institutions for such reasons.

'Dear Doctor, Please Admit'

The move to hospital birth in Edinburgh, well underway in 1925, preceded any official advice to do so. Reflecting both the long-established and miserable reputation of maternity hospitals as hotbeds of puerperal infection, and the paucity of maternity beds, in 1918 the Local Government Board advised local authorities that inpatient care should only be offered under specific circumstances.[24] Similarly, Dame Janet Campbell's 1924 recommendations to reduce maternal mortality did not include routine hospital admission.[25] However, this does not mean that there was no medical influence on place of confinement. The EIMMH justified its financial calls on its supporters not only by stressing mothers' 'warm appreciation and affection ... for the Hospital', but also by claiming that, 'placed in a district in which there is a real need for a Maternity Service',

> our Medical Staff can often repel the first onset of disease by giving skilled advice to the mothers and thus save them from the pain and misery so often due to want of care at this critical period of their lives.[26]

Earlier examinations of the medicalization of childbirth in Edinburgh have suggested a major role for antenatal clinics in encouraging admission.[27] Introduced at the ERMH in 1915, after 1917 these were administered by the city as part of its Maternity and Child Welfare Scheme. More detailed exploration has shown that early attendance at clinics was actually too patchy to produce such a large increase in admissions: even if all the clinic attendees at the ERMH's main and Leith clinics had been delivered by maternity staff in 1924, they would still have comprised less than half of all its patients.[28] The Hospice's main clinic was the exception, the result of combining antenatal care with accepting part-payments towards the cost of future admission. In 1924, when Hospice staff treated 475 women, 431 patients attended its 'High Street' clinic, and 372 patients (78 per cent) booked attendance in advance. Eleven years later approximately two-thirds of all ERMH patients did indeed attend an antenatal clinic, but there was no difference between indoor and outdoor patients in this.

Nonetheless, through their discovery and early treatment of maternal ill-health, antenatal clinics did influence hospital admission. Although the enthusiasm for admission of the large number of women sent to the ERMH for treatment (including segregated delivery) of suspected venereal disease whose tests were consistently negative can be questioned, for many women medical admission was beneficial.[29] For example, in 1924, thirty-one expectant mothers in the ERMH sample were admitted from either the clinic or their family doctor with raised blood pressure, proteinuria and oedema, that is, with a probable diagnosis of pre-eclamptic toxaemia and at risk of eclamptic fits leading to likely maternal or infant death. Although again the positive nature of the mother's choice can be questioned, the resulting improved outcomes demonstrate its wisdom. In contrast to the high pre-war mortality and morbidity, twenty-eight mothers were discharged well, and only four fitted in hospital, of whom three died.[30] In 1912 Mrs Edwards, 24, a miller's wife from Balerno, near term with her third child, had 'complained [to her doctor] of headaches and swelling of the legs, – vomiting and pain over stomach. Dr Graham told her to take Barley water and milk ... [Her] face swelled up ... – her arms and hands also became swollen'. Two days later she began to '[f]it at 5.40, Dr Graham called in about 9 pm & gave her Bromide and chloral ... Fits continued all night ... on Thursday morning ... Dr Graham sent Pat[ient] into RMH in a cab. 2 fits on journey in.' The admitting house surgeon ended his summary 'before admission reported to have had 8 fits (& how many more?) during the night. 2 fits on journey in = 10 fits+!!'. Despite energetic treatment in the hospital, including the induced delivery of a stillborn son, Mrs Edwards never regained consciousness and died eight hours after admission.[31] By contrast, in 1924 Dr Taylor of St Abbs noted Mrs Harrison's high blood pressure and albuminuria and promptly organized her admission to the ERMH. Although the 35-year-old fisherman's wife and mother of two did fit before she arrived in the hospital, her condition stabilized through immediate treatment with colonic lavage, hot packs and sedation. One week later, birth was induced, and ten days after that, she and her new daughter were both discharged 'well'.[32]

Similarly, admission for early induction or elective caesarean section for known cephalo-pelvic disproportion, typically diagnosed by a history of previous difficult or destructive delivery and antenatal pelvic assessment, was a positive choice. In contrast to 1912, when more than half the emergency admissions for obstructed labour due to disproportion ended in destructive operation, in 1924 eight women were admitted to the ERMH for pre-term induction, went on to deliver vaginally (five spontaneously), and were then discharged well with a living infant. Another eight were delivered abdominally with similar happy outcomes. The contrasting stories of Mrs Hughes and Mrs Stewart illustrate the positivity of such a decision. In 1912, Mrs Stewart, the 26-year-old wife of a ploughman, was admitted from Linlithgow after having already been at least three days in her first labour, and with '[t]he [sacral] promontory ... not able to be felt as the head [was] jammed [into the pelvis]'. Nonetheless, because a fetal heart was heard on admission, delivery by forceps was attempted in both conventional and Walcher's positions, but to 'no avail. Nothing left but craniotomy'. Mrs Stewart was profoundly shocked after her traumatic delivery, and died the day after her son.[33] In contrast, in 1924, Mrs Hughes, a labourer's wife from the Pleasance with a history of previous stillbirth following a difficult instrumental delivery, was seen before labour at the ERMH antenatal clinic. Her pelvic capacity was assessed, a rickety pelvis with a reduced diagonal conjugate was identified, and at term she was admitted for elective caesarean section. She experienced no problems, and she and her son were discharged well nineteen days after his birth.[34]

However, most women who chose inpatient delivery were problem-free. Even at the ERMH, which, as a regional centre, saw the majority of sick parturients, half its patients were admitted, delivered and discharged without any recorded problems in 1924. At the Hospice, 168 of the 269 inpatients (62 per cent) in 1924 required no treatment other than delivery, while a further 40 needed sutures only. Yet medical concern is not necessarily evident in hospital statistics: the Hospice especially was always keen to remind its donors of its supportive medical and educational regime for new mothers, and the largely physiological nature of its care.[35] In particular, the large proportion of primigravidae admitted to both hospitals suggests the possibility of an unofficial local policy of encouraging hospital delivery of first babies. Yet first-time mothers were also most likely to be affected by Edinburgh's worsening housing problems and the increase in sub-let property. The following section examines the role of Edinburgh's deteriorating housing stock in the move to hospital confinement.

'Dungeon-like Slums' and 'Furnished Rooms'

Even before World War I, Edinburgh City Council had identified areas of poor housing, principally the St Leonard's/Pleasance area and the Cowgate. The 1919 Sanitary Report noted 'the vast amount of disrepair that has accumulated during the War', and the first areas singled out for improvement were in the Old Town, where both maternity hospitals were based: the High Street – where houses were described as 'dungeon-like slum[s] devoid of almost every comfort' – the

Canongate, the Pleasance, and the George Square area.[36] Two related problems – overcrowding and subletting – were identified. A large

> shortage of dwellings [was noted] … on that account there is much overcrowding … Growing families, which in the normal course of events would have removed to larger houses, have had to remain in their already crowded abodes, and in many cases houses are shared by two or more families … Young married couples unable to obtain a house for themselves have perforce to reside with their people or take furnished rooms.[37]

In 1925, a

> room and bedcloset … with accommodation for 3 persons was [described by the Sanitary Inspector as being] occupied by 12 persons, comprising the subtenant, his wife, and family, viz.: – 5 sons aged 18 years, 16 years, 7 years and 5 weeks, and 5 daughters aged 14 years, 10 years, 4 years, and 2 ½ years.[38]

Nonetheless, the casebooks show that there was no direct association between family overcrowding and inpatient delivery. At the Hospice in 1924 domiciliary patients from the Old Town exceeded indoor patients from the same areas. Even at the ERMH, where indoor patients from these areas did outnumber outdoor, (by 15 per cent), women living in the Canongate and High Street preferred home delivery. Family overcrowding was tolerated, and mothers of large families did not usually seek inpatient care. Informants to local oral history projects emphasize this. For example, Helen Nickerson was born in 1916 and grew up in a room-and-kitchen in Leith:

> Nine o' us in the room-and-kitchen … Jenny and Aggie and Betty, all the lassies, slept in one bed, and the laddies slept in the other bed. The oldest one he slept in a sort of closet – a press … And my mother and father slept in the kitchen in the recess.[39]

Similarly, Ina Begbie, born in Tollcross (five minutes' walk from the ERMH) in 1928, remembered that '[m]y mother said I'd been her thirteenth child … quite well spread out, but in a room and kitchen that's a lot of children',[40] while her neighbour Alice Burt reported that

> nobody seemed to come back with a baby from the hospital, they all just seemed to come out of their house with a baby with them. All of a sudden the rest of the family were put out to play and neighbours took the odd one in to give them their tea … and the next thing the nurse disappeared and they all went in to see the new baby.[41]

Only one-third of the grand multiparas (women expecting a sixth or later baby) using the ERMH delivered in the hospital, and three-quarters of these had problems in either their pregnancy or delivery. Similarly, at the Hospice, only 33 of the 98 grand multiparas attending delivered indoors.

Non-familial overcrowding, the result of subletting, was a different problem, and analysis of casebook data suggests that it made a major contribution to the initial move to hospital. In 1912, at the ERMH, no married inpatients were recorded as living in shared accommodation (that is, their address was 'c/o' a third party), whilst approximately 2 per cent of outdoor patients from both the city and Leith did so: typically they were first-time mothers giving birth in their own mother's home. By 1924, 8 per cent of women in shared accommodation used the Royal Maternity dispensaries, but within the hospital 20 per cent of married patients now lived in shared accommodation, only a quarter of these with relations. Over half were primigravid, but most had unremarkable deliveries. At the Hospice, although lodgers made up only 10 per cent of the total, three-quarters delivered in the hospital. Almost all were having their first or second baby.

These patients came not from the insalubrious Old Town, but from the areas of nineteenth-century expansion – Dalry, Hillside, Gorgie and Fountainbridge – and from Stockbridge and Broughton. In 1924, 52 per cent of patients admitted to the ERMH from Broughton lived in lodgings, as did 42 per cent from Fountainbridge, 41 per cent from Dalry and 31 per cent from Hillside. Both the patients who came from Colinton were lodgers, as was one of the two from Trinity. Their landladies had considerable influence. For example, in 1930, the MOH wrote that

> [a] young married woman whose husband occupies a good position, pays 15s. a week for a furnished room. She expects to be confined shortly and has been informed that she must leave her room as the proprietrix insists that the confinement must not take place there. Prolonged anxious inquiries have failed so far to find a house.[42]

Six years before, Sister More from the ERMH dispensary had recorded that, when a pupil midwife arrived to carry out her evening check on the newly delivered Bessie Lamont, '[v]iolence [was] used towards Nurse [by the landlady]'. Sister More herself carried out the next check, but ultimately Bessie and her family were removed to Craiglockhart Poor Law Institution.[43] Choosing hospital delivery under such circumstances seems at best a neutral rather than a positive choice: nonetheless, the knock-on effects of inpatient delivery in the mid-1920s had a major influence on the continued use of hospital delivery in the 1930s.

Although the Sanitary Inspector continued to record the reluctance of the poor to leave their homes in the Old Town, squalid as they were, over the next ten years the city council began to address its housing problem, and its policy had a major impact on the geographical distribution of patients at both hospitals. Whereas in 1924, nearly 90 per cent of all Hospice patients came from central Edinburgh, in 1935, less than half of those attending the EIMMH did so. Instead, at both hospitals approximately 11 per cent of patients now came from the new council estates of Stenhouse, Craigmillar, Niddrie, Wardie and Lochend.

In contrast to the slums of the Old Town, the new houses were typically two- or three-apartment, spacious, with electric light, gas boilers, a hot water system, wash-house, tub and sink, coal cellar, drying green 'and open air all around'.[44] The estates were also provided with shopping and recreation centres, and with the support of the churches, the university settlement and the YWCA.[45] In the same spirit, the ERMH opened a branch house at Stenhouse to accommodate the pupil midwives who would attend local deliveries and provide postnatal care. If the poor quality of their old homes had forced Edinburgh's mothers into hospital delivery, then one might expect, as the ERMH evidently did, that, once settled into their new homes, the numbers of domiciliary births would once again increase. They did not. Only a fifth of new estate residents were delivered at home, and the Stenhouse branch was never much used.[46] Most mothers from the new estates continued to give birth in hospital, at this time surely making a genuinely positive decision to do so. The following section argues that they were not only influenced by their peers, but also by increasing familiarity with the medical world and its message of improving personal health.

'Onward Edinburgh' – A Changing Culture

By 1935 the habit of home confinement among voluntary maternity service users had been broken by the move away from former community support systems and the now-declining network of medical dispensaries which had previously served the population of Edinburgh so well.[47] Although Edinburgh's dispensaries declined in the 1930s, their long-term medical influence made it easier for mothers to adapt to the use of hospital care. In Leith, where there had been no maternity dispensaries, the tradition of home birth was maintained for longer, even in its new estates.[48] Additional, less direct medical influence may also have affected the choice of place of birth and enhanced the view that inpatient deliveries were better, safer or even more fashionable. Almost all the births to nurses who had previously trained in the Edinburgh Royal Infirmary and which were announced in their journal, the *Pelican*, between 1929 and 1935, took place, not in private houses, but in Edinburgh nursing homes, and one can speculate that the decisions of former colleagues influenced the attitudes of nurses working in the maternity hospitals or Public Health Department and in contact with parturients.[49] Although the MOH did not publish separate data on nursing home births, and until approximately 1930 they are difficult to identify firmly in the city birth notifications registers, nonetheless such births increased steadily throughout the interwar period. Approximately 18 nursing homes (and 300 births therein) are recorded in the city registers in 1924, but, by 1935, 28 homes can be clearly identified, where 941 births took place.[50]

In addition, a series of well-attended events organized by the Public Health Department sought to nurture a new and growing interest 'in increasing personal ... health'.[51] In 1928 Waverley Market was the site of the first Health and Hygiene Exhibition, a week-long event hosted by the Department, and combining musical entertainment by the Band of the Royal Marines with almost a hundred stands addressing such issues as the new housing (illustrated by a 'Slum House' constructed with 'materials ... taken from a demolished building ... [and] contrasted with the full-sized model of a modern house now being erected on the Prestonfield area'), dental care and 'Food and Dietetics', this stand being manned by the MOH himself.[52] At the opening of the second such event, in 1930, the Lord Provost, Thomas B. Whitson, claimed that over 120,000 people had paid their sixpences and attended the first.[53] The third and largest exhibition, 'Onward Edinburgh', which ran from 18 March to 4 April 1936, was intended to ensure that the MOH got 'the intelligent co-operation of the individual citizen' in his 'main business and desire ... the Prevention of Disease'. It particularly highlighted the role of the maternity and child welfare services, with free films on accessing medical care and bringing up children. Stands showed 'a selection of the medico-social activities of the Maternity and Child Welfare department', including 'Antenatal Hygiene', natural feeding, and the display of 'a safe and easily fitted up window balcony ... to hold a basket cot', all dovetailed with lighter entertainment in the form of music from the bands of the Coldstream Guards and the Border Regiment, keep-fit demonstrations and a daily play on the life of Florence Nightingale.[54]

The hospitals themselves sought to enhance their current status and, in the case of the ERMH, to cast off its former reputation as a shelter for the destitute to be avoided by more respectable citizens. In November 1926, in response to increasing demands for its medical services and therefore on its income, the ERMH began to plan a flag day and, on Sunday 2 January 1927, an appeal on its behalf was broadcast on the BBC.[55] Ultimately, the flag day, an extremely successful event by then in aid of the 'Maternity Hospitals in Edinburgh', was run by the Executive Committee of the Edinburgh Women Citizens Association in April 1927, and the proceeds shared with the EIMMH.[56]

The reinvention of the ERMH did not stop there. From 1927 the cover of its Annual Report emphasized to readers that

> [i]t contribute[d] to the preservation of Infant Life ... place[d] at the disposal of mothers from all parts ... the highest obstetrical skill, trained nursing and material comfort ... co-operate[d] with Local Authorities in their beneficial and vital Health Schemes [and trained] ... Medical Students and Nurses who go all over the world.[57]

In the previous year, Douglas Miller, one of its assistant physicians, proposed the publication of an annual medical and clinical report on the treatment and outcome of complicated cases, in contrast to annual reports, which focused on successful aspects of hospital care with a view to increasing financial support. Coming at a time when many hospitals drew as little attention as possible to their problem cases, these reports won the ERMH international recognition.[58] Similarly, while the EIMMH annual reports had continued to emphasize its provision of skilled but essentially low-key medical support for mothers throughout the 1920s, from the beginning of the 1930s they began to highlight its scientific work. In 1931 the focus was on its new Morgenthaler Bed for premature or delicate infants: 'an acquisition which has already made possible a more scientific and therefore more hopeful line of treatment'.[59] In following years there were references to the hospital's ongoing research into maternal mortality and morbidity arising from puerperal infection. By 1936 this had concluded 'that the problem of protection from puerperal fever is a much more difficult one to combat in the District than in Hospital'.[60]

The work of both hospitals in controlling infection is evident in their records at this time. Both segregated patients known to be infectious or believed to be at high risk of being so. For example, in 1935 all the women admitted to the ERMH following 'failed forceps outside' and whose postnatal ward is recorded, were nursed in 'ward 1 suspect room'. At the EIMMH, both new staff and future inpatients were swabbed for their streptococcal carrier status, and those who tested positive were isolated from the main hospital, carrier pupils nursing carrier patients.[61] The EIMMH research reports also advocated the strict use of masks at all times, and these can be seen in use, along with gloves, surgical gowns and sterile draping, in a series of photographs taken in the ERMH in 1936.[62] Admission instructions also emphasized the hospitals' strict control of their environment. Patients' clothes were routinely sent home ('[m]other and child have the use of Hospital garments during their stay ... Clothes for both to be brought in on day of discharge'), while visitors, potential sources of infection, were limited to '[o]ne Lady Visitor, week-days only, 2–2.30 p.m. [; h]usbands, every evening, 7–7.30 p.m. Children are not allowed to visit'.[63] Stark as these rules sound today, they did nothing to diminish the appeal of admission. Women still flocked to both hospitals to take 'advantage of the facilities and comforts ... offered'; the next section examines what these were and who they benefited.

The 'Facilities and Comforts ... Offered'

What features did women find on admission, and how did these compare with those available in their homes? Clearly the management of labour and the puerperium were priorities, and here institution casebooks can be used to make a direct comparison between indoor and outdoor patients. Perhaps the most appreciated facility was the management of pain in labour. Although in

1924 pain relief was seldom offered to women in normal labour (its use was not recorded at all at ELII, and seldom in the ERMH or its dispensaries, at the Deaconess or Hospice), by 1935 considerable change had taken place in the recorded management of labour pain, and analysis suggests this had become a major attraction for patients. This is apparent when ERMH outdoor patients are compared with their equivalents within the hospital (that is, with married Edinburgh or Leith residents booked in advance for hospital delivery, having no antenatal complications requiring hospitalization, admitted in labour and progressing to spontaneous delivery).[64] Only 4 women among 423 sampled ERMH dispensary cases in Edinburgh and Leith were recorded as receiving analgesia before delivering normally, yet 58 per cent of the hospital group (158) did so. At the EIMMH, only 29 per cent of similarly sampled inpatients received no analgesia. Staff at this hospital also recorded specifically when analgesia was not given; 154 of the 198 women whose records survive had some form of pain relief in labour. Although a local oral history informant claimed 'it was thought rather feeble to need an anaesthetic for a normal childbirth', particularly when a private practitioner could make an additional charge for its use, such a differential between indoor and outdoor use suggests that the desire for pain relief provided a major impulse towards hospital admission.[65]

A range of analgesics and anaesthetics was offered. Chloroform was popular during the second stage, sometimes in combination with intramuscular morphine for first-stage pain relief, particularly for first births.[66] It was used by approximately one-third of ERMH sample patients to have analgesia, but was less popular at the EIMMH, where only sixteen mothers in the sample used it. The ERMH was also involved in the British College of Obstetricians and Gynaecologists' trials of the Minnitt 'gas and air' machine, which allowed the supervised patient to control her own intake of nitrous oxide and oxygen, and this proved popular. Over half of the ERMH sample who had pain relief, eighty-eight women, used Minnitt machines alone, half of this group being primigravid. Only one required additional sedation: Mrs Rose Exford, a 23-year-old miner's wife from Niddrie Mains Drive having her first baby. She was admitted at 5 pm after the onset of pains eight hours earlier. By 1.25 am she was evidently sore, as she was examined vaginally and prescribed and given morphine. Three and a half hours later, she began to use the Minnitt machine, delivering a live boy spontaneously an hour after that.[67] Although the machine was being developed to increase domiciliary access to pain relief, its simple administration and control by the mother herself made it a welcome addition to hospital treatment.

Rectal paraldehyde was also being trialled at the ERMH, but was considered less satisfactory. Retention could be a problem, whilst house surgeon T. E. Elliot felt that '[t]here [was] no doubt that paraldehyde [had] a distinctly depressing action on uterine contractions' whilst failing to provide his patient with rest.[68]

Mrs Kate Low, a primigravid plumber's wife, was similarly disappointed: a '[c]ertain amount of amnesia [was] attained, but patient remembers quite a lot about the pains'. She required morphine as additional pain relief.[69] However, Staff Nurse M. C. Wright and her patient, a 24-year-old primigravida who had already been eight and a half hours in labour, considered paraldehyde 'good' (on a scale from 'excellent' to poor'), with no effect on 'conduct of labour'.[70] Delivery occurred some six hours after its administration.

While the administration of 'twilight sleep' (intramuscular morphine and hyoscine) was recorded indoors at the ERMH in 1924 on only ten occasions (1.2 per cent), by 1935 it was used in 3.2 per cent of all cases. Although it has been claimed that its use was limited, particularly in Britain, because institutions had insufficient staff to cope with the high level of patient monitoring required,[71] at the ERMH it does not seem to have been restricted in any way: seven of those in the comparison sample were given it (none as the result of the failure of a less staff-intensive treatment), of whom four were primigravid, and only one had a bad obstetric history. Lily Lewis, 34 and a chauffeur's wife, had had a 'diff[icult] instrumental' delivery of a 10-pound baby boy six years previously; in 1935 she had chloroform as well as 'twilight sleep' before spontaneously delivering a second similar-sized son.[72] Access to a readily available range of analgesia was clearly a positive reason to give birth in hospital.

Nor did inpatients 'lose' in terms of more invasive management of their labour, if not their delivery. At the ERMH, as in their homes, mobilization in labour was encouraged, particularly if progress seemed slow: when her contractions lessened following morphine, Mrs Helen Ford was encouraged to

> walk about but [only] ... succeed[ed] in ... tiring herself. On returning to the labour ward ... [she] was ... having strong contractions but considering her weary condition ... a sedative was administered following which she had five hours good sleep.[73]

Progress was not necessarily assessed by vaginal examination, and membranes were left intact, a policy which was sometimes blamed for slow progress. Dr Liston, wise after the event, recorded that 20-year-old Mrs Dora Gordon 'became distressed during a long 2nd. stage which should have been shortened by puncture of the membranes when she was examined'.[74] Nonetheless, Mrs Gordon was very much an exception; more than half of the local married women booked into the ERMH and admitted in labour delivered in less than 12 hours; only 17 per cent laboured for more than 24 hours, and only 2 per cent for more than 48 hours.[75] However, augmentation of labour was more common indoors than out: there were only three instances in the dispensaries, whereas twenty-one local, booked, married women admitted in labour at term were given uterine stimulants in the hospital. Similarly, despite this low-key approach, there was more intervention at delivery within the hospital, even among problem-free married local women. While only three were delivered by caesarean section, twenty-nine (8.3 per cent), were delivered by forceps.[76]

ERMH care not only provided effective pain relief and a more medicalized approach to delivery, but also an opportunity for recuperation, supplying both enforced rest and regular meals to women whose physical descriptions, recorded as part of the admission process in 1935, suggest they badly needed it. Although 64 per cent of women were described as healthy, or 'well-nourished good colour', 208, almost 19 per cent, were not.[77] A third of these, 6 per cent of the whole, were labelled thin, emaciated, undernourished or anaemic, although, disconcertingly, Mrs Hannah Gunn's condition was recorded as 'good, but some malnutrition'.[78] Among the sample selected as similar to outdoor patients, this increased slightly to 7 per cent. There had been 'no anorrhexia [*sic*]' in Mrs Grace Hall's home in Portobello, 'but food ha[d] been insufficient in quantity and of very limited variety'.[79] For such women the plain but regular diet at the ERMH provided a further reason for admission. Tea and bread and butter was served at 7 am, followed by milk and bread and butter at 9 am, a dinner of, typically, fish, potatoes, and milk pudding at 12.30, more tea and bread and butter at 3 pm, porridge and milk at 6.30 pm, and a supper of cocoa and bread and butter at 8 pm.[80]

By the early twentieth century, an extended period of bed rest was increasingly valued, and provided a further positive reason to seek admission.[81] In 1924, most evidence of post-delivery mobilization came from the dispensaries, where the great majority of patients apparently first got up after eight days of bed rest, before being discharged on the tenth post-delivery day. By 1935, 57 per cent of dispensary patients were recorded as first rising on the sixth or seventh post-delivery day. However, inside the hospital, only 42 per cent of delivered patients whose day of first mobilization was recorded got up in the first week after delivery; the majority, 58 per cent, stayed in bed until the second week.[82] Further, the greater supervision within the hospital ensured that this was genuine bed rest, when oral history, nursing folklore and occasional case note references all suggest that rest at home was usually a sham.[83] For example, Mrs Janet Greenwood had already been up and about in her Leith home by her seventh post-delivery day, whilst Mrs Ursula Knight, a new mother of four, unexpectedly admitted to the ERMH from Leith district for manual removal of placenta and blood transfusion, '[r]efused to stay in hospital although she was still far from well', instead leaving '[a]gainst medical advice' to resume her domestic role.[84]

Conclusion

The Edinburgh experience illustrates clearly the role of women's agency in the move to hospital birth. Admittedly the initial impetus was provided by deteriorating housing stock and the stress of living in rented accommodation, but nevertheless the early 1920s saw women with previous experience of voluntary hospital care change to inpatient delivery with enthusiasm. Their demand for beds forced the EIMMH to open a then-unfunded wing; having changed the function of newly acquired property to staff rather than patient accommodation, the ERMH struggled for sufficient space throughout the interwar period. Women were sustained in their choice first by the increasing physical rewards of admission – expert care, effective pain relief, the opportunity for complete rest and recuperation – but also by the awareness that births in hospitals and nursing homes were becoming more common. Ultimately, choosing domiciliary delivery in the new estates would be non-conformist. Concurrent with the move to hospital, and contributing to it, was a new official emphasis on personal health and responsibility for oneself, on the value of women and mothers to society. Edinburgh's maternity hospitals further encouraged this by emphasizing not their former social function as a shelter for the destitute, but rather their new scientific and life-saving role, although the decline in ERMH admissions after the opening of the maternity unit at the Western suggests that it at least may have had limited success in this. This chapter has cast further light on what was previously seen as an ideological debate about the move to hospital birth, suggesting that in Edinburgh the move was successful largely because it was driven by patient desires rather than medically enforced.

Acknowledgements

The work for this chapter was funded by the Wellcome Trust (Grant 074236/Z/04/Z), and I would like to thank the Wellcome for their support. Thanks are also due to those present at the Fourteenth Wellcome Trust Regional Forum, Glasgow, who heard an early version, for their comments; to those at the 'Perspectives on Modern Maternal Health and Healthcare, *c.* 1850–2000' conference; and to the staffs of the Lothian Health Services Archive, Edinburgh City Archives and the Edinburgh Room, Edinburgh City Libraries, for their assistance.

5 'WHAT WOMEN WANT': CHILDBIRTH SERVICES AND WOMEN'S ACTIVISM IN NEW ZEALAND, 1900–1960

Linda Bryder

The experience of childbirth has changed dramatically for most women in the Western world over the past one hundred years. There have been two major changes in that time. The first was a dramatic decline in the death rate for women in childbirth, which occurred from the 1930s. In the early twentieth century, such a death was a legitimate fear for anyone about to give birth. In New Zealand, the maternal death rate per 10,000 live births in 1927 was 44.1; by the late 1990s it was 2.5.[1] The second major change was in the location of childbirth – from home to hospital. By the 1970s, hospital birth was the norm throughout most of the Western world. Were the two changes related? Some obstetricians and others would say they were, and that modern hospitals are the safest places for women to give birth. Irvine Loudon, an historian of maternal mortality, believes that memories are short, and that almost no-one now – including doctors and midwives – remembers those past dangers and realizes that the conquest of maternal mortality since the mid-1930s has been 'one of the most remarkable achievements of modern medicine'.[2]

Not all would agree. Achievements of modern medicine came under attack from the 1970s, when epidemiological studies showed that improvements in health had more do to with nutritional status and sanitation than with medical breakthroughs.[3] At the same time, social historians were reassessing the history of modern medicine and, influenced by Michel Foucault, arguing that the rise of the medical profession had more to do with power and the social uses of that power than with so-called scientific advances. Also at that time, as part of the same questioning of authority, came the new women's movement, which was particularly interested in reproductive health, past and present. Feminist historians such as Ann Oakley interpreted the history of childbirth as the male capture of the female womb.[4] American feminist academic Sheryl Ruzek argued that obstetricians fought to keep delivery their exclusive domain, transforming what might be otherwise normal births into surgical events. In the delivery room, she claimed, the obstetrician could become the 'star of the obstetrical drama'.[5] A New Zealand feminist writer, Sandra Coney, argued in 1979 that the transfer of births from home to hospital was the result of men's 'womb envy'. In the hospital men could take control of the birth, strip women of their traditional support networks – and even pretend they were giving birth themselves.[6] This interpretation has continued, for example in an account of the history of childbirth given by Irish historian Jo Murphy-Lawless in 1998. She labelled obstetrical science as 'masculinist' and set up a model of diametrically opposed figures – male obstetricians versus women – arguing that women were victims, silenced by the patriarchal structure, though, she added, they were increasingly politicized from the 1970s as they sought to regain control of childbirth.[7]

While some of these accounts were clearly ideologically driven or politically motivated, as part of a consumer movement to promote a more women-centred birth service, they have continued to colour our view of the history of childbirth.[8] In this chapter I do not intend to contribute to the debate on whether or not hospitals have been the safest place in which to give birth. Rather, I will examine childbirth services in New Zealand from 1900 to 1960, with a view to promoting further understanding of why they took the form they did. In the early twentieth century, the government clearly envisaged midwives as integral to future maternity services and believed that not all births would be hospitalized. To what extent was the change to hospital and obstetrical controlled births by the 1950s driven by (male) obstetricians who sought to enhance their power and professional status at the expense of (female) midwives and force the changes upon women? I will argue that such a gendered perspective is too simplistic. While obstetrics was certainly a developing profession during this period, obstetricians only achieved the switch to hospitalized births with the overwhelming support of women's organizations. Once this became the norm from the 1950s, women were not rendered powerless but continued to influence the kind of childbirth services provided, again in alliance with obstetricians. This chapter examines women's involvement in determining the nature of childbirth services, and argues that, in New Zealand at least, they showed no lack of assertiveness in demanding the kind of services they wanted.[9]

A State Midwifery Service

Under a Liberal government which held power in New Zealand from 1890 to 1912, New Zealand gained an international reputation as a 'social laboratory', owing to its extensive social and labour legislation.[10] Social reforms included granting women the vote in 1893 (the first country to do so), introducing old age pensions in 1898 (the second country to do so), setting up a Health Department in 1901 (another first) and passing a Nurses Registration Act in 1901 (again, the first country to do so). In 1904 the government passed the Midwives Registration Act with the aim of improving maternity services in New Zealand.

Introducing this bill to parliament, the Premier (Prime Minister) Richard Seddon stated that the 'deaths at maternity are alarming'. His concern was directed primarily at babies; he noted that during the period 1894 to 1903, over 15,000 deaths under the age of one year had occurred and added that he was still awaiting information about the deaths of mothers. Introducing the bill into the Legislative Council, Attorney-General Albert Pitt explained that registering and training midwives would reduce infant deaths.[11] The government recognized population as a national asset, a concern about 'national efficiency' which it shared with the rest of the British Empire and indeed the Western world.[12]

In the early twentieth century, the government and the New Zealand public generally accepted that midwives would play an important role in future maternity services for most women in New Zealand, which explains the emphasis on ensuring they received adequate training. High maternal death rates were blamed, without any real evidence, on incompetent midwives. Certain stereotypes persisted, very similar to those of nineteenth-century nurses before the Nightingale reforms. Seddon maintained that some midwives 'indulge[d] a little too freely, and ... the sooner we have legislation which will ensure competent midwives – sober and especially clean midwives – the sooner you will prevent loss of life'.[13] Duncan MacGregor, Inspector-General of Hospitals and Charitable Institutions, predicted that, 'With the passing of the Midwives Registration Act the day of the dirty, ignorant, careless woman, who has brought death or ill health to many mothers and infants, will soon end'.[14]

The 1904 Midwives Registration Act provided for the registration and training of midwives in state maternity hospitals which were set up for that purpose, called St Helens hospitals. The first was opened in Wellington in 1905, and by 1920 there were seven around the country. The hospitals were run by matrons, and had no resident medical officer. Midwives were trained to handle all aspects of normal births, with doctors only called in an emergency and at the discretion of the matron. Medical superintendents were appointed, but they did not live on site and again were only summoned at the discretion of the matron. The hospitals did eventually train medical students but the training of midwives continued to take priority.[15]

The hospitals were intended for the wives of respectable working men; their husbands had to earn less than £3 (raised to £4 in the 1920s) a week for them to gain admission. In order to distinguish them from maternity homes for 'fallen women', which had been set up by various religious orders such as the Salvation Army, the women who entered St Helens contributed towards the cost of their stay. Most women stayed two weeks, which cost £3, still a considerable investment at a time when the average working-class weekly wage was £2/19s. Fees remained the same until 1929, despite a doubling in the average wage rates over that time. That year they increased to £5/5s. for fourteen days' confinement, still less than the general wage increases. The government met about half the cost of running the institutions. The hospitals also offered a district maternity service for those who chose to have their babies at home. Nurse attendance for a home delivery was £1, increasing to £2 in 1929, and for doctor attendance at delivery an extra £10/– was charged.[16]

The Health Department viewed the St Helens hospitals and a midwifery service as central to maternity services in New Zealand. An Inquiry into Maternity Services set up by the first Labour Government in 1937 noted that in a number of countries, 'the trend is towards a service in which the bulk of the normal midwifery is conducted by highly trained midwives' and that 'in such a scheme the general practitioner is excluded from all normal midwifery practice'. This was specifically the case in Holland and the Scandinavian countries 'where the maternity services are recognised to be of a very high order'.[17] The committee reported that the recommendations for a national maternity service for England and Wales put forward by the Ministry of Health, the British Medical Association and the British College of Obstetricians and Gynaecologists were 'based on the principle of midwife attendance in normal labour'. The committee's report cited the evidence of Dr Henry Jellett, formerly Master of Rotunda Hospital, Dublin, who had emigrated to New Zealand and was the Consultant Obstetrician to the Department of Health. In Jellett's view, for normal births:

> I think it is a mistake to bring in the complication of the medical man who has to attend all kinds of disease, statistics and history having proved over a period of years in other countries, and also at Home [Britain], that these cases can be attended more satisfactorily by midwives.[18]

England and Wales had introduced a national domiciliary midwifery system under the 1936 Midwives Act.

There was some medical opposition to the midwifery-run St Helens hospitals. At their instigation one doctor declared, 'These St Helens Hospitals mean pounds out of the pockets of doctors'.[19] While medical views towards St Helens appeared to soften over time,[20] doctors continued to be suspicious of a midwifery service. The New Zealand Obstetrical Society, which was set up in 1927 to represent the interests of doctors who practised obstetrics, not surprisingly advocated a doctor and hospital maternity service as opposed to a midwifery service. At a meeting in 1929 the society resolved that,

> as Dr Jellett had recently published his proposals for the future midwifery service of this Dominion, which proposals eliminate the doctors from attending cases of normal confinement, Drs North and Irving be deputed to draft a policy for the future midwifery service of their Dominion.[21]

In 1933, in the middle of the economic depression, the society commented on a Health Department scheme whereby 'in necessitous cases ... a doctor should only see a normal case once or twice during the latter period of gestation and a midwife undertake delivery etc'. Several speakers contended that this policy, 'introduced as perhaps an emergency measure, might well become the thin edge of a permanent wedge', which was after all 'an exact parallel of the English mid-wife service'.[22] In the following year the society regretted that the

> the tendency in these days of depression was for more women to be confined by midwives alone. The Society believes that for reasons of safety to mother and infant, reasonable pain relief, and elimination of future pelvic weaknesses, a doctor and a trained nurse should be present at every delivery and fear that the present tendency, now an emergency measure, might drift into a permanent custom.[23]

In 1933 Bernard Dawson, Professor of Obstetrics and Gynaecology at the University of Otago (who had qualified in medicine in England), also commented on England's midwifery based maternity services, under which he said midwives now attended 75 per cent of births compared to 58 per cent ten years earlier, and added, 'It is usual for methods adopted by England to be advocated sooner or later in her Dominions and indeed the midwife system of maternity service already has advocates in New Zealand'.[24] That same year Dr Thomas Corkill opposed a midwifery service for New Zealand. His argument was that allowing doctors to perform 'normal' deliveries would improve overall services, because, he explained, 'it is only by long personal and practical experience of the normal that reliable judgement concerning the abnormal can be acquired. There were very real dangers in a specialisation founded on an imperfect knowledge of normal practice'.[25]

However, it was not so much the medical voice which determined the form maternity services was to take under the first Labour government. Rather, it was the overwhelming evidence presented to the 1937 Committee of Inquiry into Maternity Services from women's groups which swayed the government. Women appeared to be united in their demand for hospital-based, doctor-run maternity services for all. When Dr Tom Paget, the Health Department's Inspector of Maternity Hospitals, asked Mrs McGuire, who represented a local branch of the Labour Party during the inquiry, whether she preferred a maternity hospital or a nurse service in the home, she replied, 'We think a hospital is the better'.[26] Dr Edward Lowe told the Committee when discussing maternity services, 'I find that patients are becoming more hospital-minded'.[27] He called parturient women 'patients', but so did the non-medical witnesses coming before the committee.

Hospital Births and Mothers' Views

The 1904 Midwives Registration Act which set up the St Helens hospitals was indicative of a new trend towards institutional births. At that time most New Zealand women still delivered their babies at home. In 1920, less than 35 per cent of all births occurred in hospital (defined here as an institution with two or more beds).[28] The Health Department's Director of the Division of Nursing, Hester Maclean, supported home births, explaining in 1918, 'I would like to emphasise my belief that, provided there is reasonably comfortable accommodation in the homes of the expectant mothers, the large majority of confinement cases do not need to come into hospital'.[29] Mothers increasingly disagreed. In 1936 Professor Dawson explained,

> There is a growing tendency for more and more to enter hospitals for normal confinements ... The fact that over 60 per cent of women in New Zealand are confined in hospitals clearly proves that the majority already prefer hospital treatment to domiciliary, even in perfectly normal confinements.[30]

According to the 1937 Committee, while only 15 to 25 per cent of all births in England and Wales took place in hospitals, in New Zealand 81.75 per cent occurred in hospital.[31]

Historian Signild Vallgarda, who investigated the move to hospitalized childbirth in Sweden which followed a trend similar to that in New Zealand, commented that it is hard to elicit the views of the women themselves in this process.[32] Yet in New Zealand, there is abundant evidence in the archives of the National Council of Women (NCW), the Society for the Protection of Women and Children (SPWC) and the government's 1937 Committee of Inquiry into Maternity Services, to give a clear indication of these women's views. The NCW was a non-party political lobby which incorporated 168 organizations comprising 40,000 women.[33] When a branch of the NCW set up a sub-committee to lobby the government for improved maternity services in 1936, they called it the Committee on Maternity *Hospital* Services.[34] They took it for granted that the best services would be hospital-based. The women who gave evidence to the inquiry suggested that the two most important issues for New Zealand women were the pain relief associated with hospitalized childbirth, and the fact that they felt safer in hospital. Hospitalized childbirth was linked to science and modernity, which were seen by both sexes as positive attributes in the 1930s.

The women of these organizations framed hospital births and particularly pain relief in the 1930s as a feminist issue. Pain relief in childbirth goes back to the mid-nineteenth century, though new methods were constantly developed. To take advantage of this, medical facilities and medical attendants were needed, and these were increasingly available to those who could pay. To Vera

Crowther, a British-born nurse and feminist who had emigrated to New Zealand in the 1920s and subsequently joined the Communist party, it was a class-based issue. She believed it unfair that women who were ill-nourished, overworked and mentally distraught with domestic and financial cares should suffer depletion and exhaustion of all their human powers in childbirth. She compared the movement to provide universal pain relief with the suffragettes' fight to gain the vote.[35] Crowther's was not a lone voice. The Auckland Branch of the SPWC summed up what appeared to be a widespread consensus among women in 1936 with its recommendations to the Minister of Health for improved state maternity services:

This Society is anxious that every woman, married or single, rich or poor, giving birth to a child shall be provided with the utmost attention and relief from pain which science can provide. As this can only be obtained by the services of both a Doctor and a nurse, the Society urges: 'That hospital accommodation for all classes of maternity work be extended, and that in such hospitals, resident medical officers specialised in obstetrics and gynaecology, be appointed, one of whom shall be present at every delivery'.

The report stated that the existing practice at the St Helens hospitals run by midwives, 'results in prolonged and unnecessary suffering on the part of the patient'.[36]

The SPWC representatives visited the local St Helens Hospital where they interviewed seven women who had experienced normal (uncomplicated) births: 'without exception' these women explained that only financial reasons prevented them from having a doctor at the confinement.[37] Mrs Nellie Molesworth, described by Raewyn Dalziel in her history of the SPWC as the society's 'best known figure in the 1930s', was an inspector for the SPWC from 1928 to 1941.[38] Molesworth told the Committee of Inquiry that during her time as inspector she had questioned many women at St Helens and

have heard very distressing stories of unnecessary suffering endured by these women of the poorer class and have interviewed a large number of them and in practically every case inadequate pain relief has been given. These women, unless the case is abnormal, go through the whole process of labour and delivery, conscious of acute suffering. Many of them have a Murphy Inhaler [which was a limited amount of pain relief in the form of chloroform that midwives were allowed to administer] given to them but they say it is almost useless and very often it is taken from the patient and they are told to do more to help themselves.

She also heard of 'stitches inserted by the matron or a sister without an anaesthetic'. In her opinion, 'Adequate relief should be given in all cases and definite research carried out as to modern methods of relieving pain during confinements. We think that painless maternity is every woman's right.'[39]

At this time, as noted earlier, 82 per cent of women in New Zealand were giving birth in hospital, compared to only about 20 per cent in Britain. Emily

Siedeberg McKinnon, a New Zealand-born and trained doctor who undertook postgraduate study in Britain and was later medical superintendent of St Helens Maternity Hospital in Dunedin, attempted to explain the differential rates. In accordance with New Zealand's self-image as a classless society, she argued that New Zealand women did not 'have the same sense of class inferiority' as seen in Britain, and expected higher standards.[40] These higher standards included access to hospitalized childbirth.

Yet in Britain there were moves in the same direction. In 1928 the National Birthday Trust Fund was set up to improve maternity services and specifically access to pain relief. A 1945 article in a British paper dismissed the argument that for generations women had given birth without the aid of anaesthetics, maintaining that the benefits of modern science should be available to women.[41] A survey of public opinion in the same year found many believed that there should be no class distinctions in maternity services. One commentator pointedly asked, 'What is being done to make childbirth easier? Is anything being done? Or are all our brilliant doctors and specialists still content to tell us that childbirth is a "natural function"?'[42]

It was not just pain relief that made hospitals so attractive to women in childbirth. In the early twentieth century there was a growing faith in the powers of medical science and with it the image of hospitals changed. Hospitals were no longer refuges for the poor and homeless as they had been in the nineteenth century. As Irvine Loudon noted, most women in the early twentieth century would have known someone who died in childbirth. He was writing about Britain; it cannot have been any comfort to New Zealand women to learn in 1920 that New Zealand had the second highest maternal mortality rate in the Western world. The language of the early twentieth century, when words such as 'dread' of childbirth and the 'dark hours of maternity' were common, suggests that the fear was very real. Not only death was feared, so too was long-lasting debility.[43] In Britain too, Jane Lewis has concluded from her research into the history of maternity that:

> What is clear is that women of all social classes in the early twentieth century expressed fear of childbirth in terms of both the pain and the considerable chance of subsequent health problems. Their fears were real and arose directly from the conditions of maternity they experienced. When these are understood, their demand of hospital birth becomes readily comprehensible.[44]

Nor was this simply medical propaganda to lure women into hospital. When the New Zealand Health Department advocated home births attended by midwives and offered reassurances that childbirth was 'a normal physiological process and to the healthy woman in healthy surroundings was attended with very small risk',[45] women were not convinced. Mrs Agnes Kent Johnson, who belonged to the Christchurch branch of the NCW and was a member of the Committee of Inquiry into Maternity Services, explained, 'the psychological aspect also comes in – that a woman prefers to have a doctor'.[46] The seven women interviewed at Auckland's St Helens 'expressed the feeling that it would give confidence to know a doctor would attend them ... One states that she had known a young woman who lost her baby "because she lost confidence."'[47] Doctors were the arbiters of medical science and therefore the best service included their involvement. Even the Obstetrical Branch of the New Zealand Registered Nurses' Association stated, 'Of course, it is quite the highest ideal that every patient should go through the hands of a doctor'.[48]

Women drew on professional authority to support their case. The SPWC, like its British counterpart the National Birthday Trust Fund, allied itself with obstetricians and used the Obstetrical Society to support its demands. In a 1936 letter to the Minister of Health, the SPWC cited a 1934 report of the New Zealand Obstetrical Society which, it stated, 'definitely supports our resolution' of having a doctor present at every delivery 'for reasons of safety to mother and infant, reasonable pain relief and elimination of future pelvic weaknesses'.[49]

Significantly, women's groups played a leading role in establishing chairs in obstetrics and gynaecology at Otago in 1930 and Auckland in 1949, to facilitate medical training and further research. The Auckland branch of the NCW considered the 1930 appeal 'a noteworthy advance in maternal welfare long advocated by the National Council of Women'.[50]

The leader of the fundraising was Dr Doris Gordon who, although a woman, has often been portrayed as the archetypical medical professional who sought to impose the medical model of childbirth on women.[51] Yet Gordon saw herself as firmly feminist in two respects. First, she argued with her male colleagues about the right of women to pain relief in childbirth. At her private hospital at Stratford, she continued to use the pain relief known as 'twilight sleep' (morphia and scopolamine) which had already been discredited by doctors in Britain as more trouble than it was worth – it caused disorientated mothers during labour.[52] Describing her use of twilight sleep, Gordon claimed that the stillbirth rate was much lower than at the St Helens hospitals. She stressed this point because during 1925–30, she said, the Health Department had strongly opposed the use of these drugs and had convinced the public of their dangers: 'I find that many people who previously were afraid of pregnancy are more willing to have children after they have been in my hospital and experienced "twilight" sleep methods'. She added that twilight sleep could only be given by people who were really enthusiastic about it, and that she usually spent the night in hospital when there was a case there.[53]

Second, Gordon saw the interests of the profession and women as one and the same; she said of the Obstetrical Society of which she was founder: 'Our aim was *the genuine welfare of every mother*, irrespective of colour or complexion, and her inviolable right to be treated with the same consideration as would be extended to a Prime Minister's daughter'.[54] Gordon exhorted women's groups to pressure government to set up a women's hospital and training school. She explained to Mrs Nina Barrer of the NCW that 'New Zealand badly needs one up-to-date and well controlled women's Hospital'. She maintained that cows and their hormones received more attention from the well-paid scientists of the Dairy Board than did women. She claimed that:

> New Zealand thinks of women's health solely in terms of a creditably low infantile and maternal death rate (women are assessed of their breeding values, and poorly assessed at that, for today NZ has not one special clinic for the diagnosis and cure of sterility). This Dominion does not yet realise that women have a right to POSITIVE good health, and that modern discoveries correctly taught at a Post Graduate centre would soon cure 75% of the troubles hitherto passively accepted as 'Women's lot'.[55]

She stressed that her cause was non-political: 'we can only urge Cabinet, with the united voice of all the franchise, to get on with the job [of providing a new hospital and postgraduate training centre] without any delay'. By the franchise she meant the female vote. The power of the women's voice was very much in her consciousness: 'We want all the publicity we can, but still hope to avoid flinging brickettes like the old rampant suffragettes'. She believed 'the onus will rest with the women leaders of the Dominion to push the matter'. She told Barrer that as long as she herself pushed for the new hospital, politicians would ignore the request, but that 'If hundreds of women appear to want it they will suddenly find it's their hearts desire'. She 'concentrated on the "inquiring women" knowing that, through their massed opinion, lay the road to political approval'.[56]

In November 1935 the first Labour government swept into power in New Zealand, promising social security 'from the cradle to the grave'. The commitment of the new government to social justice, and the importance it attached to building a strong population base ensured that maternity services were high on its agenda. As noted above, the Labour government set up the Inquiry into Maternity Services in 1937, which gave women a platform to express their views.

Women capitalized on the broader national concerns and used the rhetoric of 'national efficiency' to argue their case. Mrs Cassey, representing the Women's Auxiliary of the Unemployed Workers' Union, and Mrs Stewart of the Devonport Housewives' Union, told the 1937 Committee of Inquiry into Maternity Services that, 'If you want population then you must cater for them in the proper way', through a State maternity service. Mrs Cassey said,

> We believe that since the Government is definitely stating that the child is an asset to the country, then they should be prepared to maintain that asset and bring it into the world free, because it is a national and not a local problem.[57]

Mrs Grace Marshall complained to the committee about her treatment at Auckland's St Helens. This was her fourth baby – her first two had been born at home with a doctor in attendance, and the third, which had been premature, born at St Helens. The fourth, with breech presentation, was also born at St Helens. She complained that, 'during the whole confinement I was not given an anaesthetic nor was a doctor called in, the matron taking sole charge. I suffered intolerably'. She said that a medical student present suggested the use of pain relief to the matron, but he was told to be quiet and leave the room. Mrs Marshall's child was stillborn, and she exhorted:

> Surely we mothers are entitled to the services of a skilled obstetrician who would ensure the life of our babies and possible impairment of health to the mother, and an anaesthetist who would alleviate some of the suffering necessary to childbirth? My case is only one of many from what I observed while in St Helens, so why wonder at the falling birth-rate? I for one will not have any more children until proper facilities are available.[58]

Women succeeded in their goal of attaining universal free hospital childbirth services, under the 1939 maternity benefits which formed part of the 1938 Social Security Act. They were provided with fourteen days' free care in hospital at the time of delivery and the services of a practitioner of their choice. Signild Vallgarda found similar sentiments expressed in Sweden and accepted there by the Social Democrats. The new legislation in New Zealand was testimony to the lobbying powers of the women's groups. Vallgarda saw Swedish mothers dictating the trend as well, which she believed was related to the women's sense of security in hospital.[59]

Under the 1939 benefits, women could still choose to have a midwife in attendance at childbirth. The Health Department continued to employ midwives to provide domiciliary childbirth services, particularly in rural areas. However, the trend to hospitalized birth accelerated following the introduction of the benefits, for rural as well as urban women. The SPWC noted in 1939 that St Helens was booked up for two months ahead, and commented, 'Accommodation in Auckland for confinements is absolutely at a premium'.[60] The National Women's Hospital was set up in Auckland in 1946 in response to lobbying by women's groups. By contrast, over the first year following the introduction of maternity benefits, the number of Auckland St Helens domiciliary deliveries (already falling) dropped from fifty-three to nineteen. From 1946, St Helens midwives stopped providing a domiciliary service, owing to diminishing demand.[61]

Ironically, while mothers felt safer in hospital, hospitals were not a safe place in which to give birth in the early twentieth century, as has been shown by Irvine Loudon for Britain and Philippa Mein Smith for New Zealand, and as was recognized by officials within the Health Department in the 1920s when they launched a campaign to clean up maternity facilities in hospitals.[62] The major cause of death was an infection called puerperal sepsis. To combat this, the Health Department introduced stringent hygienic measures in hospitals to reduce the risk of infection, and succeeded in reducing the maternal death rate even before effective drugs were developed in the 1930s. However, by instituting a series of measures which regulated nursing procedures and called for total sterility of the hospital environment, they also helped to create a very alienating environment in which to give birth. Auckland's National Women's Hospital, located in an ex-military hospital, was symbolic of post-war regimented births.

Into the Hospitals: The 1950s

Hospitalized childbirth was becoming the norm for all New Zealand women; by 1960 93 per cent of Pakeha (European) women and 90 per cent of Maori women gave birth in hospital.[63] However, this did not mean women were the passive or silent victims of the medical model and the science of obstetrics. Women continued to have a voice in the kind of childbirth services they wanted, again primarily through their organizational networks, the NCW and the Parents Centre, a new consumer group directly related to maternity. Parents Centre president Helen Brew claimed in 1960 that this was 'the only organisation on a local or national level competent to speak on behalf of young mothers – and their husbands – in the broad field of maternity services'.[64] The first centre was set up in Wellington in 1951, and in 1957, with seven centres across the country, a Federation of Parents Centres was formed.

Jean Donnison's history of midwifery states that in North America, by the 1950s, 'childbirth was generally hospitalised and completely doctor-controlled. Typically, normal healthy women were delivered unconscious from anaesthetic, arms and legs strapped to the delivery table, the doctor performing an episiotomy and "lifting out" the baby with forceps'.[65] In New Zealand's largest doctor-controlled maternity hospital, Auckland's National Women's Hospital, forceps deliveries constituted just 15 per cent of all deliveries in 1949–50, and caesarean sections a further 9.5 per cent.[66] It is hard to know how many of the 1,148 'normal' deliveries that year received anaesthesia in the final stages of labour. In a lecture delivered in the 1940s, Dr Tom Plunkett, senior obstetrician at the new hospital, commented on the public demand for complete anaesthetics and appeared resigned to the fact that 'the parturient woman is *entitled* to … anaesthesia'. He complained that with women demanding pain relief, this would assuredly 'produce a trail of asphyxiated babies with a proportionately high mortality rate'.[67] Nor was it totally safe for mothers. A decade earlier Dawson, responding to the 'popular but ill-informed clamour for pain relief', noted that pain relief definitely contributed to the risk of haemorrhage.[68]

Parents Centre was initially called the Natural Childbirth Association, show-ing the influence of the natural childbirth movement. In a foreword to Kerreen Reiger's history of women's activism and childbirth in Australia, childbirth activist Sheila Kitzinger wrote of the natural childbirth movement that, 'Some critics still see it as a group of self-centred women, wrapped up in their own emotions, who scorn medical knowledge and are prepared to put their babies at risk as a result'.[69] Yet in the 1950s when the natural childbirth movement first took off, it was pro-moted by obstetricians primarily for the sake of the baby. Harvey Carey, the new Professor of Obstetrics and Gynaecology at National Women's, told the local press,

> Babies are healthier when delivered this way because they are not doped by the anaes-thetic and therefore breathe more easily. The trend today is away from the use of general anaesthetics. The methods most used are natural childbirth and local anaes-thetics.[70]

Pain relief made the baby sleepy and if there was a complication in the delivery, this often tilted the scales against the baby.[71] It was particularly dangerous for pre-mature babies. In 1957 Carey told a national conference of Parents Centres, 'The baby always pays some price if volatile anaesthetics are used at the time of deliv-ery. In cases of prematurity and other unfavourable circumstances, anaesthetics may adversely influence the baby's chance of survival'.[72] 'My first consideration is the baby', he said, 'I don't believe in doing anything for which the baby has to pay'. He noted approvingly in 1956 that New Zealand already had an instru-mental delivery rate of only 4 to 6 per cent, compared to 50 to 60 per cent in the United States, and went on to acknowledge the contribution made to obstetrics by Britain's Dr Grantly Dick Read, the exponent of natural childbirth.[73]

Dick Read first published his famous manual on natural childbirth in 1933; it was constantly reprinted until 1953. An advocate of natural childbirth, Read believed that women suffered pain in childbirth largely because they were afraid and unprepared. If women could be taught to relax during labour, they would not require pain relief.[74] A group of 'leading medical men' in New Zealand totally accepted Dick Read's ideas and used them when they responded to Vera Crowther's 1938 article in *Woman To-day* (referred to above). They declared that Dick Read 'show[ed] that fear of pain during childbirth ha[d] a retarding and generally serious effect on what would otherwise be a normal process'. They explained how fear 'produces tension; tension, pain; and pain, increased fear. And so the vicious circle of prolonged and difficult labour is complete'. Fear caused a woman unnecessary pain. Crowther retorted that those who feared childbirth the most were the ones who had been through it before, unrelieved by anaesthesia.[75] Feminists at this time were not persuaded by the medical argu-ments; as Dr Plunkett had noted, they believed pain relief was an entitlement.

The new psychological approach to childbirth was brought to New Zealand by Dr Maurice Bevan-Brown, a Christchurch psychiatrist, who had worked at London's Tavistock Clinic in the 1920s and 1930s. Natural childbirth, to these new psychologists, was promoted primarily in the interests of the child, not the mother. For the child's psychological health, it was vitally important for the mother to be conscious at the time of the birth. Parents Centre President Helen Brew was a speech therapist by training, and explained that in taking case histories, she had frequently observed that traumatic childbirth led to inadequate early nurture and speech difficulties, especially stammering and associated behaviour problems. For her, the goal of Parents Centre was the 'settling of our vast mental health and juvenile delinquency problems, of which a faulty mother–child relationship is indisputably the breeding ground'.[76] Her husband, also involved in Parents Centre, was a psychologist.

Along with promoting childbirth without pain relief, Parents Centre also advocated 'rooming-in', or keeping the baby by the mother's bed rather than sending it off to the nursery. The Parents Centre official historian, Mary Dobbie, wrote of her encounters with Carey. When Dobbie mentioned her interest in natural childbirth, Carey invited her to give birth in his professorial unit with freedom to try natural birth, rooming-in and demand feeding, in return for providing him with a written report, noting in particular the baby's feeding and sleeping patterns. He pointed out that in his ward she would have to do a lot of the childcare herself as nurse trainees had been withdrawn (see below).[77]

It was Carey who suggested that the various branches of the Parents Centre federate to enhance its voice as a lobby group. He also suggested a residential conference at National Women's Hospital to draw up a basic lecture series for all centres. Dobbie wrote,

> After so many rebuffs from obstetrical quarters this invitation gave a great lift to morale. There was a sense of arrival. National Women's Hospital, centre for research, trial ground of changes in obstetrical care – where better to gain a hearing from the expectant mother's point of view?[78]

The Parents Centre honorary secretary also described this conference as 'of major importance to Parents Centre'.[79]

While Carey agreed that fear was a factor in inhibiting natural childbirth, he did not favour the psychological theories of people like Bevan-Brown. He had much more practical reasons for changes in childbirth practice. The advantages to babies of childbirth without drugs have already been mentioned. Other reasons included the shortage of nurses, which favoured the move to rooming-in or mothers looking after their own babies, and perineal showering. There was also concern about infection in the 1950s, specifically the H-bug (a penicillin resistant micro-organism), believed to be spread by nurses' contact with babies. Carey also thought that panning exposed women to greater risk of infection:

> At the present time recently delivered women are not allowed to use the toilet even though they are up and about and quite fit and well. Every four hours they have to climb back into bed to sit on a sterile bed pan and then be swabbed by a junior nurse or trainee. In this way they are exposed to a greater risk of infection than if they sat on a toilet.[80]

Panning mothers in bed following the birth had emerged as part of the rules set out for nurses in 1926 to help curb infections such as puerperal sepsis, and remained on the books (the Health Department's manual, *General Principles of Maternity Nursing*, popularly known as H.-Mt.20). The Nurses and Midwives Board (NMB) appeared reluctant to consider changing the rules. Toilet arrangements thus became a bone of contention between Carey and the NMB. When Carey introduced early toileting in his so-called 'experimental' ward at National Women's, the NMB withdrew nurse trainees. Doctors complained about the 'dictatorial' attitude of the NMB in what they considered to be a 'clinical' matter, and complained about the interference between doctor and patient. Women complained too. In 1956 a meeting of the NCW, attended by representatives of fifty-six women's organizations, passed a resolution that the council request the NMB to allow more latitude for the staffing of wards in connection with research and new technology at National Women's Hospital. They added that this request came from 'responsible women', who were interested in the welfare of both patients and nurses, and were impressed with the work of Professor Carey. Women's organizations were firmly allied with the medical profession, or at least those members of the profession whom they found sympathetic to the natural childbirth movement which was increasingly gaining support among women.[81]

The NMB attempted to address the current maternity nursing shortage by revising the nurses' curriculum in 1957, to incorporate three months' maternity nursing in the training for all general nurses. Nurses now had to deliver five babies, perform twenty rectal examinations and give obstetrical anaesthesia 'to the point of rendering patients unconscious' ten times during their training.[82] This limited women's right to choose natural childbirth, as nurses needed the experience. Moreover, Dr Herbert Green, Associate Professor at the Postgraduate School of Obstetrics and Gynaeocology at National Women's Hospital, estimated that in 1960 no fewer than 12,000 rectal examinations were done each year at National Women's in the interests of nurse training.[83] Asked to justify this, the Director of Nursing explained that 'because patients have to have unpleasant things done to them, a rectal examination is one way of teaching nurses how to get patients to accept an unpleasant procedure!'[84] Green wrote to the press, 'I am glad to realise that some of the difficulties inherent in the new basic curriculum have percolated through to the people they affect most, that is the patients'.[85] He told the Parents Centre that he believed the NMB's interference was affecting patient welfare, and assured them that 'any move by organizations such as yours – who represent patients – to improve the standard of maternity services in New Zealand will meet with my unqualified support'.[86]

In their fight against the NMB and the Health Department, Carey and Green continued to look to Parents Centre and the NCW. Parents Centre decided to initiate a remit through the NCW to urge the Minister of Health 'to investigate fully the regulations covering the functioning of maternity training hospitals in regard to the rights of the individual doctor to prescribe medical treatment for his own patients'.[87] The Wellington branch of the NCW printed a report in 1960 called 'Maternity Services in New Zealand', based on wide-ranging interviews. Complaints by mothers listed in the report included 'mothers who through panic and pain "make a fuss" being [*sic*] slapped, threatened or criticised [by nurses]'. The report included as an appendix the report from the Oamaru Mother's Group, a particularly activist group. One of its complaints was

> the virtual refusal by the hospital authorities to let a mother see her doctor at the time
> of confinement except at the discretion of the nurses in charge at the time ... in many
> cases when a mother wants her doctor to be sent for she is refused by the hospital
> staff; also her contact with her doctor is restricted by the fact that she cannot see him
> to discuss any problems without a member of the staff being present.[88]

The NCW demanded an inquiry, commenting that this was an area 'peculiarly our own'.[89] The government successfully diffused the situation by setting up a Committee on Maternity Services which included a consumer representative, as demanded by the NCW, Parents Centre and the newly established National Consumer Council.[90]

Conclusion

The evolution of childbirth services in New Zealand during a crucial period of change was not simply the result of obstetricians pushing for professional control of childbirth. Government legislation, as Joan Donley has noted, medicalized childbirth by providing free and universal hospital-based childbirth services.[91] But the government responded first and foremost to pressure from organized women's groups. These women's groups were broadly based and not simply middle-class women imposing their will on the majority. Nor were they duped by obstetricians, but rather had their own ideas about the kind of services they wanted. These were based primarily on the public esteem of science and professionalism in the early to mid-twentieth century. Hospital care in itself was not enough, as shown by the constant complaints relating to the midwife-run St Helens. Once universal hospitalization was achieved, women continued to press for changes within the hospital system. When women complained of practices in hospital, it was nurses who were usually their primary target. They were the people with whom they interacted most in the hospital setting and who determined the nature of their experience. In the 1930s, women had fought for the right of pain relief in alliance with doctors; in the late 1950s, also in alliance with certain doctors, they fought for the right to refuse it, and more generally called for a less regimented and more caring environment. Yet those who publicly complained were probably a minority. Women chose to go to hospital to have their babies and many enjoyed their stay, making friends with other new mothers whilst there. Hospital births seemed to be there to stay, but mothers wanted a more homely atmosphere whilst in hospital. This was an ongoing battle, but one that was not necessarily drawn along gender lines. Women should not be viewed as passive recipients of medicalization.

6 'TWIXT GOD AND GEOGRAPHY: THE DEVELOPMENT OF MATERNITY SERVICES IN TWENTIETH-CENTURY IRELAND

Lindsey Earner-Byrne

In 1922, the southern twenty-six counties of Ireland secured political independence from Britain with the foundation of the Irish Free State.[1] The new state was no blank canvas, of course, as it proceeded to govern based on the legacy, infrastructure and legislation of hundreds of years of British rule. Nowhere was this more apparent than in the arena of public health: pre-1922 legislation relating to the medical treatment of the poor and destitute, compulsory vaccination, the registration and notification of births and deaths and the role of local government in public health were to provide the framework of the Irish Free State's approach to health. The Ireland of the early twentieth century was also focused on controlling infectious diseases, regulating midwifery (lest the country became 'the dumping ground for the inepts [*sic*] of Great Britain'),[2] and reducing maternal and infant mortality.[3]

Ireland was a predominantly rural, agrarian and traditional society, dominated by Roman Catholicism with a highly conservative moral climate. Irish public debate continued throughout the twentieth century to display suspicion of the state and central government. The Roman Catholic hierarchy was often perceived, and indeed portrayed itself as, a counterweight to the perils of undue state control or interference. The development of maternity and child health services since the foundation of the state was influenced by the legacy of a British public health culture, deep religious rivalry between Roman Catholic and Protestants, particularly in the field of medicine,[4] a predominately rural landscape and a quite unique and challenging demographic profile. This chapter seeks to analyse how these various factors intertwined to shape maternity services in twentieth-century Ireland.

In 1919, on the eve of political independence, it was publically acknowledged that Ireland was a laggard in the battle against infant mortality as:

> Nothwithstanding all the measures adopted by the [Dublin] Corporation and vari-
> ous Benevolent Societies to lower the mortality of infants, their death-rate has not
> declined to any substantial extent, whereas the infantile death-rate in England had
> declined by fifty per cent.[5]

The solution to this unfortunate Irish distinction was informed by a rationale articulated prior to political independence and current in many other European countries: the mother was the key to reducing infant mortality.[6]

> If the infant – the future man or woman – is to rebuild the nation, it must be cared
> for through its mother: feed and care for the mother, enable her to develop a healthy
> offspring, and to produce in a healthy body a healthy mind.[7]

In order to reduce both maternal and infant mortality, medical practitioners, state officials, local agencies and hospitals were in agreement that antenatal care was vital. The emphasis on antenatal care was based on a desire to protect the fetus/infant by drawing mothers out of the home and away from traditional informal birthing practices into the web of the medical system.[8] The growing belief that antenatal care could provide the crucial link in the chain of services was thus informed by an increasing conviction that the hospital provided the best site for delivery.

The emphasis on antenatal care and all the assumptions and hopes invested in it, predated 1922 and in fact formed part of the learning curve embarked on since the beginning of the notifications of births legislation. The Notification of Births Act, 1907, only came into operation in Dublin in November 1910 and the rest of the country in 1915. As in Britain, this process was greatly informed by the experience of World War I, as public health activists and government officials began to focus on the notion of reducing infant mortality as a means of offsetting war losses and providing future soldiers. As one of the chief advocates of extending the Notification of Births Act to Ireland argued in 1915: 'The war is still with us, but the great loss of adult life caused thereby makes it the more incumbent on us to do what we can to protect the infant life we have.'[9]

From the outset, public health legislation relating to maternity and infant protection had in its sights mothers of the 'poorer classes' with the intention of disseminating domestic values perceived as inherent in the middle classes. Charles Cameron, the Chief Health and Medical Officer of Dublin, noted that while the act applied to all births, it was in fact intended to facilitate the visiting of the poorer classes:

> to give advice where necessary to mothers of the poorer classes on the feeding and
> rearing of infants, but the law makes no distinction between one class and another,
> and it is, therefore, obligatory upon all classes to observe the provisions of the Act in
> that respect.[10]

The Notification of Births legislation had arguably the most profound impact on the development of maternity services.[11] The 'lady visitors' dispatched to visit the homes of newborn infants, recorded how the women had delivered (by doctor, midwife or in hospital), how the infant was being fed and whether advice was provided thus helping officialdom assess the impact of public health policy on the ground.[12] Cameron described the lady visitors of the Infant Aid Society as the 'valuable unpaid ally' to the public health mission of officialdom.[13] They also acted as advocates for improved maternal care and in particular for a focus on maternal health and nutrition. For example, in 1914 Miss C. Thornton, a Lady Sanitary Sub-Officer for Dublin argued:

> I regret to say my experience shows that in a number of cases the mothers belonging to the very poor class suffer from insufficient nourishment. If it were possible to devise a system by which it might become known that a woman was about to become a mother at a certain time, enquiry could be made into her economic condition, so as to have proper nourishment afforded. Could this be done, I have no doubt the high death-rate at present existing amongst infants would be substantially reduced.[14]

These women visitors often also documented their advice to poorer women to go to hospital for their delivery as another Lady Sanitary Sub-Officers for Dublin claimed:

> In all cases I advise the mothers to go into hospital ... and I believe I have made some converts to the theory of the impossibility of providing for a patient's safety, comfort and economy in the same measure at home in one room as in a well-equipped hospital, where they have the advantage of practical instruction in the care of the infant, and where they will be detained as along as mother and child needs medical care.[15]

The motivation for this advice was largely practical: poor mothers might get better food in hospital and some much-needed rest.

The systematic visiting of mothers upon the birth of their children facilitated a new era of encounters that would revolutionize the practice and experience of childbirth. The Notification of Births Act of 1915 prompted the first tentative cooperation between voluntary visiting groups and the maternity hospitals, which in effect constituted the linking up of hospital and the more general (and embryonic) public health system. The Infant Aid Society, a voluntary society which carried out much of the visiting on behalf of Dublin Corporation, noted that it asked for cooperation from the Dublin maternity hospitals and had met with 'a generous response'. The hospitals had:

> arranged to set apart certain days and hours each week for the attendance of mothers and children who are visited by our workers, and who may need a doctor's advice and care, and they will permit our workers to be present in order to complete their own instruction, and be better fitted to see the doctor's wishes satisfactorily carried out.[16]

These voluntary societies clearly saw part of their function to provide a link between the home and the hospital in the battle to improve infant survival.

The Notification of Birth (Extension) Act of 1915, which empowered rather than obliged local authorities to provide maternity and child welfare services, remained the cornerstone of Ireland's maternity services for the following century.[17] The Maternity and Child Welfare Act of 1918, which did so much to 'consolidate and reinforce'[18] earlier initiatives in England, was not extended to Ireland. While the powers given to Irish sanitary authorities under the 1915 act were greater than those afforded to their English counterparts,[19] its permissive nature facilitated the development of a system that varied considerably nationally. Some local authorities proved more proactive than others, which contributed to a lasting legacy of inconsistent services. The limited funding available and the financial pressures on local authorities resulted in a significant reliance on voluntary organizations. Health visiting and district nursing was often carried out by voluntary organizations such as the Lady Dudley Nursing Scheme and the Queen's Institute for District Nursing.[20]

The dawning of political independence was chaotic, costly and painful. The early years were over-shadowed by civil war (1922 to 1923) and security and stability became the priorities of the new Irish rulers. A perceptible tone of alarm and disorientation rang through the early official utterances in relation to public health services. In June 1924 the Minister for Local Government and Public Health, Seamus Burke, summed up the public health landscape: 'We have got none of these health services centralised. They are divided up between local authorities and voluntary agencies ... It is really a very difficult task to keep in touch with them all'.[21] In 1927, the Commission on the Relief of the Sick and Destitute Poor, including the Insane Poor, the first major report into health provision instituted by the new state, confirmed this impression of huge regional variation and relative legal and administrative confusion.[22]

The main initiative taken during this period of adjustment was the introduction of a system of county medical officers.[23] These medical officers were to be the administrative touchstones for central government with jurisdiction in urban and rural areas for public health, including the operation of maternity and child welfare services. The system that developed outside the capital city of Dublin grew up around these medical officers. However, the fact that not every county appointed one was an indicator of the haphazard nature of that development. The Department of Local Government and Public Health never missed an opportunity to expose the counties that had not made an appointment and to link high infant and maternal deaths to this perceived negligence.[24] By 1935, nine out of twenty-six counties still did not have a medical officer of health.[25] While it was envisaged that much of the maternity and welfare work would devolve to the public health nurse, local authorities were even slower to appreciate her value. By 1931, there were only thirteen public health nurses employed nationwide.[26]

In 1938, when reporting on the maternity and child welfare services in Dublin, the Medical Officer of Health, Matthew J. Russell, noted that due to the 'growing popularity' of hospital births, there was now 'a shortage of accommodation' in the Dublin maternity hospitals.[27] The medical profession appreciated that what was underway was a 'social revolution' with a growing 'tendency to desert the home for the institution and in fact every scheme introduced is an encouragement to that end'.[28] Indeed, state policy (such as it was) encouraged a veneration of the building in the Irish health system. From the 1930s, Marie Coleman reveals that the Sweepstake funds[29] allowed existing hospitals to develop and expand further, setting in stone the shape of the Irish health system, which became focused on 'buildings' rather than more imaginative ways of facilitating the needs of urban and rural communities.[30] Mary E. Daly has even questioned whether the Sweeps was a 'curse', as it resulted in the creation of a 'hospital service not a health care system'.[31]

Thus the hospitalization of maternity care fitted into a broader picture of institutionalizing health care. Between 1922 and 1947, the state did not extend its remit in the area of maternal health beyond providing limited funding to local authorities under the provisions of the notifications of births legislation, regulating midwifery and encouraging a move towards hospitalization of childbirth.[32] In 1927, when lamenting the 'unyielding character' of Irish maternal mortality rates, the Department revealed its limited response, decrying that: 'Notwithstanding the better equipped hospitals, the better educated physicians and more numerous and better trained midwives, the problem of safety in child birth remains unsolved'.[33] By 1930, the Department observed that 'in recent years the care of normal pregnant women has become an important part of obstetric practice'.[34] Indeed, it was repeatedly claimed that women themselves were driving this move to hospital. In 1937, for example, the Department claimed that maternity hospitals were finding 'it difficult to deal with the large numbers of women wishing to be confined in hospital'.[35]

There is little doubt that for poor women, often faced with annual pregnancies, the hospital had many advantages. It offered respite from the crushing realities of poverty and a nine to ten day rest with food.[36] Many of the women who were confined in the main Dublin maternity hospitals were drawn from the poorest areas of the city, where a confinement posed a serious financial challenge. Mrs M. Q., who wrote to the Roman Catholic Archbishop of Dublin in the mid-1920s, articulated this reality clearly:

> I write these few lines to ask you if you can for God Sake give me a little help as I have 4 young children starving with the hunger my husband is out of work for the Past 5 months and I am expecting to be confined on my fifth Baby anyday this week so I appeal to you Father for God Sake for a little help.[37]

A decade later the story had changed little for expectant inner-city mothers. In the mid-1930s, Mrs C. W. also framed her need in relation to her imminent confinement:

> Your most Gracious may i beg leave to appeal to you for a little assistance as i am expecting to become a mother very soon and i am in need of help very badly and i am in need of nourishment my husband is unemployed and i have two young children attending school i will be very grateful for any little help to help me over my confinement.[38]

These women were serviced in Dublin by the three maternity hospitals: the Rotunda Hospital (1745), the Coombe Lying-In Hospital (1823) and the National Maternity Hospital [known as Holles Street] (1894).[39] Each hospital served a catchment area in Dublin city[40] and women from outside Dublin, particularly complicated referred cases[41] or unmarried mothers who fled to the capital city in search of help and anonymity.[42] The Rotunda was the Protestant hospital, while the Coombe and Holles Street were predominantly Roman Catholic. While the religious ethos was of crucial importance to the identity of each of these hospitals throughout the twentieth century, patients of all denominations availed of their services. These hospitals provided services, without charge, to a proportion of mothers who qualified under the medical charities acts and a significant number of women were treated in return for voluntary contributions. By the mid-1940s, the three hospitals catered for 80 per cent of the city's births as either in-hospital births or on the domiciliary service. The number of hospital births increased considerably during World War II; although Ireland remained neutral and in a state of 'emergency', it was deeply affected by shortages during this period, particularly in turf. While the shift from home births to intern hospital births was undoubtedly accelerated by these shortages, the rate of home births never returned to their pre-war levels. The hospitals also worked in close cooperation with Dublin Corporation's maternity and child welfare services, acting as key drivers in the development of antenatal care. Dublin mothers were the best served in the country in terms of welfare and health provision – in or out of the hospital. Outside of Dublin, maternity services developed painstakingly slowly throughout the 1930s and 1940s. By the mid-1930s, the only other places outside of Dublin with approved maternity and child welfare schemes were the county boroughs of Cork (South), Limerick (mid-West), Waterford and Wexford (South-East). These services were linked to the main regional maternity hospitals in each area.[43] There were also approved schemes in 15 urban districts and a total of 103 voluntary associations focusing on maternity and child welfare nationwide except in Leitrim. Increasingly, the hospital became the focal point of maternity services.

In 1944, Dr Alex Spain, the Master of the National Maternity Hospital (Holles St., Dublin) declared that there was 'not a maternity service in the rest of Éire comparable to that of Dublin'.[44] He noted that the only free service available to mothers outside of Dublin was controlled by the county councils through the various county hospitals and the dispensary medical service. Spain sketched the basic contours of the maternity service that applied outside Dublin:

> our maternity service is based upon (a) the district midwife, who in difficulty calls upon (b) the dispensary doctor, who in turn may call in the help of (c) another practitioner, or may refer the case to (d) one of the hospitals provided by the local authority, or in certain circumstances to special hospitals.

In view of the fact that much of the maternity and childcare services relied on antenatal supervision, Spain's findings were particularly revealing. He found that outside of Dublin there were only four antenatal clinics, one operated by a medical officer, one attached to Erinville Hospital in Cork, Bedford Row Hospital in Limerick and one in the Lourdes Hospital in Drogheda: 'The rest of the country is entirely without specially trained ante-natal supervision'.[45] The hospital bed situation appeared even harder to gauge as most beds were provided for by the county hospitals, district hospitals or county homes and in many cases there were no beds allocated for maternity cases, in others they were effectively blocked by 'the mothers of illegitimate infants or by other waiting normal cases'.[46] Possibly of more consequence to the users of the system was what Spain described as the 'dichotomy of control', which was 'a widespread feature of our present services'. In only five counties did he find continuity of care for abnormal cases once they reached the hospital system. If, as Loudon has argued, it is not the site of delivery but the 'morale and the standard of co-operation and integration between all concerned in maternal care' that is crucial to maternal mortality,[47] then rural Irish women were at a distinct disadvantage.

Spain's critical assessment of services outside of Dublin were confirmed by the new Department of Health's 1947 white paper on health, which gave a damning summary of services since the foundation of the state. The system, it claimed:

> developed unevenly over the country as a whole and has not grown beyond the health visitor stage save in the cities and a few urban centres. In the cities the service is for all practical purposes confined to the poorer classes.[48]

It was generally conceded that Ireland could do with some of the reforming Beveridge spirit that infused Britain.[49] It was, however, strenuously argued, particularly by the Irish Medical Association (hereafter IMA) and the Roman Catholic hierarchy, that the country did not need the statist emphasis of its erstwhile colonizer polluting the waters of Irish public health. Many in the Irish medical profession looked on in horror at the development of the British National Health System.[50]

In 1943, a report on the Beveridge plan in the *Journal of the Irish Medical Association* noted that the promised 'comprehensive health service ... appears to entail the complete abolition of any form of private practice'.[51] In warning of the dangers of following England's lead, the journal evoked a history that recalled memories of degradation and pauperization under British rule:

> We have suffered much in the past from following too closely social systems which existed elsewhere. Our Poor Law System was taken lock, stock, and barrel from the already obsolescent English system, and planted in a soil which was alien to it ... Its pauperising tendency roused a hatred a hundred years ago which has hardly disappeared as yet.[52]

While the author acknowledged that the Beveridge Report was 'a revolutionary document', the recalling of a troubled history served as a warning against any attempts to transplant such a scheme to Ireland, where it would 'undoubtedly' be 'unsuitable'. Historical distortions aside, the use of the term 'pauperisation' in these medical debates seemed to refer to a type of moral degeneration resultant from physical dependency on the state. However, there is little doubt that at the heart of this concern was the fear of excessive state control and the 'pauperisation' of the medical profession and voluntary hospitals.[53]

Despite Irish neutrality, World War II exerted its own pressures on Ireland, and the infant mortality rates increased significantly, from 67 per 1,000 deaths in 1938[54] to 83 per 1,000 in 1943.[55] The paediatrician at the Rotunda, Dr W. R. F. Collis, observed:

> In spite of the war and all that it meant to England and Wales, Scotland and, let us note, Northern Ireland, the infant mortality rate fell markedly, while in neutral Éire it remained high, showing no tendency to fall till the last year or so.[56]

Ironically, however much Ireland looked with envy to Britain's more favourable mortality statistics, any attempt to follow Britain's suit in relation to maternity and child welfare was bitterly resisted.

Between 1947 and 1951, the Department of Health developed legislation for a free national mother and child scheme, for all mothers and children (up to the age of sixteen) irrespective of income. The IMA waved the 'red flag' and attempted to stoke deep-seated cultural resistance to 'all things English' by disparaging the scheme as 'largely inspired by Socialist conceptions from England and from other sources tainted with Marxian ideas, entirely alien to our traditions'.[57] In Ireland, maternity and child health services became the battleground in the war against a state medical service. Both the Roman Catholic hierarchy and the IMA[58] believed that if the mother was 'lost' to a state-funded medical system then the entire family would follow and the result would be a *de facto* National Health Service (NHS).[59] In 1947, the President of the IMA, Andrew

Ryan, claimed that the proposed medical and child health service was 'of far greater importance to the profession than any legislation that has been introduced in the recent history of medical practice in this country' because 'the doctor in general practice is going to be very badly hit'.[60]

The journal of the IMA reprinted religious sermons that warned against 'the eclipse of the individual', and argued that the most

> alarming features of the recent Mother and Child agitation was the proof it gave that some among us think God's Law – and the guardian of the Moral Law, the Church – has no place in our dealings with the Government or in the Government's dealings with us.[61]

The journal consciously attempted to construct the argument regarding increased state control of services in a moral rather than a medical framework. For example, the December 1950 editorial argued that the proposed mother and child scheme raised 'fundamental moral issues'.[62] The principal objections were to the elimination of patient choice of doctor, state control of the medical profession, a free service for those who could pay and the intention to 'educate all mothers in respect of motherhood' as this might eventually include birth control. Throughout the early months of 1952, the journal ran a series on the health services in other countries concluding that:

> We doctors and many more of the public as well do not believe that the Welfare State will offer our citizens a heaven on earth. We have but to study the social implications of that state in other countries now suffering from a pauperization of the people, with a degeneration in moral tone and a loosening of moral restraints.[63]

In this anti-state service debate, Ireland was characterized as an 'individualised society' which sought to instil 'a sense of independence and responsibility' in its citizens.[64] The irony of such statements in a country which took many ostensibly private issues out of the hands of its citizens through unequivocal legislation, for example, in relation to birth control and divorce, seemed not to present any problems for contemporaries.

A considerably revised scheme survived the controversy and was introduced under the Health Act of 1953. The mother and child scheme covered children up to the age of six weeks as opposed to sixteen years and patients were afforded a choice of doctor. Furthermore, only mothers in the lower income group were initially eligible and it was only gradually extended, until the Health (Amendment) Act of 1991 allowed all women to avail of the scheme.[65] However, in reality never more than 50 per cent of women availed of the free scheme.[66] A significant proportion of women in the middle and upper socio-economic groups were obviously opting for private services, a preference facilitated by the dual public and private health system that developed in Ireland throughout the century. This was particularly furthered by the development of the Voluntary Health Insurance Board in 1957, which Barrington described as 'a new kind of partnership between government, the medical profession and the idealized "voluntary" spirit of Irish Catholic moralists'.[67]

For much of this period, the mother was the object rather than the subject of care and medical intervention. The mother's own experience, or even her voice, was rarely considered. This was both oversight and intention. Oversight because it was genuinely believed that the mother's primary function was to ensure the survival of her infant and that it was simply a question of enlightening her in this regard. Intention because a country that prohibited birth control and lauded the large family could ill afford to consider the consequences of uncontrolled fertility on the mothers at the heart of the system.

There was an active campaign to deny women information or advice regarding their fertility. The particular Irish demographic profile is important to appreciate when considering the development and tenor of Irish maternity services. Mary E. Daly has described 'the pathology of Irish demography' as 'a low rate of marriage and late age of marriage, high marital fertility, and a very late transition to smaller families'.[68] By the mid-1930s, the Irish birth rate was higher than its nearest neighbour, England, and that of most of northern Europe and it had one of the highest marital fertility rates in Europe.[69] While Irish officials were concerned about Ireland's unique demographic profile, there was also an element of pride that Irish people retained such a high level of fertility, and a degree of complacency regarding the wider impact of high emigration, large and late families. There was little doubt that Irish women, in marrying later and maintaining one of the highest marital fertility rates in Europe, were exposed to higher risks in terms of mortality and morbidity. It is notable that Ireland was also unique in having higher male than female survival rates at any age until the 1930s; women had only marginally outstripped the male survival rate by the 1950s.[70] Mahon argues that the improvement in life expectancy can be attributed to three things: 'nutrition, public hygiene and contraception', but she notes 'the benefits of contraception accrue primarily to women'.[71] While often exaggerated, the late age of marriage in Ireland was significant when compared with other countries. In 1926 the mean age of marriage for women was 29.1 years, compared to 26.5 for England and Wales. While the difference had decreased by 1946, when the mean age for women in Ireland was 28, compared to 26.6 in England and Wales, Irish women still married later with considerably higher marital fertility rates.[72] The fact that Irish women lived in a state which prohibited contraception combined with the late marriage age left Irish women particularly vulnerable to the perils of childbirth.[73]

The first census taken after independence in 1926 revealed that of a population of 2,971,992, a massive 2,751,269 was Roman Catholic.[74] A hard core of the Roman Catholic laity, represented by organizations like the Catholic Truth Society, regarded political independence as a mandate to ensure that the values of this massive majority were represented in the new state's legislation. Thus, fuelled by the zeal of Catholic Action, the Irish Free State moved relatively quickly to ban contraception with the Censorship and Publication Act in 1929, which prohibited the sale of literature advocating the use of birth control.[75] In 1930, the Church of Ireland (informed by developments in the Church of England) no longer regarded birth control as an absolute issue, but allowed for the use of birth control in 'hard cases' and stated that contraception could be justifiable on health grounds. The 1931 Papal encyclical *Casti Connubii* 'On Christian Marriage (December 1931), however, merely spurred the Irish Catholic defence of an absolute ban on birth control. This was secured with the Criminal Law Amendment Act, 1935, which made the sale and use of contraceptives illegal. The absolute ban on contraception was instituted in Ireland precisely because of a growing international disquiet about the health implications of uncontrolled fertility: the Irish Free State sought to ensure that birth control remained a moral issue.[76] This absolute ban remained in force until the Health (Family Planning) Act of 1979.

Gillis, Tilly and Levine have argued that the medical profession and advocates of birth control have been crucial in 'shaping cultures of conception and norms of sexuality'.[77] In Ireland there were no effective advocates of birth control prior to the 1960s, instead the issue helped to cement a medico-religious alliance between Catholic doctors and the Irish Catholic hierarchy.[78] As the hospital became more central to the provision of maternity services, the ethos of those hospitals began to have a greater bearing on the experience of childbirth. There is evidence, for example, that the Protestant Rotunda maternity hospital remained the most vocal regarding the impact of repeated pregnancies on poor women. In 1944, Dr Bethel Solomons of the Rotunda was also critical when the National Maternity Hospital and the Coombe Lying-in Hospital, both Catholic in ethos, revived the procedure of symphysiotomy.[79] This procedure was no longer in use in Britain; indeed the Master of the National Maternity Hospital, Alex Spain, acknowledged that he would have performed this procedure more often were it not new to him and 'one that has to be faced against the weight of opinion of the entire English speaking obstetrical world'.[80] It appears that the Catholic maternity hospitals reintroduced this procedure from the 1940s, largely due to a belief that repeated Caesarean sections would result in physical injury to the woman and thus lead to a demand for contraception, sterilization or abortion.[81] In 1955, in an article on the treatment of disproportion, Hugo McVey explained:

> In this country we have the special circumstances of treating a population in which sterilisation and contraception are not practised. Thus a young primigravida delivered by Caesarean section for disproportion faces a lifetime of repeat operations with all the hazards of uterine rupture, adhesions and bladder injury. In gross disproportion Caesarean section is unquestionably correct, but in minor or medium degrees of disproportion if symphysiotomy allows a vaginal delivery on this and all other subsequent pregnancies, it is surely the operation of choice.[82]

Catholic doctors worldwide, particularly gynaecologists and paediatricians, were called upon to raise their voices against 'Malthusianism' and many Irish Catholic doctors regarded themselves at the forefront of that campaign.[83] In 1954, at the Sixth International Congress of Catholic Doctors held in Dublin, Arthur Barry, Spain's successor at the National Maternity Hospital, cautioned:

> Every Catholic obstetrician should realise that the Caesarean operation is probably the chief cause for the practice by the profession of the unethical procedure of steri-lization and furthermore it is very frequently responsible for encouraging the laity in the improper prevention of pregnancy or in seeking its termination.[84]

Dismissing concerns regarding the procedure in textbooks 'as sheer flights of imagination on the part of inexperienced writers', he stressed it was the best means of relieving the mild disproportion 'at no expense to the mother and child and thus you can reduce the temptation to perform many of the unethical procedures which we all so resent'.[85] In reality, the 'expense' to the women was considerable, in many cases the women who underwent this procedure in Ireland between 1944 and 1992 were left with long-term pain and other serious complications.[86]

Until 1979, Ireland's solution to any risks to women's health as a result of pregnancy was to advise abstinence. There was, however, evidence that information regarding the safe period was spreading through the middle classes in the 1930s.[87] In 1936, the first population census following political independence acknowledged the connection between class and fertility, noting: 'the more well to do the occupation the less children there are of the marriage, particularly in the earlier years of married life'.[88] However, the working-class mother, who was the chief target of maternity services, was left with a service determined not to include family planning in her health-care package. Few had the courage or con-viction to articulate the potential dangers of numerous pregnancies and births for mothers. While in 1934 Bethel Solomons (Master of the Rotunda 1926–33) coined the phrase 'dangerous multipara', in the hope of dispelling the myth that practice makes perfect in childbirth, few others would raise their heads above the medical parapet.[89]

Ireland continued to excel in the production of large families. In 1955, 40 per cent of Irish women who gave birth had done so a minimum of five times previ-ously: in 1962, there were 2,000 births to mothers that had 10 or more previous births. This figure had dropped to 55 by 1998.[90] In 1964, when writing on the issue of 'grand multipara', J. H. Young marvelled at a study carried out by J. K. Feeney, the Master of the Coombe Lying-In Hospital, Dublin which 'in a two-year period collected the amazing number of 518 women who had had seven or more vaginal deliveries ... an incidence of 12.6 per cent of all hospital deliveries'.[91] Young's study involved women on their fifth or more pregnancy at St Mary's Hospital, Manches-ter, between 1951 and 1960 and revealed that these women never made up more than 6.9 per cent of total admissions.[92] Young noted 'that Manchester cannot compete with Dublin when it comes to production of grand multiparae!'[93]

However, the voices of women who were asking when they would 'ever stop having babies' were increasingly noted in the annual reports of the hospital almoners/social workers.[94] Nonetheless, other than the testimony and lobbying of hospital social workers, there were few avenues for women's opinions to surface. The women's movement in Ireland avoided dealing with potentially 'sectarian' issues such as birth control and while the Irish Housewives Association did lobby for the free maternity and child welfare service in 1951 and the welfare of unmarried mothers in Irish institutions, there was no sustained advocacy for mothers and maternal health *per se* prior to the 1970s.[95]

In 1951, Pope Pius XII condoned, in certain cases, the use of the safe period and public opinion in Ireland appeared to slowly embrace the notion of spacing one's family and ultimately limiting family size.[96] This growing momentum resulted in the opening of the first family planning clinic in 1964 in the National Maternity Hospital. It was a measure of the growing sense that unlimited fertility was not sustainable on humanitarian grounds that the Catholic maternity hospital was the site of this new departure. The hospital explained that the clinic was 'the outcome of an increasing awareness of the real personal problems which uncontrolled fertility presented to many patients'.[97] There was considerable shock (and dismay) in Ireland when *Humane Vitae* (1968) did not offer some softening of Roman Catholic position.[98] However, the tide had turned in Ireland regardless and women began increasingly to opt for family limitation. In 1974, when women attending the Cork family planning clinic were asked how they had heard of it, they credited the Roman Catholic Bishop of Cork, who had condemned it from the pulpit and evidently given the clinic the best publicity it could have asked for.[99] Clearly, Irish Catholics were increasingly opting to practise their religion while following its moral teachings selectively, at least in the arena of 'planned parenthood'. By the 1970s, as social conditions began to improve and family size began a slow decline, the almoners could record with some relief: 'one is impressed by the youth, health and vigour of Dublin mothers compared with a decade ago … The Grande multiparae has gone!'[100]

The Health Act of 1979 allowed GPs to prescribe contraceptives to married couples for *bona fide* family planning reasons; it also incorporated a conscience clause that allowed doctors to refuse on the grounds of morality.[101] However, the legislation did not make it mandatory for health boards to supply women with family planning advice or information. In keeping with the altered legal landscape and the increasing prominence of the women's movement, women's views were increasingly sought by the medical profession.[102] In 1979, the *Journal of the Irish Medical Association* published the results of a survey of 120 recently delivered rural mothers.[103] While the survey focused on the degree to which women were informed about family planning methods and how and where they received information, it stressed that 'few mothers wanted more than four children or pregnancies after the age of forty'.[104] It revealed that 64 per cent of the women had unplanned pregnancies and that most patients were 'poorly informed'. The 1987 report into the maternity and infant care scheme noted that 48 per cent of women who used the scheme had received no family planning advice and that of those 39 per cent said that they would have liked such advice.[105] It was not until 1993 that Ireland followed the measure taken in England in 1930 to legally oblige health boards to provide family planning services and thus fully integrate family planning into maternity services.[106] The crude birth rate remained very stable in Ireland until the 1990s, after which it experienced a 'dramatic fall'. In 1949, Ireland had 21.5 babies born per 1,000 persons, by 1998 this had fallen to 14.5.[107]

Conclusion

A curious mix of religion and geography marked the development of maternity services in Ireland. The move to bring women into the net of maternity services in Ireland began in the early twentieth century with the extension of care beyond childbirth to the antenatal and post-natal phases of maternity. This process increasingly channelled women into the hospital environment, but it developed in an extremely haphazard fashion according to where a woman lived. Any attempts to reform the system were frequently frustrated by a fusion of religious and medical interests. Thus Irish women were the objects of a health system that for much of the twentieth century allowed notions of morality to limit and shape the extent of health care and frequently overlooked the wider needs of its clientele.

7 TEST TUBES AND TURPITUDE: MEDICAL RESPONSES TO THE INFERTILE PATIENT IN MID-TWENTIETH-CENTURY SCOTLAND

Gayle Davis

In recent decades, reproductive health has constituted a vibrant field of scholarship. The increasing availability of safe and effective means of fertility control – birth control and abortion – and the social politics surrounding it have comprised an important focus. Social historians have tended to locate this trend within the general programme of so-called 'permissive' measures introduced to Britain during the 'Swinging Sixties', measures that reconfigured the role of the state in issues relating to sexual morality,[1] with some consideration of the important role which the medical profession has assumed within reproductive health policymaking and the implementation of that policy.[2] Meanwhile, feminist interpretations have tended to view policy formation as a political struggle that strongly reflected the ideological prejudices of a patriarchal society,[3] and have been sharply critical of the 'medicalization' of reproductive health, which arguably left British women 'dependent on the vagaries of medical discretion and good will'.[4]

The history of infertility in modern Britain has, by comparison, been underexplored. Naomi Pfeffer's 1993 monograph *The Stork and the Syringe* remains the most comprehensive work on the subject, and provides an important introduction to medical responses to infertility, set within their wider social and political context.[5] Assisted reproduction – the use of techniques such as artificial insemination and in vitro fertilization to enhance fertility – has elicited heated debate from a range of scholars, including social anthropologists and sociologists. Interesting themes include the extent to which such 'unnatural' intervention subverts the legal and moral integrity of the family unit,[6] and its application as a strategy for positive eugenic improvement.[7]

Though multiple and occasionally contradictory definitions of female sexuality can be discerned in the historiography of sexuality and reproductive health, to a pronounced extent female sexuality has been demonstrated to have been pathologized, indeed psychiatrized, when it was perceived to deviate from a narrowly defined norm. Wilful rejections of the marital and maternal frameworks within which female sexuality was placed were commonly linked to mental instability.[8] As a key example, Sally Sheldon illustrates that the 1967 Abortion Act was 'fundamentally underpinned by the idea that reproduction is an area for medical control and expertise', with the doctor cast as the 'responsible and reassuring figure' who can be trusted to rationally decide which women merit a termination of pregnancy and to dissuade those who are not deemed to qualify.[9] The pregnant woman is depicted, in marked contrast, as being unable to make a reasoned assessment of her own situation due to her intrinsically and unhealthily emotional state. It is open to debate whether that impaired judgement is the result of pregnancy or simply femininity.

Taking mid-twentieth-century Scotland as a case study, this chapter will explore how the infertile patient was characterized and treated by the medical profession. It will consider the extent to which the infertile woman can be accommodated into the medical and political discourses found in fertility limitation. With infertile women striving to embrace their biological destiny as mothers, were they considered quite separately from women seeking to flee their maternal fate, or did they constitute a collective group of reproductive deviants?

Such was the concern that infertility and, more especially, its treatment by artificial insemination engendered by the mid-twentieth century that a Departmental Committee was appointed to investigate the issue. The terms of reference of the 1958 Departmental Committee on Human Artificial Insemination (the Feversham Committee), the impetus for which was a Scottish divorce case,[10] were:

> To enquire into the existing practice of human artificial insemination and its legal consequences; and to consider whether, taking account of the interests of individuals involved and of society as a whole, any change in the law is necessary or desirable.

The wide range of medical, legal and religious witnesses approached to give evidence, and the voluminous written and oral testimony received, provide rich insights into medical thinking and practice in 1950s Britain, and into the complex social politics and anxieties surrounding reproductive health.

This chapter will focus upon the medical testimony supplied to the Feversham Committee by Scottish witnesses, supplemented by the clinical records of the Royal Infirmary of Edinburgh infertility and gynaecological outpatient clinic, in order to explore how doctors perceived the infertile woman in 1950s Scotland. It will be considered to what extent, and in what ways, women seeking treatment for their infertility were pathologized, and whether the men involved – their husbands, the sperm donors and the doctors treating them – escaped these pathologizing tendencies.

Reluctance to Practise

A range of Scottish medical witnesses submitted written and oral evidence to the Departmental Committee on Human Artificial Insemination: a handful of individual gynaecologists and psychiatrists based in Scotland, as well as representatives from the Faculty of Medicine of the Universities of Aberdeen and Edinburgh, the Royal College of Surgeons of Edinburgh and the Department of Health for Scotland. Their evidence offers important insights into how doctors perceived and treated the infertile patient in mid-twentieth-century Scotland.

Since the Feversham Committee was established to investigate the treatment of infertility through artificial insemination, witnesses were asked to focus upon this therapy, rather than providing broader discussion of the possible therapeutic options available to the infertile patient at this time. This form of treatment was reported to have been successfully performed from the late eighteenth century, but not to have been used on any significant scale until the mid-twentieth century.[11] The method facilitated conception where it was not possible by normal sexual intercourse, either because of sterility of the husband or because of some other physical or mental disability in the husband or wife. Treatment could be performed using the semen of the patient's husband (artificial insemination with husband's semen, known as 'AIH' in medical parlance) or an anonymous donor (Artificial Insemination by Donor, 'AID'), depending on the couple's specific circumstances. In the three decades preceding the Feversham Committee, it was estimated that there had been around 2,000 births by artificial insemination in Britain,[12] though this figure could only be a rough estimate in view of the ignorance, shame and secrecy that surrounded the procedure at this time.

The Department of Health for Scotland epitomized this ignorance and secrecy by admitting to the Feversham Committee that they simply had 'no precise information about the extent of the practice or about the particular doctors' who provided it.[13] In fact, the committee's survey of those offering artificial insemination using donor semen revealed that only six doctors in Britain were providing such a service at the time of giving evidence, and that these six doctors were all based in England.[14] Some of the remaining medical witnesses claimed to have practised artificial insemination 'at one time or another', including several of the Scottish witnesses, or were currently providing insemination using only the husband's semen.[15] Their testimony was supported by a simultaneous survey of Scottish hospitals which indicated distinctly patchy use across Scotland. There was found to be no evidence of its use in the northern, north-eastern or south-eastern regions, only some private practice in the western region, and some wider use in the eastern region (in hospitals in Dundee and Perth).[16]

Reluctance to practise artificial insemination in Scotland appears to have stemmed from a complex blend of legal, practical and moral factors. Several of the doctors questioned by the committee indicated confusion as to the legal status of the practice, particularly where donor semen was utilized.[17] As one surgeon asked the committee: 'The medical profession do not at present have the right of carrying out artificial insemination by donor? Am I wrong there?'[18] Indeed, some doctors claimed to have made enquiries to the Medical Defence Union, only to be told that the organization 'would not guarantee that somebody who had had artificial insemination with donated semen could not bring a legal action' against that doctor.[19] In its submission to the Feversham Committee, the Department of Health for Scotland claimed that there was 'some uncertainty' as to the legality of the procedure, since the National Health Service had failed to issue guidelines on it, and recommended that the doctor 'seek to safeguard himself by securing the written consent of all parties to the transaction'.[20] Indeed, such uncertainty was also a feature of the legal evidence submitted to the committee. While most legal bodies considered artificial insemination a legal medical practice, T. B. Smith, Professor of Civil Law at the University of Edinburgh, argued vigorously that AID was illegal, given the 'element of deception involved' and 'the production of a bastard', and that it constituted the common law crime of fraud in Scotland and the crime of conspiracy in England.[21]

Medical witnesses also offered various practical reasons for their resistance to offering artificial insemination to patients. Dr Albert Sharman, a consultant gynaecologist, had started a clinic in the 1930s at Glasgow's Royal Samaritan Hospital for Women which was devoted exclusively to the investigation and treatment of infertile marriages, a clinic which he claimed to have been the first of its kind in the United Kingdom.[22] Although Sharman continued to undertake insemination using the husband's semen, he discontinued the practice of donor insemination at his clinic after five years, two decades prior to the Feversham Committee. The reasons he advanced were that 'success was rare', that there was significant expense involved because the practice had to be undertaken privately 'as no Hospital Board of Management was likely to countenance it', and that 'donated semen was very difficult to obtain'. Lack of success featured, similarly, in the oral evidence submitted by fellow Glaswegian gynaecologist Dr Hector MacLennan, Senior Consultant to the Department of Gynaecology at the Victoria Infirmary, who complained that patients held the 'prevalent' but mistaken idea that those 'prepared to submit to AID' would find success.[23] Given the fact that there was 'an upsurge of requests for AID when anything appeared in the Press',[24] and that this subject matter was being discussed with increasing frequency, undue patient optimism was a most unwelcome feature as far as many doctors were concerned.

Denigrating the Donor

Difficulty in obtaining semen was another significant practical problem high-lighted by medical witnesses. As Dr Sharman noted, employing a rather unfortunate – if ironically accurate – turn of phrase, 'the provision of semen' was 'entirely in the physician's hands' and involved 'considerable difficulty in obtaining suitable material'.[25] For Sharman, the solution was to approach 'personal friends and doctors', which must surely have proved an awkward business.[26] The word 'suitable' is also crucial here, for it was a question of quality even more than quantity. As Dr Audrey Freeth, who had practiced gynaecology in both Birmingham and Glasgow, noted, 'the donor situation' was 'distinctly tricky' precisely because women had to be supplied 'with a satisfactory specimen'.[27] The medical evidence submitted to the Feversham Committee suggests that semen, or more accurately its donor, was required to be 'satisfactory' in three key respects: physical, psychological and moral.

Physical fitness was one element of what might be termed the 'eugenic considerations' which lay at the heart of donor selection, a process 'designed to reduce obvious biological dangers'.[28] There was to be no history of transmissible disease or 'adverse genetical characteristics such as alcoholism, criminality, or tuberculosis'. Donors were to be of 'mature' age (30–45) so that their character could be properly assessed, of good general health and IQ, and should be married men with at least two legitimate children of their own, not only to illustrate the quality of their 'stock' but also so that their 'parental drive' would already have 'an available object'.[29]

Dr Sharman added that donors should lack 'excessively pronounced physical features' which 'might facilitate identification', indicating the fact that infertile couples often wished to be 'matched' to an appropriate donor who could produce children who resembled the husband and wife physically. Thus the semen donor's hair colour, eye colour and height were all to be considered in relation to the husband's. Some couples also requested religious compatibility, particularly in Glasgow, with its markedly higher proportion of Roman Catholics compared with the rest of the country, and some doctors expressed significant concerns over the issue of racial compatibility, worrying about the accidental use of the sperm of 'coloured gentlemen' in white couples.[30] Such was the pressure placed on doctors to 'reproduce' the husband 'by a specially chosen donor' that, as one gynaecologist stressed, couples must be warned explicitly that 'no likeness, physical or otherwise, can be guaranteed'.[31]

It was also deemed crucial to ensure that the semen donor was not related to the mother, which could 'lead to an exaggeration of all characteristics of the genetic line, including the bad ones'.[32] While this condition drew support from numerous medical witnesses as necessitating the creation of a donor reg-

ister, 'which should record the full medical history of the donors, the number
and frequency of donations, and the births resulting', these doctors also tended
to stress that such records should be 'kept centrally' with 'carefully restricted'
access, restricted even from the infertile couple in order to preserve the donor's
anonymity.[33] If the donor's identity was revealed, this might discourage would-
be donors, who were already in short supply. Psychological reasons also appeared
to necessitate a degree of secrecy. Thus, one gynaecologist feared that the donor
and maternal woman would be 'emotionally too deeply involved in procreation
to regard their relationship with detachment'.[34]

More problematic still were the potential psychological barriers to semen
donation. For some doctors, there was a lengthy list of ideal attributes, while
for others, the very fact that a man was willing to donate his semen made him
unsuitable for the task. Thus, Dr Sharman argued that 'to most balanced men
the task of donation was unpleasant'.[35] Expressing it more bluntly, Dr Hector
MacLennan explained to his patients that a donor

> prepared to give semen to a woman, whose mental and physical background is
> unknown to him, and who is prepared to father children who will be born into a
> completely unknown environment, so far as he is concerned, is a man whose ethical
> standards are so unusual as to be of doubtful value from a eugenic point of view.[36]

Such statements reveal a distinct pathologization of those men willing to act as
sperm donors.

A more subtle attempt to discredit sperm donors, expressed by numerous medical witnesses, related to their possible remuneration. A committee
of doctors representing the Royal College of Surgeons of Edinburgh declared
themselves 'at a loss to assess the motives of men who act as donors, but believed
that in most cases these must include financial gain', and emphasized their
'abhorrence' at 'the possibility that a man might make his living, or even a substantial income, out of such "donations"'.[37] Indeed, this group argued that 'there
should be no direct remuneration of the gynaecologist concerned', let alone the
sperm donor, given the technical simplicity of the procedure and the 'obvious
abuse' which could arise from financial incentives on anyone's part. In later oral
evidence to the Feversham Committee, the chairman asked them to account for
their belief 'that most cases involved financial gain', since the evidence of those
engaged in the practice of artificial insemination suggested strongly that donors
were 'often husbands of the wives who had been successfully treated' for infertility, who were thus acting 'out of gratitude, in the spirit of service to others' rather
than for financial gain.[38] When pressed, the surgeons responded: 'I do not think
we have any factual knowledge. We were judging what we believed to be the state
of affairs in the United States ... in regard to [Britain], one has heard some men-
tion of the fees paid to donors, but we have no factual evidence whatsoever'.[39]

'Infertility Games'

Such comments betray the sense that moral objections played a significant part in the formation of medical views on how to appropriately treat the infertile woman. Indeed, of those providing medical evidence, the doctors who represented the Royal College of Surgeons of Edinburgh were unusually explicit, when they referred to finding 'much that is repugnant in the practice of AID'.[40] Dr Audrey Freeth was slightly more subtle. While declaring that she 'would not send a patient [for AID] unless forced to', her strategy was to 'try and put them off it' by telling patients 'of all the difficulties and snags and point out to them the problems'.[41] Similarly, Dr MacLennan noted that a 'simple statement' could effectively call into question the suitability and motivation of the sperm donor, and that such a strategy was 'sufficient in most cases to discourage further enquiry'.[42] However, if the patient still insisted on treatment by this method, he declared himself 'quite prepared to refer her to a recognized practitioner' based in London. Making the patient travel a significant distance, at some personal expense, to obtain this form of treatment was just one of several 'obstructive' methods employed by doctors.

The group of doctors representing the Royal College of Surgeons of Edinburgh offered a further strategy to dissuade eager patients: the creation of an 'independent' panel in each region to consider applications, which would consist of 'a gynaecologist, a psychiatrist, a minister of religion, a welfare worker with experience in marriage-guidance problems, and the applicant's own doctor', who would interview both husband and wife in order principally to 'satisfy themselves that the consent of the former was both willing and sincere'.[43] By subjecting the couple to this intimidating panel of professionals, they concluded, 'it is our intention to make the whole thing rather difficult. We have not made suggestions to make it easier, quite the contrary'.[44]

Such strategies have resonances with the 'abortion games' played by British doctors a decade later, strategies adopted in order to minimize their own personal responsibility for decisions made in relation to termination of pregnancy.[45] Doctors arguably were not trained or qualified to make decisions in these areas, and thus embraced alternative strategies in order either to simplify or displace the decision-making process surrounding the provision of abortion and infertility services. Indeed, as one psychiatrist told the Feversham Committee, the judgement of psychiatrists was 'in no way enhanced because of their status as Psychiatrists. I feel that it should be stressed that psychiatrists have no peculiar right to make judgement in what is largely a moral field'.[46]

A Debasing Therapy

In addition to the decision-making process, the extent to which artificial insemi-nation was a medical procedure is indeed questionable. With its 'turkey baster' connotations, insemination was declared by some to be a 'very simple procedure' which involved the depositing of semen into the female genital tract by means of suitable instruments.[47] Thus, as was the case with abortion, some doctors may have been averse to performing AID because the procedure was 'technologically unchallenging' and potentially de-skilling.[48] Indeed, in 1950s Britain, figures like the English birth control pioneer and 'agony aunt' Marie Stopes were promoting AID as a 'home' remedy for infertility; she advised couples to avoid doctors and outlined the technique so they could 'do it themselves'.[49] It is therefore notable that none of the medical witnesses based in Scotland mentioned the possibility of couples practising the technique themselves, independently of medical involve-ment. Perhaps they believed, as one London-based AID practitioner noted, that artificial insemination took 'so much time and trouble' that there was 'practically no chance of its being carried out in back streets by unqualified people'.[50] Those few doctors who offered the therapy would have struggled to justify artificial insemination on the basis that it boosted their professional status or skill set.

An additional complication was the widespread use of AID in the agricul-tural sector.[51] Various remarks, some more disparaging than others, were voiced in the Feversham testimony on this conflation of farm and clinic. Dr Hector MacLennan noted his farming friends' extreme difficulties in finding high-quality donors, and asked the committee: 'How much more complicated is the human being than the Aberdeen Angus bull'?[52] Several of the religious witnesses to Feversham vocalized even stronger concerns on the potential of artificial insemination to degrade and dehumanize those involved by associating them with animals. As the United Free Church of Scotland (Continuing) argued, the therapy 'reduced human beings to the level of breeding animals' and should be 'confined to the farm-yard, where it belongs'.[53]

Indeed, it is worth turning briefly to the religious evidence which the Fever-sham Committee received in order to note the degree of accordance with the medical evidence received. The eight Scottish religious bodies consulted were unanimous in voicing their 'strong disapproval' of the practice of artificial insemination by donor, though some bodies were more vociferous in their con-demnation of the practice than others.[54] Most religious witnesses criticized the fact that the procedure involved masturbation, a 'vile abuse of the body' which 'in itself should be enough to show the sinfulness and the immorality of the whole process'.[55] There were also strong objections that the practice was tanta-mount to adultery and thus violated the marriage vows. Such criticisms were also found in some of the medical evidence, which supported the characterization of

AID as adulterous,[56] and which noted a disapproval of AID 'on moral, religious and ethical grounds'.[57]

While often using language of an emotional and moral nature, churchmen occasionally employed medical terminology, possibly in a conscious effort to strengthen their case. In debates surrounding termination of pregnancy, non-medical groups could be quick to recognize the power of medical language and rhetoric in fighting for their cause, whether it be to liberalize or restrict access to abortion.[58] Thus, the Free Presbyterian Church of Scotland suggested that a willing semen donor could only be regarded as 'psycho-physically or psychologically abnormal' since 'few normal men, if any, would debase themselves to donate semen'.[59] Nonetheless, churchmen did not single out the sperm donor for criticism, warning instead that everyone involved must be punished for practising 'this unnatural form of immorality' – the couple themselves, the donor who supplied the semen, and the medical man involved.[60]

While the patient was not subjected to the same level of criticism which the sperm donor received in this religious evidence, nor was she supported in her quest for motherhood. The Church of Scotland simply asked the infertile to accept 'the mysterious workings of Providence ... without resentment and in quiet trust',[61] while the Free Church urged the childless 'to recognise the Divine will' and to 'pray for submission', which would 'maintain the sanctities of the marriage bond and the joys of the marriage relationship in a way that was impossible by the [adulterous] methods of artificial insemination'.[62] On a similar note, Dr Hector MacLennan stated that barren women had 'been there since the old days, in the Old Testament', 'a tragedy as old as history', and that modern medicine was providing false hope to such women. 'It would be far better', MacLennan argued, for such patients to 'face the fact ... and be told to adopt than that she should go from clinic to clinic' with such a small chance of successful treatment.[63]

There thus appear to be distinct continuities between the language employed in, and the values which shaped, the medical and religious testimonies. As Davidson and Davis have found in so many other areas of Scottish sexuality during this period,[64] many of the Scottish churches were notoriously conservative when discussing infertility and its treatment through AID, and many doctors, it appears, were similarly minded. Medical practice on sexual matters appears to have been inhibited by Scotland's Calvinistic values, and by the traditional moral agenda pursued by the Scottish churches. Indeed, there was continuity of personnel as well as ideology between the two groups, since several of the religious groups who provided oral testimony to Feversham were represented by a combination of religious and medical witnesses, including the Baptist Union of Scotland, Scottish Committee of Catholic Union and Scottish Episcopal Church.[65]

Suitable for Motherhood?

While some members of the medical profession were more open than others in wishing to deny these patients treatment, the ways in which infertile women were characterized in the medical testimony to Feversham clearly served to illustrate their unsuitability for treatment, and to thereby justify the denial of treatment through artificial insemination. Representatives of the Royal College of Surgeons of Edinburgh noted: 'One finds most of the women who are infertile suffer from various forms of neurosis', and that steps must be taken to ensure that such women were 'genuine and honest' in their desire for such treatment.[66] Similarly, Dr MacLennan described most of the patients who approached him for this form of treatment as being 'of a highly nervous disposition', 'frustrated and introverted' and 'a bit emotionally disturbed'.[67] He stressed that he would only send patients for such therapy whose outlook was 'scientific and detached', because the remainder 'started off as a normal woman wanting a baby but ... finished up as an obsessional neurotic'.[68]

Such a transformation could surely only damage both the patient and her marriage. Thus Dr Audrey Freeth criticized the wife who 'must have a child at any price', indicating 'a lack of understanding and an emotional immaturity' that did 'not augur well for the future of that marriage'.[69] While it was natural that a married woman would wish for a family, she could want this too much and thus get 'carried away emotionally';[70] many doctors appeared to consider her wish for artificial insemination the unfortunate, selfish and damaging result. Indeed, having thoroughly denigrated the sperm donors involved, a persistent request to proceed with such a 'morally repugnant' form of treatment was taken by some doctors as the strongest indicator that a woman was not a suitable prospect for motherhood.

Case notes from the Royal Infirmary of Edinburgh infertility and gynaecological outpatient clinic during the same decade can be used to supplement the Feversham Committee correspondence.[71] While this clinical material is often of a more technical, and sometimes formulaic, nature, it provides further valuable observations from those engaged in the day-to-day work of infertility treatment. Some patient descriptions are reminiscent of the Feversham characterizations of the infertile patient as overly emotional and obsessional. Thus, Mrs E. C. was described as a 'thin, excitable patient with rather wide eyes', while Mrs M. P. 'was so anxious about interview that she came a day early. Is convinced that she has diabetes'. Mrs H. K. was noted to have been 'entirely un-cooperative' on her visits to the clinic, having been 'so upset and tearful that it was impossible to conduct a coherent conversation with her'. The cause of her agitation was reportedly that she found 'attendance at the sterility clinic embarrassing', though she expressed a wish to continue treatment 'because she wants a family so much'. Nonetheless, the clinician appears to have grown increasingly exasperated with this patient, such that, having received correspondence from her family doctor that she had fallen pregnant, his final entry in her notes concludes: 'I would be very glad if you would ask Mrs [K.] to hand into the Clinic the vaginal dilator which was given to her as it has now clearly achieved its purpose!' Mrs C. B. was spoken of in rather more complimentary tones, being 'anxious to have a family' but 'does not brood about it'.[72]

Another notable feature of these case notes is the very wide-ranging investigation that doctors appear to have conducted into the infertile patient's condition, which included consideration of her childhood and adult environments and her dietary history, as well as her menstrual and reproductive history and current bodily condition. Thus, the doctors pathologized the environment in which Mrs N. J. was raised, rather than her personally, reporting that she had a 'very unhappy' early life which included losing her mother at an early age, had been 'grossly overcrowded at home' and had 'extreme [financial] difficulty in early life'.[73] Although it is not stated explicitly, the fact that no other explanations are provided to account for her fertility problems suggests that her damaged early environment was considered a contributing factor.

While case notes can furnish us with exceptionally rich insights into medical thinking and everyday clinical practice, they are only of very limited use as a gateway to the 'patient perspective', since any patient testimony recorded in them has been heavily filtered by the hospital staff, taken out of context or edited to fit the *pro forma*.[74] Nonetheless, we get some tantalizing glimpses into the patients who attended the outpatient clinic in Edinburgh. Some of these women appear to have embodied, or adopted, the persona depicted in the Feversham witness statements, such as Mrs M. D., who 'says she is a very highly strung person'. Similarly, Mrs H. C. is noted to have asked the clinic to remove her name from their register 'as her nerves were 'getting the better of' her'.[75] Sources like diaries and letters, where one can find them, and the more 'direct' use of oral testimony, could provide valuable insight into how such patients perceived their condition and the medical treatment they received.[76]

Compliance with Science

It is important to note that the case files also contain descriptions of what might be considered to be examples of 'patient agency'. Although Mrs H. C. referred self-deprecatingly to her nerves 'getting the better of' her, she went on to note: 'I don't think there can be much wrong with me and my husband has said he won't see a Dr so there is nothing more to be done'. Such testimony highlights three important themes: the issue of which partner was to 'blame', a long-standing leitmotiv within the history of infertility; the frequency of 'defaulting', when one or both members of the married couple refused to begin or to continue with treatment; and the tussle between compliance and rebellion.

The 1950s case notes record the fact of defaulting in a range of patients, both male and female, and in some cases the stated reasons behind it. Defaulting appears to have been less common in the female patients, and was sometimes because the patient had become pregnant or had chosen to adopt an infant as an alternative strategy to achieve parenthood. In the case of Mrs E. M., a registered adoption society corresponded with the outpatient clinic to enquire whether this patient might make a suitable adoptive parent. Her consultant responded that Mrs M. 'was a co-operative patient and I would recommend her as a suitable candidate to consider'.[77] While it was not uncommon for patients to exercise some agency in these medical encounters, by resisting the doctor's attempts to diagnose and treat them, or insisting that the fault lay instead with their partner, such patients hardly won the respect of their doctors. 'Co-operation' was the favoured strategy.

Returning to the Feversham testimony, the honesty of patients was also discussed. The moral compass of infertile patients was called into question even in cases of artificial insemination using the husband's semen. Dr Sharman noted his belief that such a practice should be legal, and that he provided the service to patients, but cautioned that many doctors practising this technique simply asked the female patient 'to bring along a specimen of the husband's semen', without requesting proof that this was indeed her husband's semen *and* that he had consented to the procedure.[78] While Sharman acknowledged that many husbands were 'co-operative', sometimes phoning or writing to him, he mused that 'the woman could bring along a substitute semen if she so felt', which would be difficult for the doctor to prove; in short, doctors were 'injecting it in good faith'. Although the committee appeared interested to know that it was not common practice to obtain the written consent of the husband in such cases, a member of the committee retorted that this point was surely 'only a theoretical one' since any woman who would 'go to the trouble of bringing the semen of a man other than her husband' would 'surely try ordinary methods of adultery'. Sharman responded defensively that he was merely offering 'a highly theoretical point', but that he had 'no doubt ... from the way an occasional woman talked to him, that she did indulge in adultery'.[79]

Damaging the Damaged

As well as attracting patients and donors who were considered morally or psychologically 'damaged', numerous witnesses alleged that the treatment itself was destructive. Dr Sharman noted the 'danger of psychological damage to the patients, both husband and wife', 'either through the inevitable interference with their sexual relations or through the consciousness of reproductive inferiority'.[80]

Various measures were suggested in an attempt to reduce this risk, including a 'careful initial selection of cases' and attention paid to patients' reactions to the treatment. Alexander Kennedy, Professor of Psychiatry at the University of Edinburgh, argued that 'difficult psychological situations' would inevitably arise from this therapy, given its questionable legal status and the 'deception or misrepresentation' inherent in it.[81] Dr John McDonald, a Registrar in Perth, suggested that artificial insemination was problematic for any less than perfect marriage, for the birth of a child by this procedure would constitute 'a standing reminder' of 'already disturbed family relationships'.[82] He added that the patient 'may even feel that she is committing adultery with the doctor'.

Particular criticism was aimed at 'AIHD' (artificial insemination by husband and donor), the practice of inseminating a woman with a mixture of semen from her husband and an anonymous donor. This practice appears to have been adopted in the hope that the couple would believe that they had conceived naturally, but the extent to which the procedure was psychologically beneficial or damaging was debated vigorously in Feversham Committee proceedings. One doctor's technique involved not telling the husband when he was totally sterile, but to have a 'heart to heart talk' with his wife and then to ask her to keep that information to herself.[83] As he put it, 'I told the wife she was not to go home and blurt out the whole truth of the matter ... I saw marriages going on the rocks, ruin and divorce, through telling the husband'. The husband was instead told that he was 'impaired' but that there was 'hope with treatment or in time things might remedy themselves', thus any resulting pregnancy using AIHD might be passed off as resulting from marital intercourse.

Such doctors noted that the procedure of mixing sperm might mitigate some of the psychological dangers inherent in donor insemination, including damage to the self-esteem of infertile husbands and the 'stigma of "test-tube" origins' in resulting children.[84] However, the majority of medical witnesses expressed deep concern that the procedure led to 'unnecessary confusion and ambiguity', made the 'accurate' keeping of records 'impossible' and was fundamentally dishonest to place the couple in a position where they did not know whether or not the husband was the father of their child.[85] Such therapeutic measures, and the 'secrets and lies' inherent in them, throw into sharp relief the hypocrisy of the medical profession in characterizing the infertile woman as somehow 'duplicitous'.

Conclusions

A valuable snapshot of medical thinking and practice is offered by the evidence presented to the Feversham Committee. A lack of experience is apparent in those giving evidence, for a range of legal, practical and moral reasons, but strong views were nonetheless expressed by these medical professionals. Indeed, one might ask precisely who these patients, real or imagined, were who formed the subject of the impassioned medical testimony of the Scottish doctors.

As in the history of fertility limitation, in fertility initiation there was a pronounced tendency to pathologize the infertile woman, considered diseased not simply by virtue of her imperfectly functioning reproductive system, or even because of a perceived association with psychological impairment, but because it was psychologically and morally questionable to seek out artificial insemination by donor as a form of treatment. A wish to receive this form of therapy was the very proof that you were not a healthy and appropriate candidate for motherhood. As feminist historians have stressed, maternity has long been considered the 'female norm',[86] but some women could want this too much, such that they became frustrated, obsessional and precisely the wrong sort of person to 'function well as a parent'.[87] Thus, the infertile woman seeking treatment by artificial insemination was arguably considered to be as reproductively 'deviant' as the woman seeking a termination of pregnancy in mid-twentieth-century Scotland. Doctors appear to have discouraged or refused to offer this form of treatment where it conflicted with their own moral sensibilities, and used various strategies to repel eager female patients, including robustly critiquing the health of willing semen donors and subjecting patients to intimidating scrutiny. Even those patients who resigned hope of bearing their own child and opted instead for adoption were required to be sufficiently unemotional and 'cooperative' to gain the support of their doctors as appropriate candidates for parenthood.

Historical sources such as these – Departmental Committee testimony and hospital case notes – allow us rather effectively to capture the medical perspective on infertility and its treatment. The 'patient' perspective is more difficult to capture, as is so often the case in the histories of medicine and sexuality. Thus, the voices of the infertile patient, married couple and semen donor are all but silenced in these records; we are, instead, offered 'interpretations' of these individuals, and rather damning interpretations in most cases, despite emanating from the supposedly 'rational' and 'detached' doctors.

The Feversham evidence indicates that the infertile woman was not by any means the only pathological element of the procedure. Indeed, one could say that every element of artificial insemination by donor was pathologized by mid-twentieth-century doctors: patient, sperm donor, the doctor (on occasion) and the very procedure itself.[88] A rather more paternalistic attitude was displayed towards the husband, with concerns that he had not consented to such a treatment and might thus be deceived by an adulterous wife, or that his self-esteem simply could not cope with the knowledge of his reproductive inadequacy. Perhaps a high rate of defaulting in male patients, as is suggested by the outpatient case notes, encouraged doctors to be gentle.

Less concern was expressed where female patients were concerned. There was an explicit questioning of what motivated those women seeking insemination treatment, with perceived risks of dishonesty due to the level of desperation that many felt to be pregnant, and concerns over the further damaging of these already vulnerable women. The motives of the willing semen donors were questioned even more vigorously, with utter incredulity in some medical quarters that the inducement could be anything more than financial, and in others the firm belief that a willingness to donate one's sperm to a complete stranger was itself a sign of psychological damage.

Ultimately, such beliefs tended to be based on a slim evidence base of medical experience, or none at all. The sexual sciences have long straddled the uneasy ground between legitimate research and titillation, with suspicion continuing to linger that professional respectability is somewhat tainted by involvement in sexual matters. Given the low-tech nature of artificial insemination as a procedure, and its agricultural associations, involvement in this sphere of activity did nothing to boost a doctor's skill or reputation. And with the motives of everyone else involved in the artificial insemination procedure being called into question, why should the doctor escape that interrogation.

Acknowledgements

I am indebted to the Wellcome Trust for their financial support of the research upon which this chapter is based, and to Roger Davidson, Mark Jackson and the volume and series editors for their intellectual support.

8 WOMEN'S EXPERIENCES OF THE MATERNITY SERVICES IN BERKSHIRE AND OXFORDSHIRE, *c.* 1970–1990

Angela Davis

During the 1970s and 1980s, the effect of interventionist procedures was an object of study for many of those investigating maternity care. Sally McIntyre has described how the mid-1970s witnessed a vigorous public debate about obstetric practices: '[I]t seemed as though a dam of hitherto latent antagonism to the obstetric profession had burst, flooding medical, nursing and midwifery journals, the quality and popular press, television and, ultimately, parliament, with debate and controversy about obstetric practices'.[1] Within this context the feminist sociologist Ann Oakley conducted a study of women's views of first-time motherhood based on interviews with fifty-five first-time mothers during their pregnancies, labour and deliveries, and experiences at five and twenty weeks postpartum, in the late 1970s. She found pregnant women were undergoing a hitherto unknown level of monitoring: 100 per cent of the mothers in the sample had taken drugs of one kind or another in pregnancy, 100 per cent had blood and urine tests, 68 per cent were given ultrasound, 19 per cent X-rays and 30 per cent had other tests. The average number of antenatal visits was thirteen.[2]

The increasing medicalization of pregnancy and childbirth is a well-known story,[3] but the aim of this chapter is to tease out the experiences of women themselves in order to consider the complexity of their responses. The chapter's findings are therefore based on seventy oral history interviews with women from Berkshire and Oxfordshire.[4] Whilst in many ways maternity care in this period was subject to national (and indeed international) trends, such as the virtual cessation of domiciliary delivery, the counties under discussion were notable for often being at the forefront of developments. The area's maternal mortality, infant mortality and perinatal mortality rates were generally below the national average. These advances came in part from a forward-looking medical profession encouraged by the presence of a prominent teaching hospital in Oxford, but also because the locality attracted influential middle-class intellectuals such as the birth educator Sheila Kitzinger.[5] However, the area itself was not homogenous and the Berkshire and Oxfordshire interviewees chosen for this study were evenly distributed amongst different locations in the counties – rural, urban and suburban. These are the villages of Benson and Ewelme in south Oxfordshire; the Wychwood villages in west Oxfordshire; the twenty-four square miles near Banbury in north Oxfordshire covered by the *Country Planning* (1944) survey;[6] the market town of Thame which lies in the east of the county; Oxford city centre; and the contrasting suburbs of industrial, working-class Cowley and Florence Park in east Oxford and professional, middle-class North Oxford and Summertown in north Oxford. In addition, two villages in the neighbouring county of Berkshire – Crowthorne and Sandhurst – were included, to enable the comparison of provision of maternity care in Oxford city, Oxfordshire and Berkshire, which was an aim of the wider project.

Women's experiences of maternity care were also determined by where their children were born. After 1970, women principally attended either midwife-led units in maternity hospitals or small local hospitals, or consultant-led units in larger general hospitals. For example, midwife-led units were in operation at Wallingford Community Hospital in south Oxfordshire and the Maternity Hospital in Wokingham in Berkshire. In Oxford there was also the GP unit, attached to the John Radcliffe Hospital, where women were delivered by their GP or community midwife. Women who chose to attend these smaller units did so because they felt they were more intimate than large hospitals and they were often closer to where they lived, making it easier for family to visit. In terms of consultant-led units, most Oxfordshire women attended the John Radcliffe Hospital in Oxford, but there were also women who went to other consultant-run units in general hospitals in neighbouring counties, such as Reading's Royal Berkshire Hospital and Aylesbury's Royal Buckinghamshire Hospital. Amongst the Berkshire residents, Reading's Royal Berkshire Hospital was predominant, but women also attended Frimley Park Hospital in Camberley, in neighbouring Surrey. Women who were deemed at risk (due to factors such multiple births, parity or ill-health) were recommended to attend consultant-led units, but other women would also choose them, particularly for first babies, as there was not the provision of services such as epidural anaesthesia available in midwife-led units.

The remainder of this chapter will be formed of two main parts. The first part will consider the interviewees' experiences and attitudes towards five practices that were common during the period (but were also the subject of some debate): ultrasound scans, episiotomy, induction, epidural anaesthesia and caesarean section. But, second, it will also examine women's accounts of their relationships with the hospital staff who attended them. The chapter will conclude that it was not simply technical advances women reacted against, but the way in which they were employed.

Ultrasound Scans

Ultrasound was first used in obstetrics and gynaecology by Ian Donald in Glasgow in the mid-1950s to diagnose a range of conditions including twins, fibroids and ovarian cysts.[7] From its introduction, concerns were raised about its safety due to the association between maternal exposure to x-rays during pregnancy and subsequent childhood cancer.[8] However, Donald and his team concluded that, at the diagnostic levels they were proposing to use, there was no evidence of harmful effects of ultrasound.[9] By the later 1970s and 1980s, ultrasound was also being regularly employed to determine gestational age as it was recognized that uncertainties regarding gestational age were associated with higher rates of perinatal mortality and morbidity.[10] Whilst it was acknowledged that errors, both systematic and random, were to be expected in such an application, and were found to be dependent on factors such as the growth rate of the dimension under consideration, it was viewed that these problems were outweighed by the fact that ultrasound was a painless, non-invasive and apparently safe technique.[11]

Five of the women interviewed expressed doubts about ultrasound. Two, Andrea and Tara, had ultrasound scans which they felt were inaccurate. Andrea's experience reflected both ultrasound's growing use and its limitations. She had three children in 1978, 1981 and 1984. She had an ultrasound scan with her third child and was sceptical whether it really was beneficial: 'And in fact that was the only one they actually queried the dates on. But I knew my dates were right'.[12] Andrea felt her knowledge of her own body had been challenged by the use of technology which ultimately was itself discredited. Tara also had a story of a scan which was proved wrong. She had her first child in 1988 by emergency caesarean and had hoped to deliver her second baby, born in 1990, vaginally. However, 'they did one of those scans ... And they told me the baby was actually quite large ... And so I was a bit scared thinking this baby was, you know, going to be quite substantial'. As a result of the scan Tara opted for an elective caesarean, but found the experience 'nerve wracking and immediately the baby was delivered I got really, shockingly depressed'. In actuality Tara's daughter was 'tiny'. She was 'five and a half pounds', and Tara concluded: 'I would probably have been wiser to try and deliver her normally but what do you know?'[13] Hermione felt ultrasound scans contributed to a general medicalization of pregnancy and childbirth which she disapproved of.[14] For Sandra it was not the scan itself but the way that it was administered that she criticized. Sandra had not minded having a scan with her first child in 1976, but was unhappy with the way her consultant gave her the results. She explained:

> I had a scan and they said, 'Oh, alarm bells, the baby is not growing,' ... that was Friday, and, 'We want you to come in on Monday. The baby might have brain damage because it's not growing'. I was told that by myself. I drove myself home. My husband

was away. It was ghastly ... So from that point of view it was awful. I think there was an arrogance from the doctor.[15]

Nonetheless, despite these women's doubts about the medical benefits of ultrasound scanning, with Pippa even fearing they could be harmful,[16] by the end of the period it had become an established part of antenatal care. In total thirteen interviewees gave accounts of ultrasound scans.[17] For those who had them in the 1970s it was usually if there were concerns about the baby or if a multiple birth was suspected. During the 1980s they were increasingly becoming the norm. The routine nature of ultrasound scans also meant that by the end of the period they had become a rite of passage for many women, and when some first felt they were really pregnant.[18] For example one of the interviewees, Cynthia, who had her only child in 1993, said, 'certainly until I had my first scan I really had this sort of notion that it wasn't real'.[19] One study of prenatal testing published in 1995 under the auspices of the Institute of Epidemiology and Health Services Research at Leeds University showed a 99 per cent uptake for ultrasonography.[20] However, women's reasons for undergoing the scans were rather different than those intended by the maternity services. The study's authors concluded that ultrasonography was valued for nonmedical reasons and chosen even by fully informed people who eschewed prenatal diagnosis.[21] Women welcomed the opportunity to see their unborn child, but they seemed rather less enthusiastic about ultrasound's medical uses.

Episiotomy

Contemporary studies revealed that the increasing technologization of pregnancy was then magnified when it came to childbirth itself. While induction may have received the most attention during this period, episiotomy was the most commonly performed obstetric operation after clamping of the umbilical cord.[22] In the UK, clinicians viewed episiotomy as an emergency procedure until the 1960s, but its use then rapidly increased and by the 1970s was routine in many consultant units.[23] In their 1982 review of the literature surrounding episiotomy, the epidemiologists David Banta and Stephen Thacker noted there were four reported benefits of episiotomy. First, that a clean, straight incision was easier to repair and healed better than a tear. Second, that fewer third-degree lacerations followed an episiotomy. Third, that episiotomy prevented fetal brain injury because it reduced the pressure of the fetal head on the pelvic floor. Fourth, episiotomy shortened the second stage of labour and therefore helped prevent damage to the pelvic floor. However, Banta and Thacker found the data on the benefits of episiotomy to be very poor and offered no convincing argument to support the routine use of the procedure.[24] In addition, in an analysis of 24,439 deliveries between 1980 and 1984 carried out at Oxford's John Radcliffe Hospital, during which period there was a large decline in the use of episiotomy, the study's authors found that the reduction in the episiotomy rate and an increase in the proportion of women with an intact perineum had no increase in the incidence of adverse outcomes.[25]

Sheila Kitzinger and Rhiannon Walters conducted a study of episiotomy based on 1,795 questionnaires that were given out by 40 National Childbirth Trust (NCT) teachers between March 1979 and March 1980.[26] They found significant differences in the experiences of those women who did and did not receive an episiotomy. For example, women who had episiotomies reported experiencing more pain at the end of the first week; they were more likely to find it difficult to get or maintain a position in which they could comfortably breastfeed; and they were more likely to experience pain on intercourse.[27] The studies conducted by the NCT at this time had a particular research agenda. The organization had been set up in 1956 under the name of the Natural Childbirth Association to campaign for a more natural approach to childbirth. After a period of internal conflict it became a charitable trust changing its name to the NCT in 1961. By the 1970s, the NCT was publicly challenging interventionist procedures.[28] Nonetheless, their research provides an interesting point of comparison with the oral history material.

Pain also featured prominently in the descriptions of episiotomy given by the women interviewed for this study. Each of the nine interviewees who remembered having an episiotomy said that it was painful.[29] Sandra had her first child in 1976 and 'got a really sore bottom from all the operations, stitches'.[30] Dawn had her son in 1979 and recalled that when he was about a day and a half old she had difficulty feeding him because she had so many stitches she could not sit.[31] But it was not only the pain of episiotomy that had stayed with the interviewees. They also recalled their unhappiness that episiotomies were carried out routinely; and that women were not informed about the procedure. Carol had her first baby in 1979 and her account of episiotomy reflects both these points.

> And I think it was routine as well, to give you an episiotomy on your first. And so, because he was being born so quick, I had no injection, to numb the pain. And they said, 'just a little snip'. And ... nobody told me they did that routine. They just did it. And it was just ... felt like a pair of shears ... just cutting into you. It was the only time out of all five children that I let out a scream. Coz that was just really painful. And shocking as well, coz they didn't tell you.[32]

Carol's complaints about her episiotomy were centred on the fact that she was not involved in the decision-making. While episiotomy was in itself inherently painful for women, they were also critical of the lack of say they had in its use.

Induction

As well as episiotomy, induction and acceleration of labour were also routine procedures during the 1970s and 1980s. Induction through artificial rupture of the membranes and/or the use of oxytocin administered by an intravenous drip was at its peak in the 1970s and was perhaps the most controversial issue surrounding childbirth at this time. Much research into induction was conducted, but it was largely concerned with its possible effects on the physical health of mothers and their babies and whether induction lengthened labour or shortened it. Proponents of induction argued it reduced perinatal deaths by preventing babies going beyond term,[33] but others argued it was being overused.[34] In contrast, Ann Cartwright, in her study of induction published in 1979, sought to examine what women themselves thought about induction. Cartwright, a statistician and socio-medical researcher, took a feminist perspective. She interviewed mothers from a random sample of 2,182 live births about their experiences of childbirth.[35] She found that despite a higher rate of pain relief among women who were induced, levels of pain were similar, indicating that induced labour was intrinsically more painful. Many women found the mechanics of induction restricting and induced labours more often resulted in an assisted delivery.[36] Cartwright argued her study showed, therefore, that 'mothers and babies were less healthy and happy when labour was induced'.[37]

The oral history interviews conducted for this article revealed a somewhat more nuanced picture. Nineteen interviewees said they were induced.[38] Five women felt they had benefited from induction.[39] For example, Patsy had two children in 1970 and 1972; comparing the births, she spoke of the great improvement with her second child. He was 'induced early because of the problems I'd had with [my first son], so he was induced and, of course, I had no problems whatsoever and I think I probably only stayed twenty-four hours before I came home'.[40] While it would be an overstatement to say women were pleased to be induced, it is important to note that some women felt they benefited from the procedure.

Indeed, reflecting the contemporary uncertainty surrounding induction, many interviewees' accounts indicate their doubt about whether induction or acceleration of labour was beneficial, detrimental or of no consequence. Liz's third baby was induced in 1980 and she was unsure about the procedure. She had not been induced with her first two pregnancies, but was with her third as she had not put on weight. She was told,

> 'You'd better come in tomorrow and we'll put you on a drip'. And I'd never had a drip before. And I thought no, I just want to do it the way I know ... So ... the doctor came round and said, 'Oh we'll have to put you on that drip anyway'. And I [thought] ... 'Ooo you nasty man'. Oh and he wasn't gentle at all when he ... coz I went red ... the midwife was so sympathetic. She was lovely. So I think he ... I think he broke the waters, that's what he did. He put me on the drip and then that.[41]

Liz's account touches on a number of different issues that were present in maternity care during the 1970s – the change in practice over time, the division between doctors and midwives and the power relations between them and their patients. However, it would be wrong to consider maternity care at this time as simply a case of helpful midwives versus uncaring doctors. Josie's labour was accelerated with her first baby in 1985, but she felt this was a result of an unsupportive midwife. She recalled the birth as being a 'nightmare'. The midwife had intimidated her and made her feel very nervous. As a result she felt the labour was prolonged causing her to have to be put on a 'drip'.[42]

However, whilst six of the interviewees were unhappy their labours had been accelerated or induced and doubted whether this was really for their benefit,[43] a greater number were accepting of the judgements made by health professionals. These women believed that even if induction caused them some discomfort, the decision to induce was taken in the best interests of their babies.[44] For example, describing the birth of her son in 1967, Anna explained: 'I was actually overdue then, so they decided they needed to induce the labour. So I was induced'. Nonetheless, her experience did mirror those of those women from Cartwright's study in that the induction resulted in a long labour and a forceps delivery. She said the labour 'seemed to go on forever, thirty-six hours or something like that, I mean not in active labour all the time. They finally delivered me by forceps'.[45] Anna recalled her feelings of being induced in a very different way to the women in Cartwright's study, though, and she was not critical of the staff who attended her. This difference may have resulted from the passing of time, or perhaps because she herself was a doctor and therefore sympathetic towards the health professionals, or because she felt in control of the events that transpired. In a 1999 study of women's views about their birth experience based on 519 questionnaires given to women on their second post-natal day, the article's authors (a research midwife, consultant in feto-maternal medicine and lecturer in midwifery) found that women who felt in control during the intrapartum period were more satisfied with their labour. However, this did not necessarily require women to feel personally in control, but equally could result from their belief that the hospital staff were in control.[46] Anna's happiness with her care may have resulted from her sense the staff were in control, encouraged by her trust in her medical colleagues.

Viv was also positive about her experience of being induced with her second child at Reading's Royal Berkshire Hospital in 1971. Whilst she could have presented the birth as a traumatic event – she had high blood pressure, a trolley system was in operation at the hospital and her labour was long – instead Viv said the hospital was 'fantastic' and told the story in a light-hearted manner, remembering how spent her time 'getting up and wandering and chatting to everybody else'.[47] Bev similarly presented her experiences as amusing rather than distressing. She was overdue with both her children, born in 1987 and 1990. When asked whether this resulted in her being induced Bev joked that the hospital unsuccessfully tried to induce both babies, but it did not work.[48] Perhaps it was possible for these women to present their experience in a light-hearted manner because of their ultimate faith in their attendants and because they remembered it as a positive experience.

Whether or not a woman was induced depended on practices of the hospital in which she was delivered. A survey of consultant obstetric units in 1989–90 reported the overall induction rate was 17 per cent, but rates for individual units varied between 4 per cent and 37 per cent.[49] Kaye, a midwife in Oxfordshire during the period, discussed the different policies towards induction at the various hospitals where she worked.

> At St Thomas's [London] where I did my obstetrics, you know, the consultants would routinely induce people when it suited them sort of thing, not at weekends, and I thought that was all wrong. So yes I thought it was, you know, much more natural the way they did things at the smaller hospitals and the midwives were, you know, skilled in normal deliveries without using episiotomies routinely and that sort of thing.[50]

She continued: 'At the Royal Bucks [Royal Buckinghamshire Hospital] it wasn't very good. The doctors sort of interfered unnecessarily and if a labour wasn't going as fast as they'd like they'd stick a drip [in] ... to speed things along'.[51] Kaye also explained that she turned down a job at Oxford's John Radcliffe Hospital because, 'their induction rate was so high at the time which I thought was terrible. It was something like thirty-seven percent. This was in the mid-1970s'.[52] As Kaye intimates here, rates of induction were higher at consultant-led hospitals, like the John Radcliffe Hospital or Royal Buckinghamshire Hospital, than midwife-led units.[53]

It was therefore some women's perception that their care was determined by hospital policies and practices rather than medical need. For example Mildred, who had her second child at the Royal Buckinghamshire Hospital in 1969, was told she could not be induced at the weekend as there were not enough staff around.[54] Tasha had her daughter at the John Radcliffe Hospital in Oxford in 1972.

> At the time, the hospital idea was that babies were induced. And [my daughter] was induced a day early, to suit the hospital regime. And when I'd said, '13th?' Coz she was due on the 14th. The consultant said, 'oh yes well I suppose we could delay it and not have it on the 13th because that's an unlucky day, no doubt'. 'No, no,' I said, 'it wasn't that. That's early' ... They were saying you know, you pick apples from the tree before they're ripe and you store them and everything and it's perfectly okay. And ... yeah ... you were brainwashed.[55]

Some interviewees presented themselves as being bemused, rather than angered or distressed, that the births of their children had become so 'unnatural'. There

was a similar trend amongst those women who had undergone elective caesareans. Geraldine's youngest daughter was born in 1989 by caesarean section
because she was a breech baby. She explained that:

> the obstetrician that handled it said, 'right, no I don't deliver ... I don't deliver breech
> babies vaginally so you're ... you'll have to have a caesarean section'. And I remember
> thinking how weird it was that sitting in front of him. He got out his diary and he
> said, 'What do you say the 29th of March. Is that okay?' And I thought ... I think it's
> weird.

Geraldine did not say she was unhappy that her consultant had decided when
the baby should be born; rather, she accepted it, concluding the story by saying,
'That was it really.'[56] Georgie had her second baby in 1975. She not only acqui-
esced to the consultant planning the caesarean before the due date of her baby
because he was going away, she actively encouraged it. She recounted the story:

> he said, 'Right, I'm going on holiday in September when the baby's due'... so he said,
> 'Well, what about if I deliver the baby before I go away', so I said, 'Well, what date?'
> He said, 'Twenty-seventh of August,' I said, 'Brilliant, that's brilliant'. He said, 'Oh
> you want it early?', I said, 'It's not that, it's just that I would rather have the baby young
> in his school year than old, and if he's born in September he will be old in his school
> year and if he's born in, it, it will be young in its school year'.[57]

Georgie's experience demonstrates that women could be as keen supporters of
medical intervention in their pregnancy and birth as their attendants.

Epidural Anaesthesia

The oral history interviews revealed a similarly complex picture surrounding
women's experiences of epidural anaesthesia. Eleven women recalled having
epidurals.[58] Four were very positive.[59] For example, Dawn had an epidural with
her first baby in 1979 after being recommended to do so because the baby was
breech. She said it worked incredibly well and therefore she elected to also have
an epidural when she later had twins in 1981.[60] Five had more ambivalent experiences.[61] Harriet told an unhappy account of her birth with her twins in 1986.
With hindsight she felt she should have chosen to have an elective caesarean.
Nonetheless within her generally negative account she spoke positively of her
experience of epidural anaesthesia.[62] In contrast, two women felt the epidural
itself was the cause of their difficult births. Carmel's epidural was not successful
and therefore coloured her whole experience. Carmel had a caesarean with her
first baby in 1977 and said, 'the actual birth wasn't great really'. She blamed the
effects of the epidural, explaining: 'In those days they couldn't get the, they didn't
get the dose, now they can fine tune it. But it really, I mean, completely numbed
my whole body I think ... So that wasn't great'.[63] Ellen had an epidural with her

first baby in 1975, but not with her next five. She said the side effects of the epidural wearing off were worse than the pain of birth itself.[64] These mixed views of the procedure extended to those women who had not had epidurals. Jean was upset that she had been unable to have an epidural at Wallingford Community Hospital where her baby was born in 1987 because, as a midwife-led unit, it did not have the facilities to offer epidural anaesthesia.[65] In contrast, Bonnie had been offered an epidural when she had her second child in 1981 but refused because of the bad reports she had heard. She said that many of her friends who had undergone epidurals complained about subsequent back problems and she had not wanted to take this risk.[66]

The consequences of having an epidural were often not separated from the birth process more generally in interviewees' accounts. Epidurals were rarely presented as turning points in women's stories of birth, either leading to an 'easy' or 'difficult' birth, but rather just another procedure to be undergone. For example, describing the birth of her first son in 1983, Pippa associated epidural anaesthesia with the process of being induced and fetal scalp monitoring. One followed on from the other:

> It hadn't started naturally the night before, and I spent most of the day there and nothing much happening ... and then they wired me up and ... a lot of pain but not much happening ... got really, really tired ... and eventually I had an epidural ... which sort of did speed things up ... and that had worn off and I did, sort of, push him out.[67]

The various procedures women underwent were therefore often not differentiated in their recollections and may explain why they could find it difficult to recall what had happened during their labours. Neither was the birth seen in isolation from what followed. Patsy had her first son in 1970. She said her 'pregnancy was fine, but the birth was difficult and I had to have an epidural'. She felt this difficult labour then affected her ability to bond with her baby:

> It was quite dramatic and he went off into one of these little incubator things, mainly because he was just, I suppose, tired really because it was quite a difficult birth and I didn't, I somehow felt that he had to be damaged and I just didn't want to know, I didn't want to go down and feed him, I didn't want to know.[68]

When reflecting back upon the births of their children the different interventions interviewees underwent often became inseparable – they were not viewed as distinct procedures. Therefore what was important to Patsy as she recalled her son's birth was that her traumatic experience led to her feelings of depression; she felt this then affected her relationship with him. She was concerned less with what made the birth difficult than with its consequences.[69] While good or bad experiences of epidural anaesthesia were recalled as being significant by the interviewees, this was framed less in terms of the procedure itself and more by what they felt were its effects.

Caesarean Section

The ambivalence with which the women remembered their experiences of epidural anaesthesia was also seen in their accounts of caesarean section. Sixteen interviewees said that they had caesareans.[70] Three recalled their experience as principally a negative one.[71] For instance Pam, who had her first baby in 1977 said,

> It wasn't an easy birth. I had to have a caesarean, and the wound got infected, so it was a difficult time really. And I had to stay in hospital and I couldn't feed, so it was a difficult time.[72]

In contrast Katherine was the most positive. Her first child was born in 1983 in Frimley Park Hospital. Like Pam she had a traumatic birth. She explained how 'suddenly the distress [signal] went out and they, you know, did all sorts of things and it was an emergency caesarean by the evening'. However, while recalling her experience of the birth of her son as frightening, she then added that she did not regret having a caesarean, stating, 'I was glad because he was a big baby'.[73] Most of the interviewees recalled their caesareans with mixed feelings.[74] Tara had both her babies (born in 1988 and 1990) by caesarean section, the first being an emergency caesarean and the second elective. It is interesting that as she compared the births she recalled the emergency caesarean as the better experience.

> But the first time had been an emergency caesarean ... When they just ... put you out completely so that was in a way easy for me. What I didn't realize was the second time it was an elective caesarean and I had to be wide awake ... at the time it was happening and it was far worse. And I sometimes think that if I'd known it was going to be like that I would have terminated the pregnancy. But you live and learn, don't you?[75]

Tara's lack of knowledge of the differences between an emergency and elective caesarean and the type of anaesthetic she would receive indicates how women could still feel uninformed about what could happen during their labours.[76]

In her 1992 study of caesarean section which was based on interviews with fifty women who had emergency caesareans,[77] Edith Hillan, a midwife, found women did not feel that they received sufficient explanation of the procedure prior to the section and were left confused by the events and how the decision to operate was reached.[78] Bonnie's first baby was born in 1978. She said women were not told in advance about caesarean section and she had not known it involved an operation. She was extremely traumatized on being given the news when she arrived at hospital that she would have to have her baby 'cut out'.[79] However, it was not simply a lack of information about what happened before the birth of their babies which women found distressing. Aftercare was also extremely important in determining how they recalled their experiences. Bev had both her children, born in 1987 and 1990, at St Peter's Hospital in Chertsey, Surrey, rather than her local hospital Frimley Park. Bev had been treated at St Peter's Hospital for ongoing fertility problems and was therefore advised to give birth there; she had suffered from a series of seventeen miscarriages before children were born. Bev had spoken entirely positively about her antenatal care and felt without technological advances she would never have been able to have children: 'I am grateful for science'.[80] She also felt that she was well-prepared for a caesarean. However, Bev was critical of what happened after the birth:

> I felt up to that point, I was given everything I wanted and listened to. But after he was born, when things went a little bit squiff ... I felt like I wasn't in control at all. Now whether that was my mental state or whether that was ... how things really were, I don't know...I wouldn't like to say. I felt I was like ... in a German concentration camp. The nurse was 'Get up. Do this. Do this. Do this'. You know. The baby was ... you know, I was manhandled to feed him. And ... I wasn't well.[81]

A caesarean section is major surgery and in consequence it featured prominently in the birth stories of women who underwent the procedure. However, it is noteworthy that the events leading up to the operation, and indeed the experiences that followed it, could be remembered as being equally important.

Relationships with Hospital Staff

Bev's complaints about the aftercare she received illustrate the second main focus for women's complaints about their maternity care – the hospital staff. It is also noteworthy that nurses, midwives and doctors all featured within the interviewees' accounts and all could receive criticism. Women's unhappiness with their attendants had been exposed by contemporary research. In a study of women's experiences of rupture of the membranes in labour in the late 1980s the NCT found: 'One of the most important aspects of labour – if not the most important – is having good attendants ... The letters women wrote are full of references to the crucial role of the midwife at the time of childbirth'.[82] Reviewing the survey material, they concluded: 'Whether the birth was normal or more complicated and requiring medical intervention, an understanding, caring midwife made all the difference from the woman's point of view'.[83] Frustration with the shift system in hospitals was a recurring theme in the respondents' accounts and they indicated that understaffing had the greatest effect on the quality of support they received, rather than the approach of the individual midwife.[84] In her study of induced labour based on 614 reports of pharmacologically induced labours written by women who had attended NCT classes, Sheila Kitzinger found similar criticisms of the hospital staff.[85] The respondents' reports revealed that women felt they lacked information and that asking questions risked them being considered 'difficult'.[86] Kitzinger concluded: 'The most unequivocally positive and the most unequivocally negative reports showed that length of labour is irrelevant, but that the quality of emotional support in labour and choice as to pain relief are of primary importance'.[87]

The oral history interviews revealed many of the same complaints. Lynne's account epitomized both how technological advances could not offset the effects of poor relationships with health professionals; and how interventions were exacerbated by a lack of support from hospital staff. She described the birth of her only child in 1973:

> So the hospital was very well equipped and so on but, I don't know, the weekend [my son] was born the obstetrician, oh I don't know it was just terribly lengthy you know the whole thing, being in labour for about nearly a day and then them deciding that he should be born by caesarean and then I think the nurses were quite tough, he was then taken off to a nursery and you know they would bring him out to a tight strict schedule and all that sort of stuff and it took ages to get him sort of sorted.[88]

Women could therefore feel that whilst they received good medical care, the emotional care was lacking. Carmel had her first baby at the West London Hospital in 1977. She said the hospital had been 'trumpeted far and wide' because it had featured in Sheila Kitzinger's *Good Birth Guide*. However, Carmel was not so enamoured with the hospital and felt the *Guide* had been too concerned with what was happening at the 'top', namely speaking to 'consultants and senior nursing staff', and not what happened 'at the grass roots'. She said, 'They weren't there on a Sunday night which is what happened to me with, you know, your bog standard midwife who couldn't really care less'.[89]

Midwives and nurses featured most prominently in the interviewees' accounts, reflecting the fact they were the health professionals women most frequently came into contact with, but women also levelled similar criticisms against their consultants and other doctors (as seen above in Sandra's account of ultrasound and Liz's account of induction).[90] Katherine recalled what happened when she returned to the maternity unit at Frimley Park Hospital after her baby was born for her six-week check:

> when I got in the doctor took one look at me and said, 'I don't see postnatal'. Sort of, you know, I just felt awful. And the nurse actually was very kind ... And in the end he had to and he was a bit brutal. So, it was just a horrible experience. And the nurse, but the nurse, I think the nurse realised how horrible he was and she was terribly nice to me. But, you know, it wasn't her fault.[91]

Women also suffered from the belief on the part of some health professionals (including nurses, midwives and doctors) that they, rather than the women they were attending to, knew best. Women's knowledge of their own bodies was disregarded. Josie explained what happened at the birth of her second baby in 1989.

She recalled that she arrived at the hospital about half past six in the morning. She told the staff that she felt the baby was coming, but they ignored this and told her it would not be until the afternoon. She eventually persuaded them to take her down to the delivery room and her son was born at half past seven. A similar course of events occurred with the birth of her twins in 1991. Again she entered hospital early in the morning, but was told by the hospital staff she would not deliver them until lunchtime, despite her protestations to the contrary. She was taken to the delivery suite to have an epidural as it was a multiple birth, but by the time the anaesthetist arrived the first baby had appeared. Josie could not understand why the hospital staff had not believed her when she had told them the baby was coming.[92]

Not only were women not listened to, they could be deliberately kept uninformed. Carol had her first baby in 1979. She explained what happened afterwards at a hospital appointment during her second pregnancy the following year.

> I went up to the hospital and she said, 'Oh I see here your first baby had to be resuscitated'. And I said 'Pardon?' She said, 'Yeah, he had to be resuscitated. They gave you the Pethidine too close to the birth'. And nobody told me. You know I told you they wouldn't let me out? Now I wonder if that's why they wouldn't let me out. You know, there was so much cover up in them days, you know. They didn't tell me I was going to be cut. They didn't tell me the risks of Pethidine. They didn't tell me that my son needed resuscitating, after the birth. And they didn't tell me that's why they wanted to keep me in, I presume. You know, and it was so bad. I was sixteen and vulnerable. You know I just feel that it was a really horrible experience.[93]

However, it was not only young or first-time mothers who were left powerless in relation to the hospital staff. Pippa was a university-educated middle-class mother in her thirties when her third child was born in 1988. She was an active campaigner for mothers and involved in a number of parents' groups. However, she found herself bullied by her midwife and was still so upset by the experience that she cried whilst recalling it.

> I had a sort of natural birth ... without pain relief et cetera. And another big baby. She was about ... she was nine pounds one ounce. But no sort of complications. Great to have a girl. And ... then everything was hunkey dorey. But after the birth ... I just shook and they'd sort of cleaned me up and put me on this trolley thing, and given me a glass of water, which had spilled in the bedding. And this woman came in and screamed at me ... I mean, the porter was shocked. 'You've spilt the water everywhere. Now I'm going to have to change your ... ' you know change the bedding. And I nearly wrote afterwards, coz it was my last chance to have a ... a sort of more pleasant experience and she sort of ruined it then. I was very upset. I always felt. I was really upset, I'm still upset now. It's funny isn't it? It was really upsetting.[94]

The most frequent complaint made by interviewees about their time in hospital was the absence of continuity of care. It is noteworthy this was also true for the women I had interviewed about their experiences of motherhood during the period 1945 to 1970.[95] Dawn had her first baby at the Royal Berkshire Hospital in Reading in 1979. She had no criticisms of the birth itself and felt she had received excellent care. However, she said that after the birth she never saw the same nurse twice and thought the hospital was like a baby factory.[96] Katherine levelled the same complaints against Frimley Park Hospital in Camberley where she had her first child in 1983. She said:

> It was a variety of different sort of nurses that would come in and look after you and some of them were very jolly and, 'Oh, yes, you should be up doing this'. And then there were some going, 'Oh, no, no, no, you shouldn't be doing this, that and the other'.[97]

Katherine's account indicates that the lack of continuity of care not only made it harder for women to establish relationships with their attendants, but also meant they received mixed messages from them.

Contemporary surveys had found a very different experience of childbirth amongst those women who had had home births. In 1974 Jean Robinson, a patients' rights advocate and founder member of the Association for Improvements in the Maternity Services (AIMS), published an essay in *The Times* based on the letters of women and men who had written to her about their experience of birth. She found:

> Descriptions of home births by mothers – and fathers – were moving and even lyrical. The new baby was introduced to brothers and sisters in happy and secure circumstances which some parents believed affected their future relationship, breastfeeding could be established unhindered by rigid hospital regulations, and comments from several mothers suggested they felt a closer bond with the baby born at home than those born in hospital.[98]

In a study of home birth based on sixty-five letters in response to advert in NCT newsletter in 1975,[99] Sheila Kitzinger discovered that women appreciated the way in which one midwife cared for them not only during the labour, but for ten days after the birth.[100] Nevertheless, she concluded that respondents were worried about the safety of a home confinement, especially since they were frequently warned of the dangers by obstetricians.[101]

Such a picture also emerged from the oral history interviews. Margaret's children were born at home, in 1969 and 1970, and she explained that she faced a lot of pressure to go into hospital.[102] Kaye was a midwife in Oxfordshire and talked at length about how she felt birth had become too interventionist in large consultant hospitals during the 1970s and that she favoured the midwife-run smaller units which enabled a more 'natural birth'. However, she said:

> I was never that happy with home births because you just never know what might happen and I only did seven in my three years in Oxford and I'd done none before

that whatsoever. So although there weren't any problems with them, I still felt it was a pointless risk.[103]

Indeed, the issue of home birth was the one area in which the contemporary survey material diverged from the accounts of the oral history interviewees. The oral history material is less supportive of home birth and more critical of ideas about natural childbirth more generally. There are two main problems with the evidence which prevents a true comparison. First, many of the contemporary studies were carried out by the NCT and often conducted amongst its members or through its newsletters. As noted above, the NCT campaigned for a more natural approach to childbirth. The organization's aims would likely influence their research findings. Second, only a small minority of the women interviewed for this study (five out of seventy)[104] had a home birth, reflecting the tiny numbers having home births in the general population at this time. As a result, their views on the place of birth were based on their preferences rather than their actual experiences. As Campbell and Macfarlane have noted, this situation is problematic, because:

> apart from those who have been dissatisfied, women tend to express a preference for whatever type of delivery they have had. This, coupled with findings which show that a sizeable proportion of women feel that they are given little or no choice about where to give birth, means that survey questionnaires asking women to make hypothetical choices about places of birth which they have no experience may elicit responses which are difficult to interpret.[105]

A very different picture emerged during my prior research conducted with women who had their children between 1945 and 1970. Many of these earlier interviewees had experienced home birth and had spoken of great satisfaction with the experience and their preference for home over hospital delivery.[106] The pace of change is astonishing. In the ten years from the mid-1960s to the mid-1970s, home birth had gone from being viewed as something normal to something extraordinary. For the interviewees who had their children between 1970 and 1990, being delivered at home by a midwife was no longer considered mainstream, but something eccentric. For example, when I asked Jean whether she had thought about having a home birth, she replied: 'No, I'm not that adventurous. No'.[107] April told me: 'I didn't want to have children at home, I just thought that was something hippyish'.[108] Very few women recalled they wanted home births but were prevented by doctors, or that the fear of medical complications stopped them choosing a home birth. Only Amelia said she had asked to have a home birth but was refused, because as she was over thirty, she was too old.[109] Rather, the interviewees presented home birth as a subject that was never even an option. For example, Bev said, 'home births was another thing that sort of didn't occur to me'.[110]

The activities of the NCT could also elicit a similarly half-hearted response. Geraldine had her two children in the late 1980s. She said she knew about the NCT, but 'thought they sounded rather earnest. And I didn't want to get involved with them at that time'.[111] Geraldine's scepticism is particularly interesting as she later became very active within the NCT. Her turnaround was not a reaction to a bad birth experience, but because she came to value the social side of the NCT in enabling women to make friends with other mothers. There were also women who felt they had been misled by the natural childbirth movement into expecting a 'natural' birth which they did not then enjoy. For example Sheilagh, who had her children in the early 1970s, felt that the NCT encouraged women to have unattainably high expectations of birth, which meant they could feel like failures when these were not realized.[112] Commenting on the lack of preparation she had received for a caesarean in the early 1980s, Tara thought the NCT was to some extent at fault. She explained:

> Before I had the baby we went to the NCT classes. I suppose lots of people tell you they went to NCT classes. We had to pay for those ... But it wasn't very expensive. And they're really in favour of natural childbirth. And I think that they should've realized that me being very small and thirty-three already it was not going to be a natural childbirth situation.[113]

Harriet had decided to deliver her twins vaginally but now believed she should have had a caesarean section. She believed she had been swept up by the feeling in the mid-1980s that natural childbirth should be promoted.

> I think I thought, well, no, no, I think I ought to give it a try. So, don't be unreasonable. You know, I'm not just going to go along with what the doctors say. But if the NCT and everyone else I'm talking to seems to say 'Well, you know it's a just try and see what happens'. And I was fairly determined that that was what I was going to do.

However, Harriet now felt that 'if I knew what I know now and I went through afterwards, I think I probably shouldn't have tried to deliver them normally'.[114] Harriet's comments indicate that while interviewees could be critical of the care they received in hospital, their complaints do not imply that they were opposed to technical interventions. Indeed, with hindsight, some could feel that a greater degree of medical involvement during their pregnancy and birth would have been beneficial to them.

Conclusions

It is clear that levels of intervention in pregnancy and childbirth did dramatically increase during the 1970s. This was not unquestioningly accepted and voices criticizing these practices increased and intensified, as was evident in the debates around obstetric practices seen in the late 1970s and 1980s and the campaigns of bodies such as the NCT. However, analysing women's own accounts of these changes indicates they had a rather ambivalent response to the developments that occurred. While they did report unhappiness with some of the interventions they underwent, this seemed as much a criticism of the lack of information they received, the lack of choice they felt they had and their dissatisfaction with the hospital staff, as of their dislike of the procedures themselves. Indeed, women could feel they received excellent medical care, but criticized their treatment by hospital staff. It is striking that these are the very same complaints that I found amongst the women I interviewed for the period 1945–70. Women were still unhappy at their treatment by self-important health professionals who believed that they, rather than their patients, knew best. Women still felt they were left uninformed about the procedures being carried out and that their emotional needs were not being met. Complications and interventions were still recalled as less troubling to women who felt comfortable with and supported by their attendants. It seems it was less the interventions women were critical of, and rather it was the culture of the maternity units where they took place.

Of course, the increasing use of technology was not insignificant. Procedures such as induction, episiotomy or caesarean section did play a role in determining women's satisfaction with their care. However, when reflecting back upon their experiences from their current perspective, it is poor interpersonal relationships and their consequences that feature most prominently in the interviewees' accounts. In consequence, I would like to argue that historical accounts of maternity care which have focused simply on what was being done to women can miss the importance of subjective factors such as their knowing and liking the person who was doing it. Interviewees who objectively had similar birth experiences, for example the same length of labour, technical interventions or pain relief, could recall them very differently. Those women who said they knew and trusted their attendants, and believed they acted in their best interests, remembered their care more positively.

9 FROM *MULLER* TO *JOHNSON CONTROLS*: MOTHERS AND WORKPLACE HEALTH IN THE US, FROM PROTECTIVE LABOUR LEGISLATION TO FETAL PROTECTION POLICIES

Allison L. Hepler

Alice Hamilton, the path-breaking woman who created the field of industrial toxicology in the United States at the beginning of the twentieth century, was also a physician, factory inspector, a professor at Harvard's School of Public Health and a lifelong part-time resident of Hull House, the Chicago settlement house started by Jane Addams. She was a progressive, and one of the early experts in industrial lead poisoning, travelling to various cities throughout the nation. And in 1917 she spoke about the effects of lead poisoning in women workers. Speaking before Pennsylvania's Industrial Welfare and Efficiency Conference, Hamilton praised the increased entrance of women into nontraditional jobs in industry, but expressed a popular reservation about such moves: 'It will be no boon to women if it demands that they are to enter trades which are not fitted for them and do work which will injure their health'. Like many progressive reformers of the period, she was concerned about protecting the health of women in factories, but interestingly, she qualified her position:

> I am myself in favor of employing women in all such work so long as the danger is not one to which her sex is peculiarly liable; so long as the danger is one which a man faces equally, I think there is no reason why a woman should not face it also.[1]

In 1917, most workplace reformers focused their attention on the dangers of women working long hours. Why did Hamilton also want to examine specific hazards to reproductive health?

The short answer is because she was a scientist who preferred precise solutions. And she was a feminist who supported women's equality in many ways. But Hamilton was also a realist. She saw the effects of industry's long hours on all workers, but recognized that wage-earning mothers had families to care for, and believed that shorter factory hours would allow women time for both jobs. Also, as a strategist, Hamilton believed that laws protecting women from industrial excess were a 'foot in the door', eventually paving the way for shorter workdays for all workers, a goal of many reformers during this period. Hamilton's work during her long life formed the core of industrial toxicology in the first half of the twentieth century, and therein lies her historical significance. She is generally not remembered for her support of what would later be called 'fetal protection policies', but her view represents a small and, in retrospect, significant step toward these policies, which began to emerge in the second half of the century.

The more important question is, 'how and why did sex-based workplace policies shift in the twentieth century?' This chapter argues that a combination of factors, such as feminism, business imperatives and medicine, are inextricably linked elements in shaping workplace health in the twentieth-century United States, and also in reflecting prevailing ideas about motherhood. Workplace health policies 100 years ago promoted a definition of motherhood that was very broadly conceived – motherhood was not only about childbearing, but also child rearing, and assumed broad social and community responsibilities for all women, wage-earning or not, mothers or not. This was also true in society. Women could not vote, for example, because many believed that the 'man of the house' also spoke for his wife and family. A woman's role in society was to bear and raise children, and to maintain the household and moral standards of the community. Employment policies on working women's health and safety, therefore, reflecting the gender and class norms of this period, most commonly limited the hours that women could work, in part so that they would have time and energy to be a good mother.

By the second half of the twentieth century, ideas about motherhood, more specifically about women's role in society, began to change – motherhood was not the goal of all women, but rather only one part of some women's lives. In the workplace, this more narrow understanding of motherhood theoretically expanded women's employment opportunities, notably by recognizing that not all women were mothers but that some were, and those women merited protection in the workplace from hazards specific to reproduction.

While this chapter is not a legal history, per se, two US Supreme Court decisions bracket and represent this shift in thinking about motherhood. In *Muller* v. *Oregon* (1908), the court ruled that all women were mothers or potential mothers and that the state had a legitimate obligation in compelling employers to protect them from harm in the workplace, usually by limiting their hours in the workplace and/or placing lifting restrictions on them. In 1991, the high court, in *UAW* v. *Johnson Controls*, decreed that policies that kept all women out of jobs deemed risky to motherhood were illegal sex discrimination.[2]

This chapter traces this shift in the context of workplace health and motherhood, examining the basis for protective labour legislation in the early twentieth century, analysing how and why these laws shifted and, finally, discussing the social and political implications of *Johnson Controls*, because it raises some interesting historical parallels as well as important differences. While feminists in 1991 generally applauded the ruling in *Johnson Controls* for its recognition of equal treatment for women workers, I argue that it was, and still is, a double-edged sword. This is not to say, however, that the politics of difference offers a better deal.

Muller v. *Oregon* and Protective Labour Legislation

Curt Muller was a laundry owner in the state of Oregon who employed women to work at his shop in defiance of a 1903 state law limiting the number of hours that women could work to ten per day in factories and laundries. When the case reached the US Supreme Court in 1908, the high court had struck down a similar New York state law that limited the hours of bakery workers. In its 1905 *Lochner* v. *New York* ruling, the court concluded that the state law unconstitutionally infringed on workers' freedom of contract rights. One critical difference, however, was that bakers were men. Where women were involved, different standards applied. In *Muller* v. *Oregon*, the Supreme Court ruled that because women were at a physical and social disadvantage in the workplace and could not adequately protect themselves against the ruthlessness of the industrial world, the state had the right to protect them with workplace limitations. The court's decision also assumed that all women were mothers or potential mothers, another reason for the state to step in: government has an interest in protecting the future of the race, said the court. Evidence from scientists and physicians citing the strain of modern industry on women further persuaded the court.[3]

Examining this case through the lens of workplace health and safety, one can appreciate what it may have meant to be a woman worker at that time and also understand the motives of reformers – many of whom called themselves feminists – who supported such legislation. Some reformers saw the gendered laws as a strategy that would lead to future health and safety legislation. Others believed that in many cases, the life of a wage-earning mother was one of fatigue and poverty. These women often came home from the factory to face several hours of housework and cooking and childcare. True then and true today is the reality of women's 'double duty' or 'second shift'. Women played a key role in maintaining family and community, reformers said, and while in an ideal world women workers would have a more balanced life, the reality was that many were working themselves to death. And to be fair, protective labour legislation advocates also proposed minimum wage rules to compensate for the shorter hours, even though, in 1923, the Supreme Court ruled that establishing a minimum wage unfairly restricted a worker's freedom of contract rights.[4]

While some feminists of the time viewed the *Muller* decision as discrimina-tory, particularly the National Woman's Party, public health organizations and bureaucrats staffed by reformers were also devoted to women's rights, and saw protective labour legislation as essential in boosting the status of women work-ers. The most public battle over the nature of protective labour laws occurred in debates over the Equal Rights Amendment, which was first introduced into Congress in 1923. This proposed Constitutional Amendment to eliminate discrimination based on sex would, for all practical purposes, invalidate virtu-ally all state protective legislation if enacted.[5] In the decades to come, feminists would disagree publicly and passionately about the impact of sex-based labour legislation on women's rights. Both sides agreed on the ends, just not the means. Looking back at this debate, it is helpful to see it as portentous and still partly unresolved – are workplace rights best advanced through the special treatment of women or by treating women the same as men, exposing them to both equal protection and equal risk? With respect to workplace safety and health, sex-spe-cific protective laws, primarily in the form of limiting hours, prevailed and did not include much in the way of specificity.[6]

This is not to say that employers did not pinpoint specific health and safety problems. Quite the contrary, the trajectory of the occupational safety and health in the twentieth century was to become more precise in solving prob-lems. In part, this was due to employer incentives to keep accident and illness rates low to keep their workers' compensation premiums low. Also, by looking at particular processes, employers could more reasonably hold workers responsible for their own health – you must be ill because you did not wear the respirator correctly, says the employer, and that is not our fault.[7]

For women workers, the increased specificity could have served to increase their participation in workplaces that had previously been prohibited to them, but it did not, in part because the major policymaker and advocate for women in the workplace was the Women's Bureau, housed in the US Department of Labor, and it supported protective labour legislation as a way for women to escape longer hours of exposure to hazards. Established in 1920, the Women's Bureau deserves more attention in its historical promotion of better health for all workers. At a time when most workplace health and safety regulation was conducted at the state level, the federal offices of the Women's Bureau reached a national audience, and also provided a context for some of the workplace legisla-tion that came out of the New Deal in the 1930s. While the bureau focused its energies on female-dominated industries and its research was aimed at improv-ing the lives of working women, investigators continually pointed out the need for its recommendations to be equally applied to male workers. The bureau exhibited a remarkable combination of specificity and environmentalism. For example, its research on the many occupational diseases that affected women in the workplace also affected men. The bureau wanted to eliminate hazards for women not by prohibiting women from dangerous jobs but by cleaning up the workplace, which would benefit men as well. The bureau also noted the inconsistencies and selectivity used to restrict women from working conditions they had long faced at home, such as tedious heavy labour.[8] Nevertheless, during this period, women's work lives were governed primarily by sex-specific state laws in a professed effort to protect motherhood in society.

Wartime Changes

Changes wrought by World War II supported the Women's Bureau's contention that women were not necessarily weaker because of their sex. Foreign policy imperatives meant that employers now needed women to perform any number of jobs previously closed to them. Protective labour laws were suspended in many states for the duration of the war and the federal government did its part to persuade women that defence-related jobs in industry were now particularly suited to stereotypically female work and physical characteristics – riveting was like sewing, women's small hands were just the thing for packing bullets. Many workplace sites were re-engineered to meet the needs of women, but workers discovered that some of these changes also benefited individual men (who also came in different sizes and shapes and levels of strength). Workplace policies generally did not differentiate mothers from other women workers.[9]

By the end of World War II, state protective labour laws were back in place but they seemed even more glaringly discriminatory and arbitrary. Nora Stanton Barney, granddaughter of women's rights pioneer Elizabeth Cady Stanton, remarked that a woman could legally carry 75 pounds in Massachusetts, but in California, she would be prohibited from carrying more than 10 pounds up a flight of stairs. Aside from the dubious assertion that women in California were somehow weaker than their sisters in New England, Barney wondered how mothers were to carry their children in California.[10] In this, of course, Barney was only exposing the long-standing double standard and hypocrisy inherent in protective legislation for wage-earning women. But it also illustrates the variety and number of actual women workers who were now in the paid workforce and how they negotiated their working conditions. Indeed, historians Nancy Gabin and Dorothy Sue Cobble have described the ways in which women workers in the 1950s 'alternated between the poles of special protection and equal treatment'.[11] Double standard or no, many women workers accommodated their work to their real-life double duty, while other women, especially those in heavily male, unionized occupations sought equal opportunity and shunned sex-specific protective laws. But there was ambivalence. Even for women in traditionally male occupations like the automobile industry, protective labour laws might allow working mothers time off to take care of family responsibilities.[12]

In addition to the blanket state-wide prohibitions on women's labour in the post-war period, employers began to focus on gender-specific hazards. In 1952, General Motors implemented fetal protection policies – barring fertile women from working in areas with high lead exposure – in its foundries and later in its manufacturing and battery plants. At the time, General Motors based its decision on prevailing scientific and medical evidence, noting lead's deleterious effects on women's reproductive capacity.[13] In fact, since the late nineteenth century, medical experts knew that women who worked with lead suffered more stillbirths and spontaneous abortions.[14] Alice Hamilton was not the only scientist who had noticed this. By the 1920s, they understood that lead was stored in mothers' bones, and that fetuses drew calcium from those bones. Interestingly, scientists also knew that lead affected male fertility. But it was the continued exposure of women and developing fetuses that began to concern employers. Specific evidence of fetal harm began to emerge. Lead present in women prior to pregnancy also created risks, said public health scientist Anna Baetjer, writing in 1947, since it appeared that 'lead stored in the bones ... may be released subsequent to exposure'.[15]

Actually, General Motors may have been more worried about an issue that would be at the forefront of Johnson Controls' radar screen – tort liability not covered by workers' compensation. Workers' compensation insurance, devised and regulated by each state, protected employers from injury lawsuits brought by workers and in return provided for injured workers, but did not cover harm to their families. In 1946, a federal court permitted a suit on behalf of a child who had been injured by a physician during an emergency delivery following a car accident. The judge wrote that a viable fetus was not part of the mother, although any rights conferring to the fetus only occurred after it was born alive. Subsequent cases in the late 1940s and 1950s expanded this notion of limited fetal rights to injury sustained before viability, and raised the specter of infants damaged due to prenatal exposure to a workplace hazard suing their mothers' employer.[16] New scientific evidence and economic imperatives were now affecting employer policies regarding women workers and their role as mothers.

The 1960s and the Rise of 'Equal Treatment' and Feminism

In general, employers treated male and female workers differently, relying in part on state protective laws but also on company policies common in this period. Historians like Eileen Boris and Alice Kessler-Harris have documented the very common sex-specific disparities in terms of wages, promotion opportunities and marriage bars, for instance. These were challenged in the 1960s, raising anew conflicting ideas about women and workplace health, not only among those women workers who 'alternated between the poles of special protection and equal treatment', but also among feminists in a resurgent women's movement. Increasingly, the pendulum began to shift toward 'equal treatment'. Supporters of the equal treatment of women in the workplace were, if forced to choose, also less interested in fetal rights.[17]

Federal legislation helped promote equal treatment. Title 7 of the 1964 Civil Rights Act specifically outlawed employment discrimination based on race or sex. It also established the Equal Employment Opportunity Commission (EEOC) to adjudicate discrimination claims.[18] Nicholas Pedriana has examined the early history of the EEOC in the context of protective labour legislation. He documents an early and inconsistent interpretation of how federal law prohibiting sex discrimination in employment was to play up against state protective laws that did indeed discriminate against women. A series of decisions by the federal agency, headed primarily by policymakers sympathetic to state protective labour legislation, nevertheless leaned toward equal treatment of women in employment advertisements, for example. The agency wobbled, says Pedriana. On the one hand, it posted a number of discriminatory practices that had clearly been based on stereotypes about women workers that were now illegal under the new law. On the other hand, the EEOC refused to back them up with its rulings, leaving it up to federal courts as to whether federal law or state law would prevail in these cases.[19]

Nevertheless, the die was cast, according to Pedriana. Frustrated by the EEOC's inaction but heartened by the legal structure that had started to crumble protective laws, feminists, some of whom had been involved with strengthening the EEOC, formed their own organization in 1966, the National Organization for Women, and promptly devoted much of its activism on behalf of equal treatment of women in the workplace. It pushed the EEOC toward favouring equal treatment over protection, and by the end of the decade, EEOC had intervened in two court cases on behalf of eliminating state protective laws that imposed weight-lifting limits on women. And, by 1973, only six states, down from forty-six, had any form of sex-based state protective labour laws; by 1976, only one, Nevada.[20] These laws were not generally replaced by any statewide fetal protection policies. This would be left up to individual employers. Indeed, the closest state laws came to fetal protection policies were those that allowed some sort of accommodation for pregnant women to be temporarily transferred to alternative assignments, but left it up to employers to decide what was 'reasonable'. Two states, however, California and Connecticut, did prohibit employers from demanding sterilization as a condition of employment. This meant that employers who then tried to keep fertile women out of certain jobs would be practising illegal sex discrimination. In a sense, these state laws effectively outlawed fetal protection policies ten years before the Supreme Court acted, although no one filed a claim under these laws.[21]

The Civil Rights Act did not directly address pregnancy and childbirth. Pregnancy-related discrimination cases posed different employment issues but activists came at the issue from the same two perspectives: was pregnancy one of many 'temporary disabilities' and therefore similar to other temporary conditions that affected men and women alike, or was pregnancy to be seen as something unique to women and therefore deserving of special treatment? In 1978, the Pregnancy Discrimination Act avoided having to make that distinction by simply amending the Civil Rights Act to prohibit employers from discriminating against women who take time off for pregnancy or maternity-related matters.[22] Nothing in this Act regulated fetal protection policies.

As legislation and case law during this period moved toward an 'equal treatment' understanding of women in the workplace, other social and political changes began to make women's rights more visible to the public. In addition to employment rights, women's activism to end discriminatory practices in banking, marriage and divorce, and housing brought about significant changes in all women's lives and indeed, throughout society. 'Equal treatment' seemed dominant. But probably no issue raised more controversy than women's health, specifically reproductive health, and here is where an 'equal treatment' approach was of limited value and also where fetal rights became politicized.[23]

Others have written extensively about the political and social impact of legalized abortion in this country after the 1973 decision in *Roe* v. *Wade*, but for the purposes of this chapter, suffice to say that reproductive health received increasing attention by the public, including employers and lawmakers. Activism against abortion rights increasingly included calls for fetal rights, and it became even more of a political and scientific issue, in addition to a moral issue. Feminists who linked abortion rights with women's rights promoted women's health over that of the fetus.[24] The women's movement along with federal legislation brought about significant advancements for women in the workplace; women wage earners became less identified by their maternity, even as calls for fetal rights gained traction.

Fetal Rights and Fetal Protection

Fetal rights as a policy issue emerged beginning in the 1980s with news of an epidemic of cocaine-addicted babies. While Cynthia Daniels and others have noted the flawed nature of the research behind this conclusion, physicians and social workers nevertheless supported and encouraged the prosecution of women who abused drugs or alcohol during pregnancy and even supported a charge of manslaughter or murder in the case of a stillbirth. By the early 1990s, estimates of between 200 and 400 women had been charged with fetal abuse of some sort, although, when challenged in the courts, nearly every case had resulted in dismissal or acquittal. Nevertheless, writes Daniels, public health campaigns presented the issue as one-sided and aimed at demonizing women, despite evidence that alcohol and drug abuse also adversely affected sperm.[25]

For employers who needed its women workers, the presence of known reproductive hazards in the workplace presented a somewhat different problem, less moral and more economic. Temporarily transferring confirmed pregnant workers out of potentially hazardous working conditions was doable, but protecting workers from prenatal or pre-pregnancy exposure to known hazards was more difficult, especially since scientists and health activists concerned about working conditions were making some disturbing, if somewhat contradictory, discoveries. While some scientists worried that the emphasis on equal treatment had hindered sex-specific research on women's exposure to dangerous workplaces, nearly all agreed that simply removing women from hazardous workplaces did not guarantee a safe workplace. One researcher found an increased risk of birth defects not only in the offspring of female hospital operating room personnel but also in the children born to unexposed wives of male operating room workers.[26]

Several events in the 1970s triggered studies of male reproduction. In 1977, male workers involved in the production of the pesticide DBCP (dibromochloropropane) became aware of sterility problems; researchers later found increased rates of spontaneous abortion in the spouses of those workers. Despite research on a number of occupational exposures that demonstrated associations between paternal exposure and fetal health problems, fetal protection policies for male workers never became standard. According to Daniels, studies of paternal effects were routinely criticized because they did not control for maternal exposure (although she notes that studies of maternal exposure seldom if ever controlled for hazards experienced by fathers), and were therefore seldom used by employers.[27]

By the late 1970s, employers were avoiding the issue of workers altogether and focused on the fetus instead. Policies differed: demanding proof of women's sterility, prohibiting all women of childbearing age from certain jobs or prohibiting only pregnant women from hazardous work. At least fifteen Fortune 500 companies and numerous hospitals in some way excluded fertile or pregnant women from some jobs deemed dangerous to the fetus. In addition to Johnson Controls, this list included Shell Oil, Exxon, DuPont, American Cyanamid, Eastman Kodak, Monsanto, Union Carbide, Dow Chemical and Firestone Tire. One observer correctly predicted that fetal protection policies would become the major occupational health issue of the 1980s, and indeed, legal challenges increased during this period.[28] The most highly publicized case involved five women workers at an American Cyanamid paint plant in West Virginia who, in order to keep their jobs, underwent surgical sterilization. The factory closed a year later, leaving these women without jobs in this rural area, although they successfully sued the company on sex discrimination charges.[29] Employers, relying on science, albeit selectively, and in part responding to increased interest in fetal rights from some circles, had begun to implement fetal protection policies in the workplace.

Feminist Health Activism

Workers affected by fetal protection policies attacked them on a variety of fronts, usually without help from the federal government, the Pregnancy Discrimination Act notwithstanding. According to Rachel Roth, the EEOC simply sat on about 100 discrimination charges in the 1980s. Unionized workers also tried arbitration and collective bargaining, as well as appeals to state human rights commissions and even stockholder resolutions.[30]

Feminist health activists and women workers also fought back by bringing their concerns to the public. When women began to be eliminated from workplaces due to reproductive risks, many women workers and health activists raised the question of equal risks to men who worked in these places. Activists working on behalf of women workers, such as the Coalition for the Reproductive Rights of Workers, challenged industry to re-think its traditional gender assumptions about risks 'peculiar to female workers', often sponsoring courses and workshops along with the variety of Committees on Occupational Safety and Health groups across the country. A number of scientific conferences were held in the mid-1970s that focused on women and workplace health. At a 1975 American Academy for the Advancement of Science symposium, participants debated the biological risks to women of childbearing age in the workplace, pointing out the growing number of health risks to male workers.[31]

In 1976, the Society for Occupational and Environmental Health, federal government agencies and the March of Dimes sponsored a conference, 'Women and the Workplace', that was attended by workers, industrial hygienists, union representatives, federal scientists and policymakers and some employer physicians. While many speakers focused on the reproductive hazards to women, conferees tried to push speakers and conference organizers further. Health activists recognized women's 'double duty' in the home and workplace and their limited access to day care, the low number of women who worked in union-protected jobs and the work-related stress associated with low-paying, dead-end jobs. Several women who met at that conference – calling themselves the 'Women's Political Action-Occupational Health Caucus' – delivered a statement to the sponsors and organizers strongly critical of the 'narrow view this conference had toward women' as well as the conference's 'emphasis on technical terms and presentations' that limited access to their own understanding of the issues.[32]

At that conference, Oil, Chemical and Atomic Workers Union President Anthony Mazzochi urged participants to trust the workers: 'They weren't trained epidemiologists, but they knew just by casual observation – not knowing anything about statistics mind you – that an abnormal number of people died of a particular cancer ... or had various infirmities'. Typical was a heated exchange that took place at the same conference, where workers repeatedly criticized scientists (in government primarily) for focusing on 'statistics, figures, and dates' about worker health, these being 'things they don't have any feelings about'. Not surprisingly, a representative from the DES Action Network scolded scientists who ignored 'emotional feelings' of patients. Other women activists called the scientists' attitudes 'condescending' and 'paternalistic'. At the time, sympathetic scientists pointed out that employers would not respond solely to workers' emotions, and pleaded with workers to 'talk to us' in order to provide good data.[33]

Federal health and safety law offered limited guidance for workers or employers. In 1970, Congress enacted the Occupational Safety and Health Act and an agency (OSHA) to oversee the nation's workplaces. Since its inception, it has inspected workplaces and issued fines, and its research arm, the National Institute for Occupational Safety and Health, has developed various standards for toxic materials, but OSHA has not been the watchdog that labour hoped it would be. In the first decade, OSHA enacted several standards, provided funding for labour organizations for education and training and identified three substances – lead, ethylene oxide and the pesticide DBCP – as reproductive hazards, but its charge from the Reagan administration in the 1980s was to minimize the regulatory burden on employers.[34] Thus, a growing number of workers, feminists and health activists criticized employers and government agencies for their general inattention to workplace health and their overemphasis on fetal protection.

Fetal Protection Workplace Policies

Johnson Controls relied on OSHA's lead standard. Before being taken over by Johnson Controls in 1978, Globe Union's battery division had a voluntary fetal protection policy against lead exposure in place. It informed female workers of the risks, encouraged them to contact a physician and urged at-risk employees to transfer to other parts of the plant. Citing growing medical evidence about lead toxicity in fetuses but acknowledging disagreement over the implications of the evidence, Globe Union was nevertheless worried about the long-term effects on any of its female workers who became pregnant.[35]

Johnson Controls, a Milwaukee-based company with sixteen battery plants at the time, continued the voluntary programme until 1982, by which time eight employees in high-exposure areas and with high lead levels had become pregnant; in fact, they had higher lead levels than OSHA-recommended levels for adults. The company then implemented an involuntary policy, interestingly, one that was very similar to American Cyanamid's, which allowed only sterile or post-menopausal women to work in the high-exposure areas of the plant. It is worth noting that lead levels at the plant were said to be fully in compliance with the lead level exposures established by OSHA for adults, but it is not clear when those exposure levels were achieved. The United Auto Workers (UAW), which represented workers at the plant and had prior experience fighting these policies, finally turned to the federal courts, and filed suit under Title 7 in 1984.[36]

In defending itself, Johnson Controls not only relied on scientific evidence – some of which, ironically, was supplied by the United Auto Workers – that pointed out how lead in a pregnant woman's body poisoned the fetus's brain and nervous system (while ignoring union evidence about harm to sperm), but it also planted itself firmly in the pro-women's rights camp. The company, said corporate executives, was actually promoting gender equality by acknowledging women's childbearing ability: 'Johnson Controls wants to employ women. We have many women in good-paying, responsible jobs. What we do not want to do is put their children in jeopardy'.[37] In its pro-motherhood and pro-natalist guise, however, Johnson Controls was treating all women as potentially pregnant and did not trust any of its female employees of childbearing age to remove themselves from harm in the workplace. It was also consistent with the pro-life positions taken by the Concerned Women of America and the US Catholic Conference, both of which submitted briefs in support of the company.[38]

Also creating a climate for fetal protection policies was the growing fear of liability. In 1975, Exxon medical director Norbert Roberts announced his company's concerns in what would become a widely quoted comment. Speaking specifically about benzene, Roberts announced:

> Our recommendation probably will be that women of child-bearing age should not be exposed ... until the facts are in. If we don't take such action, we may be in trouble scientifically; and if we do, we may be in trouble legally. But we'd rather face the EEOC than a deformed baby.[39]

Despite this potential reality, Johnson Controls de-emphasized this defense, although it did come up in oral arguments.[40]

As the case made its way through the courts, workers continued to make the same arguments that health activists had made in the 1970s, namely, that both male and female workers – mothers and fathers – were at risk. In Bennington, Vermont, two women workers were able to work in areas of the plant only because they had been sterilized. Neither woman had the procedure done in order to keep their job, but both admitted that it allowed them to leave lower paying jobs in order to work at Johnson Controls, which paid substantially higher wages in the small rural town. One woman, however, was pressured into sterilization despite her husband's vasectomy. Another woman of 50, who was still fertile, was moved out of the leaded area of the plant when the involuntary policy was put in place. While Johnson Controls continued to pay her her former wages, she was disadvantaged when it came to promotions. All of these women, as well as organizations like the American Civil Liberties Union, were dismayed and angered at the plant's unwillingness to trust fertile women to make decisions for themselves.[41]

Similarly, women's health activists resisted the idea that women should be identified only by their reproductive capacity. Fetal protection policies were discriminatory, stated toxicologist Jeanne Stellman, because they assume that 'just because a woman *can* bear children, it is presumed that she *will* bear children – the perpetual pregnancy myth'. Protecting women from lead poisoning while ignoring risks to men neither 'safeguard[ed] human reproduction nor prevent[ed] the children already born from suffering the effects of lead'.[42]

The United Auto Workers also pointed out that lead was harmful to men in the plant. In fact, Johnson Controls' own health and safety monitor in the Vermont plant said that they ought to be protecting the men as well as the women. To be fair, said union officials, Johnson Controls had implemented several systems to reduce individual exposures, from a central vacuum system to individual respirators and uniforms that stayed at the plant. Nevertheless, lead particles continued to get into clothing and occasionally, the vacuum system failed. The United Auto Workers also pointed out what even conservative Justice Antonin Scalia noted, namely, that these policies were blatantly selective. 'Fertile women', according to the United Auto Workers brief, 'are not likely to be excluded wholesale from jobs as childcare workers, nurses, or dental assistants ... even though those jobs involve exposure to fetal hazards'.[43]

The federal discrimination suit filed on behalf of workers at Johnson Controls challenged the court to uphold equal treatment for women workers, and to view motherhood as a choice, not a mandate.

UAW v. *Johnson Controls*

On 20 March 1991, the US Supreme Court ruled that fetal protection policies were illegal. Johnson Controls' exclusion of all women from the workplace because some of them were pregnant or may eventually become pregnant violated Title 7 of the Civil Rights Act, specifically the elements of the Pregnancy Discrimination Act. Congress, said the court,

> indicated that the employer may take into account only the woman's ability to get her job done ... and that the decision to become pregnant or to work while either being pregnant or capable of becoming pregnant was reserved for each individual to make for herself.

Since Johnson Controls had presented no evidence that fertile women were not as capable as men in producing batteries, the company's 'professed moral and ethical concerns about the welfare of the next generation' were not a sufficient basis for legal discrimination. Moreover, the court reminded Johnson Controls that it did not express interest in the unborn children of its male workers.[44]

What impact did *Johnson Controls* have in the workplace? The modern feminist spirit that had been so outraged by the implications of *Muller* was cheered by *Johnson Controls*. In contrast to *Muller,* the court recognized that just because a woman could have a baby did not mean that she would. Furthermore, she could make informed decisions about the risks involved and not be subjected to employment policies that discriminated against women, especially since excluded jobs often brought higher pay. Writing in 1997, Cynthia Daniels praised the decision, citing the court's rejection of traditional assumptions about women, motherhood and work. The 'truly equitable workplace', she writes, recognizes and incorporates difference by requiring that '*all* of the needs specific to pregnant women [are] addressed by workplace policies, not just those that pose a liability risk to employers'.[45] Rachel Roth, in the context of her research into fetal rights, also praised the decision because of its rejection of traditional gender assumptions. She saw a potentially more far-reaching and positive possibility, one that would pass along, at least in part, the costs of a clean workplace to consumers, thereby making the larger community responsible for workplace health.[46]

More germane to this discussion is how courts have used *Johnson Controls* to limit employer responsibility for occupational safety and health. Indeed, nothing in the 1991 decision required employers to make the workplace equally safe for male and female workers, pregnant or not. The court simply ruled that employers could not exclude only women workers from a dangerous workplace. Did this decision actually result in an 'equality of misery'? Were women and men now equally free to harm themselves without recourse to their employer? Nothing in the decision forced employers to clean up the workplace for everyone.[47]

One year after the decision, a group of researchers offered a number of different possible strategies available to employers, including the following: (1) Informed consent. Such policies would fully inform the affected women workers of the risks involved in continuing to work in high-exposure areas and place responsibility back on the workers. It is not clear whether, if women were to move elsewhere in the plant, they would receive the same pay. Presumably that would be a collective bargaining issue, assuming the plant is unionized. (2) Clean up the workplace and implement suitable environmental engineering and personal protective equipment and/or reduce the lead levels in the plant. (3) Robotics. This, of course, would keep all workers from harm in this area of the plant, but would also keep many well-paying jobs (many of which were in rural areas where good jobs were hard to come by) out of reach. (4) Move overseas. In the US, countless manufacturing plants have moved overseas due to the nation's relatively high level of regulation over workplace conditions. Johnson Controls closed its battery manufacturing plant in Bennington, Vermont, in 1994, but since it merely consolidated its manufacturing elsewhere within the US, it is not likely that the court's decision was the reason.[48]

Other observers have reached contradictory conclusions. In the months immediately following the decision, journalist Susan Faludi argued that the ruling simply shifted responsibility for hazards to the women workers themselves, requiring them to sign waivers, a criticism of informed consent policies. She also noted that employers still do not trust their female employees; 'doctor's notes' are required by some. Others in the health care field, reporting a few years later, have actually noticed employers cleaning up the workplace. It is likely that both conclusions are true.[49]

In 1996, Suzanne Samuels analysed a number of lower court rulings that relied on *Johnson Controls* in the five years since the decision, and found some surprises. In subsequent lower court decisions, judges have tended to misinterpret the Supreme Court's ruling in a number of important ways. For instance, in contrast to the decision reached in *Johnson Controls*, some courts have incorrectly ruled that workplace policies that discriminate against pregnant workers are not necessarily illegal because the policy only affects pregnant women, not all women. Also, courts have used the decision to promote the 'special treatment' of women in the workplace rather than the 'equal treatment' approach clearly delineated in the *Johnson Controls* case.[50]

Another aspect of motherhood that the *Johnson Controls* case chose not to address is, of course, the question of fetal rights. Nothing in *Johnson Controls* prohibited a child born alive from suing his or her mother's employer based on injuries sustained *in utero*. While some scholars have scoffed at the likelihood of tort liability, they admit that workers' compensation insurance covers employees, not their unborn children. To date, no cases have come forward.[51] While *UAW* v. *Johnson Controls* had enshrined the concept of 'equal treatment' for women in the workplace and acknowledged that childbearing was only one part of some women's lives, its legacy remains unclear.

Conclusion

For historians, it might be helpful to see the 1991 decision as the other end of a continuum, a very broad view of motherhood in the early twentieth century that had become a much narrower one at the end of the century. Instead of the broad social responsibilities assumed by the Court in *Muller*, motherhood as a social role became more limited to childbearing. This evolution enshrines the goals of modern feminism and its promotion of equality and individualism. Treating women as individuals rather than as categories obviously carries us forward as a society. And, with respect to industrial health, it also brings responsibility. In 1977, scientist Andrea Hricko reinforced this notion, saying:

> Women have to be aware of the hazards they are exposed to so they can make judgments; so they can decide whether they want to cut down on their caffeine consumption; so they can assess what kinds of hazards they are exposed to at work. We are not going to have protection other than that which we feel we need for ourselves, and which we are willing to go after.[52]

But there are other consequences of this more narrow understanding of motherhood in the workplace. First, it runs the risk of ignoring the very real consequences of industrial health. Women's health activists like Alice Hamilton throughout this period kept an eye on the larger picture. Not only did they insist that a cleaner workplace benefited all workers, male or female, fertile or not, they also recognized how outside forces – in the home, in the community – also had an impact on workers' health. Tying workers' health to that of their offspring or potential offspring can keep that focus more broad-based and more amenable to alliances.

Second, despite the demise of fetal protection policies in the workplace, the shift toward fetal rights over maternal rights in our country has remained, and it carries risks to be aware of. The Supreme Court grants a woman autonomy over her own body with respect to abortion, yet laws also seek to criminalize a pregnant woman who drinks too much or uses drugs. Also, tying women to their reproductive capacity can be (and has been) used to limit women's choices. Too often, 'different' has been translated as 'inferior'.[53]

Still, the changes described in this chapter suggest that the history of women's political, economic and legal rights is not the only window into gender norms. Workplace health has also acted as a mirror to society, carrying its own social signals. It also provides a different way of understanding how workers have negotiated their work lives in the midst of conflicting values, laws and policies. Mothers and fathers have always had to do this when trying to make a better life for their children.

NOTES

Bryder and Greenlees, 'Western Maternity and Medicine: An Introduction'

1. Sir D. Baird, 'The Evolution of Modern Obstetrics', *Lancet*, 276:7150 (10 September 1960), pp. 557–64.

2. A. Oakley, *The Captured Womb: A History of the Medical Care of Pregnant Women* (Oxford: Basil Blackwell, 1984), pp. 2, 250; see also A. Oakley, 'The Medicalized Trap of Motherhood', *New Society*, 34 (18 December 1975), pp. 639–41, and A. Oakley, *Women Confined: Towards a Sociology of Childbirth* (New York: Schocken Books, 1980) where she 'speculates[s] about the ways in which women's treatment as mothers is associated with their oppression as women': Introduction, p. 1.

3. Oakley, *The Captured Womb*, p. 274.

4. Ibid., pp. 254–5.

5. J. W. Leavitt, *Brought to Bed: Childbearing in America 1750–1950* (New York and Oxford: Oxford University Press, 1986), p. 3.

6. Ibid., pp. 4, 5.

7. S. B. Ruzek, *The Women's Health Movement: Feminist Alternatives to Medical Control* (New York: Praeger, 1978), p. 117.

8. See S. Wells, *Our Bodies, Ourselves and the Work of Writing* (Stanford, CA: Stanford University Press, 2010); L. Umansky, *Motherhood Reconceived: Feminism and the Legacies of the Sixties* (New York and London: New York University Press, 1996). For its dissemination to New Zealand for instance, see L. Bryder, *Women's Bodies and Medical Science: An Inquiry into Cervical Cancer* (London: Palgrave Macmillan, 2010), pp. 109–11.

9. W. R. Arney, *Power and the Profession of Obstetrics* (Chicago, IL, and London: University of Chicago Press, 1982). On Arney, see C. G. Borst, 'The Professionalization of Obstetrics: Childbirth becomes a Medical Specialty', in R. D. Apple (ed.), *Women, Health, and Medicine in America: A Historical Handbook* (New York and London: Garland, 1990), pp. 204–6. For instance, he was still cited in the introduction and in three chapters in H. Marland and A. M. Rafferty (eds), *Midwives, Society and Childbirth: Debates and Controversies in the Modern Period* (London: Routledge, 1997), pp. 12, 35, 246, 269.

10. J. Lewis, *The Politics of Motherhood: Child and Maternal Welfare in England, 1900–1939* (London: Croom Helm, 1980).

11. Ibid., pp. 134–5.

12. J. Lewis, 'Mothers and Maternity Policies in the Twentieth Century', in J. Garcia, R. Kilpatrick and M. Richards (eds), *The Politics of Maternity Care: Services for Childbear-*

ing Women in Twentieth-Century Britain (Oxford: Clarendon, Oxford University Press, 1990), p. 20.

13. J. Lewis, '"Motherhood Issues" in the Late Nineteenth and Twentieth Centuries', in K. Arnup, A. Lévesque and R. Roach Pierson with the assistance of M. Brennan (eds), *Delivering Motherhood: Maternal Ideologies and Practices in the 19th and 20th Centuries* (London: Routledge, 1990), p. 12.

14. Ibid., p. 14.

15. S. Arms, *Immaculate Deception: A New Look at Women and Childbirth in America* (Boston, MA: Houghton Mifflin, 1975); G. Corea, *The Hidden Malpractice: How American Medicine Treats Women as Patients and Professionals* (New York: Morrow, 1977); B. Ehrenreich and D. English, *For Her Own Good: 150 Years of the Experts' Advice to Women* (New York: Anchor Press, 1978); M. Harrison, *A Woman in Residence* (New York: Random House, 1982); E. Martin, *The Woman in the Body: A Cultural Analysis of Reproduction* (Boston, MA: Beacon Press, 1989); A. Rich, *Of Woman Born: Motherhood as Experience and Institution* (New York: Norton, 1976); D. Scully, *Men Who Control Women's Health: The Miseducation of Obstetrician-Gynecologists* (Boston, MA: Houghton-Mifflin, 1980); N. Stoller Shaw, *Forced Labor: Maternity Care in the United States* (New York: Pergamon Press, 1978); B. Katz Rothman, *In Labor: Women and Power in the Birthplace* (New York and London: W. W. Norton, 1982); B. Katz Rothman, *Recreating Motherhood: Ideology and Technology in Patriarchal Society* (New York: W. W. Norton, 1989).

16. R. E. Davis-Floyd, *Birth as an American Rite of Passage* (Berkeley, CA, and London: University of California Press, 1992, 2nd edn, 2003), p. 5.

17. W. Mitchinson, *Giving Birth in Canada, 1900–1950* (Toronto: University of Toronto Press, 2002), p. 367.

18. J. H. Wolf, *Deliver Me From Pain: Anesthesia and Birth in America* (Baltimore, MD: Johns Hopkins University Press, 2009), p. 196.

19. M. Tew, *Safer Childbirth?: A Critical History of Maternity Care* (London: Free Association Books, 2nd edn, 1998), p. 10.

20. Ibid., p. 20.

21. J. Murphy-Lawless, *Reading Birth and Death: A History of Obstetric Thinking* (Cork: Cork University Press, 1998), p. 19.

22. Ibid., p. 20.

23. Ibid., p. 22.

24. J. Donley, *Save the Midwife* (Auckland: New Women's Press, 1986); E. Papps and M. Olssen, *Doctoring Childbirth and Regulating Midwifery in New Zealand: A Foucauldian Perspective* (Palmerston North: Dunmore Press, 1997).

25. H. Marland, 'Childbirth and Maternity', in R. Cooter and J. Pickstone, *Companion to Medicine in the Twentieth Century* (London: Routledge, 2000), pp. 559–74, on p. 567.

26. 'Introduction', V. Fildes, L. Marks and H. Marland (eds), *Women and Children First: International Maternal and Infant Welfare, 1870–1945* (London and New York: Routledge, 1992), pp. 1–2.

27. L. Marks, *Metropolitan Maternity: Maternal and Infant Welfare Services in Early Twentieth Century London* (Amsterdam: Rodopi, 1996), p. 5.

28. A. Susan Williams, *Women and Childbirth in the Twentieth Century: A History of the National Birthday Trust Fund, 1928–1993* (Stroud: Sutton, 1997).

29. K. M. Reiger, *Our Bodies, Our Babies: The Forgotten Women's Movement* (Carlton South: Melbourne University Press, 2001).

30. See also A. Nuttall, 'Maternity Charities, the Edinburgh Maternity Scheme and the Medicalisation of Childbirth, 1900–1925', *Social History of Medicine*, 24:2 (2011), pp. 370–88; A. Nuttall, '"Because of Poverty Brought into Hospital ...": A Casenote-Based Analysis of the Changing Role of the Edinburgh Royal Maternity Hospital, 1850–1912', *Social History of Medicine*, 20:2 (2007), pp. 263–80.

31. See also A. Davis, 'A Revolution in Maternity Care? Women and the Maternity Services, Oxfordshire *c.* 1948–1974', *Social History of Medicine*, 24:2 (2011), pp. 389–406.

32. Cited by J. Barrrett Litoff, 'Midwives and History', in Apple, *Women, Health, and Medicine in America*, pp. 443–58, on p. 446; B. Ehrenreich and D. English, *Witches, Midwives and Nurses: A History of Women Healers* (Oyster Bay, NY: Glass Mountain Pamphlets, 1973).

33. J. Donnison, *Midwives and Medical Men: A History of the Struggle for the Control of Childbirth* (London: Historical Publications, 1988); first published as *Midwives and Medical Men: A History of Inter-Professional Rivalry and Women's Rights* (London: Heinemann Educational Books, 1977), p. 174.

34. Donnison, *Midwives and Medical Men*, p. 208.

35. Ibid., pp. 208–9.

36. Tew, *Safer Childbirth?*, pp. 7, 20.

37. C. G. Borst, *Catching Babies: The Professionalization of Childbirth, 1870–1920* (Cambridge, MA: Harvard University Press, 1995), p. 11.

38. T. McKeown, *The Role of Medicine: Dream, Mirage or Nemesis?* (London: Nuffield Provincial Hospitals Trust, 1976).

39. I. Loudon, 'Midwives and the Quality of Maternal Care', in Marland and Rafferty (eds), *Midwives, Society and Childbirth,* pp. 180–200, on pp. 196–7 (his emphasis). I. Loudon, 'Obstetric Care, Social Class, and Maternal Mortality', *British Medical Journal* (*hereafter BMJ*), 293 (1986), pp. 606–8; I. Loudon, 'Maternal Mortality: 1880–1950. Some Regional and International Comparisons', *Social History of Medicine*, 1:2 (1988), pp. 183–227; I. Loudon, *Death in Childbirth: An International Study of Maternal Care and Maternal Mortality, 1800–1950* (Oxford: Clarendon Press, 1992); I. Loudon, 'The Transformation of Maternal Mortality', *BMJ*, 305 (1992), pp. 1557–60.

40. Mitchinson, *Giving Birth in Canada*, p. 159.

41. Leavitt, *Brought to Bed*, p. 192.

42. M. M. Grehan, 'Professional Aspirations and Consumer Expectations: Nurses, Midwives and Women's Health' (PhD dissertation, University of Melbourne, 2009), pp. 254, 312.

43. Loudon, *Death in Childbirth*, p. 227.

44. Mitchinson, *Giving Birth in Canada*, p. 7.

45. See also W. Mitchinson, 'Agency, Diversity, and Constraints: Women and the Physicians, Canada, 1850–1950', in The Feminist Health Care Ethics Research Network, S. Sherwin (co-ordinator), *The Politics of Women's Health: Exploring Agency and Autonomy* (Philadelphia, PA: Temple University Press, 1998), pp. 122, 127, 146 note 3.

46. Mitchinson, *Giving Birth in Canada*, p. 10.

47. See also S. Al-Gailani, 'Teratology and the Clinic: Monsters, Obstetrics and the making of Antenatal Life in Edinburgh, *c.* 1900' (PhD dissertation, Cambridge University, 2010).

48. Fathers have only recently entered the stage of maternity histories: See J. Walzer Leavitt, *Make Room for Daddy: The Journey from Waiting Room to Birthing Room* (Chapel Hill, NC: University of North Carolina Press, 2009); L. Bryder, 'Tensions in the Birthing Room: Fathers and Childbirth during the Second Half of the Twentieth Century', paper

delivered to *Past Tensions: Reflections on Making History, New Zealand Historical Association Biennial Conference*, University of Waikato, Hamilton, 16–18 November 2011.

49. R. Arditti, R. Duelli Klein and S. Minden (eds), *Test-Tube Women: What Future for Motherhood?* (London: Pandora Press, 1984). See most recently, S. Dubow, *Ourselves Unborn: A History of the Fetus in Modern America* (Oxford: Oxford University Press, 2011). On abortion, see L. Reagan, *When Abortion was a Crime: Women, Medicine and the Law in the United States, 1867–1973* (Berkeley, CA: University of California Press, 1997); L. Gordon, *The Moral Property of Women: A History of Birth Control Politics in America*, 3rd edn (Chicago, IL: University of Illinois Press, 2007) among others.

50. On race and childbirth history in Western countries see, for example, P. Jasen, 'Race, Culture, and the Colonization of Childbirth in Northern Canada', *Social History of Medicine*, 10:3 (1997), pp. 383–400; H. Mountain Harte, 'Home Births to Hospital Births: Interviews with Maori Women who had their babies in the 1930s', *Health and History*, 3:1 (2001), pp. 87–108; A. Harris, 'I wouldn't say I was a Midwife': Interviews with Violet Otene Harris', *Health and History*, 3:1 (2001), pp. 109–23; V. L. Kennedy, *Born Southern: Childbirth, Motherhood, and Social Networks in the Old South* (Baltimore, MD: Johns Hopkins University Press, 2010); and A. D. Danzi, *From Home to Hospital: Jewish and Italian American Women and Childbirth, 1920–1940* (Lanham, MD: University Press of America, 1997).

1 Grehan, 'Safely Delivered? Insights into Late Nineteenth-Century Australian Maternity Care from Coronial Investigations into Maternal Deaths'

1. See for example, R. Linn, *Angels of Mercy: District Nursing in South Australia 1894–1994* (Norwood: Royal District Nursing Society of South Australia Inc., 1993); B. Abel-Smith, *A History of the Nursing Profession* (London: Heinemann, 1960); M. A. Nutting and L. L. Dock, *A History of Nursing; the Evolution of Nursing Systems from Earliest Times to the Foundation of the First English and American Training Schools for Nurses* (New York: G. P. Putnam's sons, 1907–1912); S. A. Tooley, *A History of Nursing in the British Empire* (London: S. H. Bousefield, 1906); F. Meyer, 'Medical Practice in Australia', in British Medical Association (ed.), *The Book of Melbourne, Australia 1935* (Melbourne: British Medical Association, 1935), pp. 73–88.

2. See K. Fahy, 'An Australian History of the Subordination of Midwifery', *Women and Birth – Journal of the Australian College of Midwives*, 20:1 (2007), pp. 25–9; L. Barclay, 'Australian Midwifery Training and Practice', *Midwifery – Journal of the Australian College of Midwives*, 1 (1985), pp. 86–96; N. Purcal, 'The Politics of Midwifery Education and Training in New South Wales during the last Decades of the 19th Century', *Women and Birth – Journal of the Australian College of Midwives*, 21:1 (2008), pp. 21–5; A. D. Summers, ''For I Have Ever so Much More Faith in her Ability as a Nurse': The Eclipse of the Community Midwife in South Australia, 1836–1942' (PhD dissertation, Flinders University, Adelaide, 1995).

3. M. Grehan, 'Professional Aspirations and Consumer Expectations: Nurses, Midwives, and Women's Health' (PhD dissertation, University of Melbourne, 2009), p. 145.

4. Australian Government, Department of Foreign Affairs and Trade, at http://www.dfat.gov.au/aib/island_continent.html [accessed 20 May 2011].

5. These figures are compiled from Victoria's *Parliamentary Papers*, specifically the Statistical Registers.
6. Grehan, 'Professional Aspirations and Consumer Expectations', p. 152.
7. Ibid., p. 153.
8. L. Frost, *No Place for a Nervous Lady: Voices from the Australian Bush* (Melbourne: McPhee Gribble, 1984), p. 176.
9. Grehan, 'Professional Aspirations and Consumer Expectations', p. 128.
10. J. McCalman, *Sex and Suffering: Women's Health and a Women's Hospital* (Melbourne: Melbourne University Press, 1996).
11. These data are calculated using a combination of the *Statistical Registers of Victoria* (Censuses) and summaries of the Women's Hospital's Midwifery Books in McCalman, *Sex and Suffering*, pp. 370–1.
12. *Coroners Act 1890* (Vic). 54 Vict, no. 1077, at http://www.austlii.edu.au/au/legis/vic/hist_act/ca1890120.pdf [accessed 24 July 2010].
13. J. Rangelov, 'The Port Phillip Magistrates 1835–1851' (PhD dissertation, Victoria University Melbourne, 2005), p. 211.
14. Public Record Office Victoria (hereafter PROV), VPRS 24/P0000, unit 494, 1886/302. Proceedings of Inquest into the Death of Jane Renton at Harrietville.
15. Women could be involved if they happened to be a licensed victualler. Under Section 16 of the *Coroners Act 1890* (Vic), licensed victuallers were required to house a body for post mortem and to accommodate the subsequent inquest or inquiry.
16. *Courts and Criminal Justice – Inquest Records, Public Record Office of Victoria* (Guide no. 71, at http://www.access.prov.vic.gov.au/public/PROVguides/PROVguide071/PROVguide071.jsp [accessed 1 June 2007].
17. *Coroners Act 1890* (Vic), s 6. Magisterial Inquiries did not have this power.
18. Generally, newspapers carried reports of inquiries into maternal deaths in columns reporting on all inquests conducted in a given locality. Occasionally, cases were reported in greater detail, but the extent of reporting varies enormously.
19. M. Knight, *Inquest Index-Victoria 1840–1985* (Hampton: Macbeth Genealogical Services, 2000). It consists of around 240,000 inquests conducted in Victoria from 1840 to 1985.
20. Not until the *Midwives Act 1915* (Vic) was passed were there requirements for the reporting of a death in childbirth, but even this did not apply to doctors under the Act. Dr Wendy Pollock, an Australian midwifery and intensive care nursing academic, argues that capturing maternal death data continues to be problematic. See W. Pollock, 'Critically Ill Pregnant and Post-natal Women in Victoria: Characteristics, Severity of Illness, and the Provision of Acute Health Services' (PhD dissertation, The University of Melbourne, 2008).
21. For example, the cause of death is sometimes recorded as the locality where it occurred. In three cases examined, investigations into male deaths listed 'ruptured uterus' as the cause of death.
22. Taxonomies changed over time. By the 1890s, 'haemorrhage' was used in place of 'flooding'. Notably 'fitting in parturition' or eclampsia is listed once only. Eclampsia is a manifestation of very high blood pressure in pregnancy. Its precursor, pre-eclampsia, is known to occur in 1–2 per cent of the maternity population. Pre-eclampsia deaths may have been categorized as Bright's disease, dropsy or even epilepsy in accordance with medical understandings of the time.

23. The abortion deaths resulted from infection. In the twenty year period examined, only one case (that of Florence Waddilove 1883/1496) was listed as 'blood poisoning' *and* 'childbirth'. Termination in that case was suspected to have taken place at seven months' gestation. For more on abortion, see S. Swain and R. Howe, *Single Mothers and their Children: Disposal, Punishment and Survival in Australia*. (Melbourne: Cambridge University Press, 1995). For more on the consequences of abortion, see McCalman, *Sex and Suffering*.

24. M. Grehan, 'A Most Difficult and Protracted Labour Case', *Provenance – Journal of Public Record Office Victoria*, 8 (2009), pp. 63–74.

25. *Argus*, 15 October 1881, p. 13. The accuracy of Jamieson's assessment that maternal deaths in Victoria were 'excessive' is hard to assess, given the deficits in the reporting system, but it is possible to compare his mortality figures with the maternal mortality ratio (MMR) in Australia today. The MMR is the number of reported maternal deaths per 100,000 births. Jamieson's 1874 (MMR 981/100,000) and 1880 (1112/100,000) figures are far greater than Australia's 2010 MMR (8–12/100,000). It is probable that Jamieson's statistics were an underestimate of the real incidence of maternal mortality in the late nineteenth century, given that many maternity related deaths were not recognized and not reported. For more on current MMRs, see *Trends in Maternal Mortality 1990–2008: Estimates Developed by WHO, UNICEF, UNFPA, and The World Bank* (2010). It is sobering to note that Jamieson's 1880 estimates correlate with the 2010 MMR for Afghanistan, Sierra Leone and similar countries. For more on maternal morbidity, see W. Pollock, E. Sullivan, S. Nelson and J. King, 'Capacity to Monitor Severe Maternal Morbidity in Australia', *Australian Journal of Obstetrics and Gynaecology*, 48 (2008), pp. 17–25. I thank Dr Pollock for her valuable input into interpreting MMRs.

26. *Argus*, 26 January 1883, p. 9. That year, there were 27,541 registered births in Victoria. See also G. Strachan, 'Present at the Birth: "Handywomen" and Neighbours in Rural New South Wales 1850–1900', *Labour History*, 81 (2001), pp. 13–27; T. Pensabene, *The Rise of the Medical Practitioner in Victoria*, Australian National University, Health Research Project Monograph no. 2 (Canberra: Australian National University, 1980); Swain and Howe, *Single Mothers and their Children*.

27. *Argus*, 24 February 1880, p. 7.

28. *Argus*, 6 April 1882, p. 6.

29. PROV, VPRS 24/P0000, unit 596, 1892/529, Proceedings of Magisterial Inquiry into the Death of Elisabeth Welsh at Langi Kal Kal. Evidence is presented as recorded, without adding grammar.

30. PROV, VPRS 24/P0000, unit 560, 1890/355, Proceedings of Inquest into the Death of Ann Hayes at Hardie's Hill, Buninyong.

31. PROV, VPRS 24/P0000, unit 497, 1886/554, Proceedings of Inquest into the Death of Mary O'Connor at Inglewood Road, Sandhurst.

32. PROV, VPRS 24/P0000, unit 507, 1886/1525, Proceedings of Inquest into the Death of Margaret Jones at Derinallum. Whether Mrs Edgar was a midwife was not stated.

33. PROV, VPRS 24/P0000, unit 600, 1892/956, Proceedings of Inquest into the Death of Alice Elisabeth Richardson at Rhyll, Phillip Island.

34. PROV, VPRS 24/P0000, unit 423, 1881/649, Proceedings of Inquest into the Death of Mary Ann Kilmartin at Gigarre East.

35. *Herald*, 5 February 1892, p. 5.

36. PROV, VPRS 24/P0000, unit 545, 1889/644, Proceedings of Inquest into the Death of Margaret Pitt Martin at Footscray.

37. Grehan, 'Professional Aspirations and Consumer Expectations', p. 141. Up to the 1920s in Victoria, under the related legislation, it was possible for a woman to take up midwifery practice without any training in a maternity hospital. According to a survey of the midwifery field in the mid-1920s by the inaugural Professor of Obstetrics at the University of Melbourne, almost a third of private maternity hospitals in Victoria were run by women without a certificate in midwifery. See Grehan, 'Professional Aspirations and Consumer Expectations', p. 237.

38. Only eighty nurses completed training in the twenty years from 1861 to 1880. Grehan located thirty-three certifications from 1861 to 1873 inclusive and Jamieson (*Argus*, 26 January 1883, p. 9) reported thirty-four completions from 1873 to 1880. In this period, the average yearly number of registered births was 428,000. Thus it is unlikely this innovative local model in the care of women had much impact on standards of maternity care.

39. Up to the 1880s, newspaper editorials criticized female midwives as well as herbalists, dentists and other people untrained in medicine who attended maternity cases. From the 1880s, criticism of female attendants appears to have abated. See Grehan, 'Professional Aspirations and Consumer Expectations', p. 148.

40. See S. Curtis, 'Midwives and their Role in the Reduction of Direct Obstetric Deaths during the Late Nineteenth Century: The Sundsvall Region of Sweden 1860–1890', *Medical History*, 49 (2005), pp. 321–50; I. Loudon, *Death in Childbirth: An International Study of Maternal Care and Maternal Mortality, 1800–1950* (Oxford: Clarendon Press, 1992), p. 388.

41. 1886/302, Proceedings of Inquest into the Death of Jane Renton.

42. In the 1860s it was thought that giving birth while squatting, or on all fours, encouraged rupture of the perineum. See *Australian Medical Journal*, 6 (1861), p. 224.

43. PROV, VPRS 24/P0000, unit 642, 1895/599, Proceedings of Inquest into the Death of Mrs Alice Rochford at Cheritta.

44. Ibid.

45. 1889/644, Inquest into the Death of Margaret Pitt Martin. The use of abdominal binders to encourage the uterus to shrink had fallen out of favour by the 1850s.

46. 1889/644, Inquest into the Death of Margaret Pitt Martin.

47. *Argus*, 8 May 1889, p. 9. The sense is that the rumours inferred possible negligence by the midwife, although this is not stated.

48. W. Balls-Headley, 'Antiseptic Midwifery', Reprint from *Medical Journal of Australia*, 15 July 1888, p. 7. Dr Ball-Headley Pamphlets, University of Melbourne Special Collections.

49. 1881/649, Inquest into the Death of Mary Ann Kilmartin.

50. 1889/644, Inquest into the Death of Margaret Pitt Martin; 1886/1525, Inquest into the Death of Margaret Jones; 1886/554, Inquest into the Death of Mary O'Connor.

51. *Argus*, 3 February 1892, p. 7.

52. McCalman, *Sex and Suffering*, p. 47.

53. 1886/554, Inquest into the Death of Mary O'Connor.

54. *Kilmore Free Press*, 27 May 1886, p. 4.

55. *Argus*, 28 August 1881, p. 10. The records of this inquest were not located because the file bearing Mrs Pollovineo's name held files relating to a male death. This occurred in three of the inquest records examined.

56. *Argus*, 22 January 1883, p. 7.

57. See Grehan, 'A Most Difficult and Protracted Labour Case', pp. 69–70; Grehan, 'Professional Aspirations and Consumer Expectations', p. 147.

58. Two deaths reported in newspapers as subject to inquest involved the administration of drugs: laudanum and chloroform. These are the deaths of Mrs Mary Jane Stones (*Argus*, 21 March 1885, p. 11); Mrs Jessie Missen (*Argus*, 29 April 1896, p. 7). These deaths are not listed in Knight's *Index*. Two other deaths were categorized as erysipelas (Group A beta haemolytic Streptococci infection) following delivery of a baby at term; one of these files was missing.

59. Horse travel was complicated in itself in these circumstances. Draft horses (work horses, not race horses) were what most rural dwellers owned. A draft horse, in good condition, could canter a distance of 50 km in approximately four hours. At night, the speed travelled depended on how well a horse could navigate in the dark. I am indebted to Max Marriott for his knowledge on horse travel in late nineteenth-century Victoria.

60. 1892/529, Inquiry into the Death of Elisabeth Welsh.

61. PROV, VPRS 24/P0000, unit 595, 1892/425, Proceedings of Inquest into the Death of Elizabeth Cook at Annandale.

62. *Camperdown Chronicle*, 25 December 1886, p. 2. Mrs Jones may have been a diabetic, given the reference to the 'enormous' sized infant.

63. 1881/649, Inquest into the Death of Mary Ann Kilmartin.

64. Grehan, 'Professional Aspirations and Consumer Expectations', p. 145.

65. Ibid., p. 146.

66. The author observed this mechanism still to be in use in 1985 in the jungle areas of Panama, where older women sat themselves on the abdomen of women to hasten labour.

67. D. Porter, *Health, Civilization and the State: A History of Public Health from Ancient to Modern Times* (London: Routledge, 1999), p. 143.

68. McCalman, *Sex and Suffering*, p. 56.

69. Grehan, 'A Most Difficult and Protracted Labour Case', on p. 68. The condition of a body was reported upon in each examination.

70. 1890/355, Inquest into the Death of Ann Hayes.

71. 1886/302, Inquest into the Death of Jane Renton.

72. PROV, VPRS 24/P0000, unit 415, 1880/165, Proceedings of Inquest into the Death of Nannie William Thomas at Long Gully, Sandhurst.

73. 1889/644, Inquest into the Death of Margaret Pitt Martin.

74. 1886/554, Inquest into the Death of Mary O'Connor.

75. *Herald*, 11 January 1892, p. 2.

76. *Argus*, 9 January 1892, p. 8.

77. PROV, VPRS 24/P0000, unit 502, 1886/1016, Proceedings of Inquest into the Death of Georgina Elisabeth Graham at the Melbourne Hospital.

78. *Age*, 6 February 1892, p. 10.

79. 1895/599, Inquest into the Death of Mrs Alice Rochford.

80. *Age*, 6 February, p. 10.

81. 1892/529, Inquiry into the Death of Elisabeth Welsh.

82. Sweetnam was correct. Practically speaking, a caesarean section, then a new and risky operation, was necessary. Fetal destruction in utero was the only option.

83. *Camperdown Chronicle*, 22 December 1886, p. 2.

84. 1889/644, Inquest into the Death of Margaret Pitt Martin.

85. *Argus*, 21 March 1885, p. 11. As this inquest file is missing, it is unclear where Thompson obtained her certificate, or if she signed her deposition. The deceased was administered one and three quarter ounces of laudanum.

86. *Argus*, 21 March 1885, p. 11.

87. *Argus*, 7 July 1885, p. 6.
88. *Argus*, 17 July 1885, p. 7.
89. *Age*, 6 February 1892, p. 10.
90. *Age*, 6 February 1892, p. 10.
91. *Argus*, 8 May 1889, p. 9.
92. 1895/599, Inquest into the Death of Mrs Alice Rochford.
93. J. Jamieson, 'Childbirth Mortality in the Australian Colonies', *Transactions of the First Intercolonial Medical Congress of Australasia*. Adelaide, August–September 1887, p. 272.
94. Grehan, 'Professional Aspirations and Consumer Expectations', p. 164.
95. P. Grimshaw, 'Gendered Settlements', in P. Grimshaw, M. Lake, A. McGrath and M. Quartly (eds), *Creating a Nation* (Ringwood, Victoria: McPhee Gribble, 1994), p. 194.
96. Grehan, 'Professional Aspirations and Consumer Expectations', pp. 197–8.
97. Ibid., p. 241.
98. Ibid., p. 318.

2 Al-Gailani, 'Pregnancy, Pathology and Public Morals: Making Antenatal Care in Edinburgh around 1900'

1. G. F. McCleary, 'Safer Motherhood', *The Times*, 30 September 1937, p. 51.
2. Ibid., p. 51.
3. P. Thane, *The Foundations of the Welfare State* (London: Longman, 1982), p. 102.
4. For antenatal care: A. Oakley, *The Captured Womb: A History of the Medical Care of Pregnant Women* (Oxford: Basil Blackwell, 1984). For the politics of motherhood *c.* 1900: L. Bryder, *A Voice for Mothers: Infant Welfare and the Plunket Society, 1907–2000* (Auckland: Auckland University Press, 2003); R. Cooter (ed.), *In the Name of the Child: Health and Welfare 1880–1940* (London: Routledge, 1992); A. Davin, 'Imperialism and Motherhood', *History Workshop Journal*, 5:1 (1978), pp. 9–66; A. Digby and J. Stewart (eds), *Gender, Health and Welfare* (London: Routledge, 1996); D. Dwork, *War is Good for Babies and Other Young Children: A History of the Infant and Child Welfare Movement in England* (London: Tavistock, 1987); C. Dyhouse, 'Working-Class Mothers and Infant Mortality in England, 1895–1914', *Journal of Social History*, 12:2 (1978), pp. 248–66; V. Fildes, L. Marks and H. Marland (eds), *Women and Children First: International Maternal and Infant Welfare* (London: Routledge, 1992); J. Lewis, *The Politics of Motherhood: Child and Maternal Welfare in England, 1900–1939* (London: Croom Helm, 1980); L. Marks, *Metropolitan Maternity: Maternal and Infant Welfare Services in Early Twentieth Century London* (Amsterdam: Rodopi, 1996).
5. See above, n. 4. For international perspectives: R. G. Fuchs, *Poor and Pregnant in Paris: Strategies for Survival in the Nineteenth Century* (New Brunswick, NJ: Rutgers University Press, 1992), pp. 112–25; A. Klaus, *Every Child a Lion: The Origins of Maternal and Infant Health Policy in the United States and France, 1890–1920* (Ithaca, NY: Cornell University Press, 1993); J. McCalman, *Sex and Suffering: Women's Health and a Women's Hospital: The Royal Women's Hospital, Melbourne 1856–1996* (Carlton: Melbourne University Press, 1998), pp. 153–65; R. Meckel, *'Save the Babies': American Public Health Reform and the Prevention of Infant Mortality* (Baltimore, MD: Johns Hopkins University Press, 1990); W. Mitchinson, *Giving Birth in Canada, 1900–1950* (Toronto: University of Toronto Press, 2002), pp. 104–57; W. Schneider, *Quality and Quantity:*

The Quest for Regeneration in Twentieth-Century France (Cambridge: Cambridge University Press, 1990), pp. 55–83.

6. G. F. McCleary, *The Maternity and Child Welfare Movement* (London: P. S. King, 1935); C. Hanson, *A Cultural History of Pregnancy: Pregnancy, Medicine and Culture, 1750–2000* (Basingstoke: Palgrave Macmillan, 2006), p. 8; Meckel, *'Save the Babies'*, p. 162; H. McHold, 'Diagnosing Difference: The Scientific, Medical and Popular Engagement with Monstrosity in Victorian Britain' (PhD dissertation, Northwestern University, 2002), pp. 235–72; Oakley, *The Captured Womb*, pp. 46–50.

7. Ann Oakley's still-authoritative account first recovered Ferguson's involvement, but underplayed the following generation of Edinburgh obstetricians' efforts to integrate his contribution into the history of antenatal care: Oakley, *The Captured Womb*, p. 50; 'Memorial to Dr Haig Ferguson', *British Medical Journal* (hereafter *BMJ*), 3831:1 (1934), p. 1049; R. W. Johnstone, 'Fifty Years of Midwifery', *BMJ*, 4644:1 (1950), pp. 12–16.

8. A. Nuttall, 'Maternity Charities, the Edinburgh Maternity Scheme and the Medicalisation of Childbirth, 1900–1925', *Social History of Medicine*, 24:2 (2011), pp. 370–88 assesses the impact of the scheme on maternity care in the city and highlights the long-term contributions of voluntary agencies.

9. Johnstone, 'Fifty Years of Midwifery'; F. J. Browne, 'The Initiation and Development of Antenatal Care', in J. M. Munro Kerr, R. W. Johnstone and M. H. Phillips (eds), *Historical Review of British Obstetrics and Gynaecology 1800–1950* (Edinburgh: E. & S. Livingstone, 1954), pp. 145–57; J. Sturrock, 'Early Maternity Hospitals in Edinburgh', *British Journal of Obstetrics and Gynaecology*, 65:1 (1958), pp. 122–31.

10. See especially Oakley, *The Captured Womb*.

11. Ibid., p. 28.

12. T. Bull, *Hints to Mothers* (London: Longmans, Green, 1877), p. 49.

13. L. Reid, 'Childbirth', in S. Storrier (ed.), *Scottish Life and Society: Scotland's Domestic Life* (Edinburgh: John Donald, 2006), pp. 440–57, on p. 443.

14. Johnstone, 'Fifty Years of Midwifery', p. 13.

15. R. Mander and A. Nuttall (eds), *James Young Simpson, Lad o' Pairts* (Scottish History Press, Edinburgh, 2011).

16. Obituary of A. R. Simpson, *BMJ*, 2885:1 (1916), p. 572–4, on p. 572.

17. For biographical details on Ballantyne: *BMJ*, 3240:1 (1923), pp. 213–6; H. Russell, *J. W. Ballantyne M. D., F.R.C.P.Edin., F.R.S.E. 1861–1923* (Edinburgh: Royal College of Physicians of Edinburgh, 1971).

18. *Scotsman*, 8 February 1911, p. 7. On temperance in Scotland: T. C. Smout, *A Century of the Scottish People* (London: Fontana, 1987), p. 144.

19. On alcohol and degeneration theory: W. F. Bynum, 'Alcohol and Degeneration in Nineteenth-Century European Medicine and Psychiatry', *British Journal of Addiction*, 79:4 (1984), pp. 59–70.

20. Obituary of A. R. Simpson, *British Weekly*, 13 April 1916, p. 31.

21. *British Weekly*, 1 February 1923, p. 397. Stefan Collini uses the term 'public moralists' for a broad spectrum of largely metropolitan intellectuals: S. Collini, *Public Moralists: Political Thought and Intellectual Life in Britain, 1850–1930* (Oxford: Clarendon Press, 1991). I use it here more narrowly to refer to individuals involved with such groups as the National Council for Public Morals.

22. C. Lawrence, 'The Shaping of Things to Come: Scottish Medical Education 1700–1939', *Medical Education*, 40:3 (2006), pp. 212–8, on p. 217.

23. For Ballantyne's teratology: McHold, 'Diagnosing Difference', pp. 235–72; S. Al-Gailani, 'Teratology and the Clinic: Monsters, Obstetrics and the Making of Antenatal Life in Edinburgh *c.* 1900' (PhD dissertation, Cambridge University, 2010).

24. On pathology museums: S. Alberti, *Morbid Curiosities: Medical Museums in Nineteenth-Century Britain* (Oxford: Oxford University Press, 2011). On embryology: F. Churchill, 'Chabry, Roux, and the Experimental Method', in R. Giere and R. Westfall (eds), *Foundations of Scientific Method: The Nineteenth Century* (Bloomington, IN: Indiana University Press, 1973), pp. 161–205. On alienism and anthropology: C. E. Russett, *Sexual Science: The Victorian Construction of Womanhood* (Cambridge, MA: Harvard University Press, 1991), p. 68.

25. J. W. Ballantyne (autobiography) Acc. 13189, MS National Library of Scotland (hereafter NLS Acc. 13189), vol. 18, fol. 151.

26. J. W. Ballantyne, *Manual of Antenatal Pathology and Hygiene: The Foetus*; and *The Embryo* (Edinburgh: William Green, 1902; 1904).

27. Al-Gailani, 'Teratology and the Clinic'.

28. NLS Acc. 13189, vol. 18, fol. 59.

29. J. W. Ballantyne, *Expectant Motherhood: Its Supervision and Hygiene* (London: Cassell, 1914), p. xiv.

30. J. W. Ballantyne, 'On Antenatal Therapeutics', *BMJ*, 1998:1 (1899), pp. 889–93, on pp. 889, 893.

31. Ballantyne, *Manual: The Foetus*, p. 15.

32. 'Some Economic Aspects of Antenatal Pathology', *BMJ*, 2060:1 (1900), p. 1547. On abortion debates around 1900: J. Keown, *Abortion, Doctors, and the Law: Some Aspects of the Legal Regulation of Abortion in England from 1803 to 1982* (Cambridge: Cambridge University Press, 1988), pp. 49–78.

33. On debates over midwives' registration: J. Donnison, *Midwives and Medical Men: A History of the Struggle for the Control of Childbirth* (London: Historical Publications, 1977), pp. 159–74.

34. Schneider, *Quality and Quantity*, p. 73.

35. Ballantyne, *Expectant Motherhood*, pp. 236–77.

36. Ballantyne, *Manual: The Embryo*, p. 466.

37. Ballantyne, 'On Antenatal Therapeutics', p. 890; T. C. Allbutt, 'Address on Tuberculosis', *Practitioner*, 70:1 (1903), pp. 145–54, on p. 153.

38. NLS Acc. 13189, vol. 18, fol. 147.

39. G. Jones, *Social Hygiene in Twentieth-Century Britain* (London: Croom Helm, 1986); F. Mort, *Dangerous Sexualities: Medico-Moral Politics in England since 1830* (London: Routledge, 1987).

40. J. W. Ballantyne, 'A Plea for a Pro-Maternity Hospital', *BMJ*, 2101:1 (1901), pp. 813–4. He dropped the prefix 'pro' (Greek 'before') for the Latin 'pre' to avoid confusion: Ballantyne, *Manual: The Foetus*, p. 465.

41. RMH Annual Reports, Lothian Health Services Archive, Edinburgh (hereafter LHSA) LHB 3/7; A. Nuttall, '"Because of Poverty Brought into Hospital …": A Casenote-Based Analysis of the Changing Role of the Edinburgh Royal Maternity Hospital, 1850–1912', *Social History of Medicine*, 20:2 (2007), pp. 263–80.

42. For the history of the RMH: Nuttall, '"Because of Poverty"'.

43. *Scottish Medical and Surgical Journal*, 10:1 (1902), p. 151. Surviving admissions records for the period before 1876, however, show that it was not uncommon for women to be admitted more than one week before they gave birth: W. P. Ward, *Birth Weight and*

Economic Growth: Women's Living Standards in the Industrializing West (Chicago, IL: University of Chicago Press, 1993), p. 37.

44. RMH Hamilton Ward Casebook, LHSA LHB 3/17/19.
45. J. W. Ballantyne, 'Valedictory Address on Hospital Treatment of Morbid Pregnancies', *BMJ*, 2454:1 (1908), pp. 65–71, on p. 70.
46. The Salvation Army opened shelters for single pregnant women and a maternity hospital in London in the 1880s: A. Higginbotham, 'Respectable Sinners: Salvation Army Rescue Work with Unmarried Mothers, 1884–1914', in G. Malmgreen (ed.), *Religion in the Lives of English Women* (Bloomington, IN: Indiana University Press, 1986), pp. 216–33; R. G. Kunzel, *Fallen Women, Problem Girls: Unmarried Mothers and the Professionalization of Social Work, 1890–1945* (New Haven, CT: Yale University Press, 1993).
47. 'Memorial to Dr Haig Ferguson', *BMJ*, 3831:1 (1934), p. 1049.
48. Lauriston Home Annual Reports (Edinburgh: The Darien Press) Acc.6313, NLS (hereafter NLS Acc.6313), 1913, fol. 12; 1914, fols 9–10.
49. E. Lundberg and K. Lenroot, *Illegitimacy as a Child Welfare Problem* (Washington, DC: US Department of Labor, Children's Bureau, 1920), p. 14.
50. NLS Acc.6313, 1912, fols 7–9.
51. Annual reports included statistics about applicants to the home between 1908 and 1919, during which time 711 women and girls were given shelter. Most were between 18 and 23, with the youngest aged only 13. The majority of applicants were employed in domestic service, while a significant number came from their own homes and were in no settled work.
52. NLS Acc.6313, 1916, fol. 9.
53. NLS Acc.6313, 1912, fol. 8; 1913, fol. 4.
54. NLS Acc.6313, 1909, fol. 4; 1912, fol. 4; 1913, fols 10–11.
55. NLS Acc.6313, 1914, fol. 5.
56. Ballantyne, 'A Plea for a Pro-Maternity Hospital', p. 813.
57. 'Discussion on Fatal Cases of Jaundice in a New-born Child', *Transactions of the Edinburgh Obstetrical Society*, 38 (1912), pp. 296–301, on p. 299.
58. D. Dow, *The Rottenrow: The History of the Glasgow Royal Maternity Hospital, 1834–1984* (Carnforth: Parthenon Press, 1984).
59. 'Diet in Pregnancy', *BMJ*, 2129:2 (1901), pp. 1187–88, on p. 1188.
60. Confidential Report of Finance Committee, RMH, 11 June 1913, LHSA LHB 3/26/10.
61. Letter from J. W. Ballantyne to Sub-Committee, RMH, 9 June 1913, LHSA LHB 3/26/8.
62. J. W. Ballantyne, 'Mother Welfare in Pregnancy and Infant Health', *Edinburgh Medical Journal*, n.s.:18 (1917), pp. 348–60, on p. 350.
63. M. Milne Murray, *Practical Training in Midwifery*, LHSA LHB 3/26/6; RMH: Confidential Report to Directors, RMH, 13 July 1908, LHSA LHB 3/26/7; LHSA LHB 3/26/10.
64. Ballantyne, 'Valedictory Address', p. 70.
65. RMH Annual Report, 1907, LHSA LHB 3/7.
66. J. W. Ballantyne, 'Pre-Maternity Hospital Practice: A Series of Thirty Cases of Morbid Pregnancy Treated in the Royal Maternity Hospital, Edinburgh, during the Autumn Quarter of 1908', *Journal of Obstetrics and Gynaecology of the British Empire*, 15:2 (1909), pp. 169–86, on p. 177.
67. NLS Acc.6313, 1908, fol. 4.

68. NLS Acc.6313, 1909, fol. 4. On unmarried mothers' resistance: Kunzel, *Fallen Women, Problem Girls*.

69. J. W. Ballantyne, 'An Address on the Nature of Pregnancy and its Practical Bearings', *BMJ*, 2772:1 (1914), pp. 349–55, on p. 355.

70. LHSA LHB 3/17/19; Marks, *Metropolitan Maternity*, p. 17.

71. J. H. Ferguson, 'Some Twentieth-Century Problems in Relation to Marriage and Child-birth', *Transactions of the Edinburgh Obstetrical Society*, 39 (1912), pp. 3–39.

72. J. W. Ballantyne, 'Antenatal Clinics and Prematernity Practice at the Edinburgh Royal Maternity Hospital in the years 1909–1915', *BMJ*, 2875:1 (1916), pp. 189–92, on p.189. The cooperation of health visitors would elsewhere become vitally important for increasing attendance at maternity clinics: Marks, *Metropolitan Maternity*, p. 265.

73. Ballantyne, 'Antenatal Clinics', p. 190; J. W. Ballantyne, 'Note on an Antenatal or Preg-nancy Clinic at the Edinburgh Royal Maternity Hospital', *BMJ*, 2908:2 (1916), pp. 420–1.

74. Ballantyne, 'Antenatal Clinics', p. 190.

75. Ibid.

76. J. W. Ballantyne, 'Alcohol and Antenatal Child Welfare', *British Journal of Inebriety*, 14:3 (1917), pp. 93–116, on pp. 98–9.

77. For increasing antenatal clinic attendance: RMH Annual Reports, 1900–1923, LHSA LHB 3/7.

78. Ferguson, 'Some Twentieth-Century Problems', pp. 4–5.

79. Davin, 'Imperialism and Motherhood', pp. 44–6; S. Grayzel, *Women's Identities at War: Gender, Motherhood and Politics in Britain and France during the First World War* (Chapel Hill, NC: University of North Carolina Press, 1999), pp. 112–14.

80. M. M. Smith, 'Some Observations on an Inquiry into Still-Births Occurring in Manches-ter since 1905', *Public Health*, 21:2 (1908), pp. 15–22, on p. 22; Edinburgh Hospital for Women and Children: Elsie Inglis Memorial in Scotland, 1918, LHSA LHB 8/11/1; *Midwife*, 4 October 1913, p. 284.

81. Sub-committee on Antenatal Pathology, 1919–1925, National Archives, Kew, Medical Research Council Child Life Investigation Committee Files, FD1/3870.

82. A. Routh, 'Antenatal Pathology', *BMJ*, 2768:1 (1914), p. 170.

83. G. Newman, *Infant Mortality: A Social Problem* (London: Methuen, 1906); W. L. Mackenzie, *The Medical Inspection of School Children: A Textbook for Medical Officers of Schools, Medical Officers of Health, School Managers and Teachers* (Edinburgh: William Hodge, 1904); D. Armstrong, 'The Invention of Infant Mortality', *Sociology of Health and Illness*, 8:3 (1986), pp. 211–32.

84. Supplement 532, *BMJ*, 2792:2 (1914), p. 4.

85. W. L. Mackenzie, *Report on the Physical Welfare of Mothers and Children: Scotland* (Liv-erpool: Carnegie UK Trust, 1917).

86. Nuttall, 'Maternity Charities', p. 370. By 1917 there were seven clinics altogether.

87. 'Maternity and Child Welfare Scheme Agreement', 12 June 1918, LHSA LHB 3/25/7.

88. LHSA LHB 3/25/7.

89. *First Annual Report of the Maternity and Child Welfare Department* (Edinburgh: Turn-bull & Spears, 1919), p. 18, Edinburgh City Archive Public Health Committee Files, SL 27/1/2. On national developments: Lewis, *The Politics of Motherhood*, pp. 89–113.

90. RMH Annual Report 1916, LHSA LHB 3/7. Alison Nuttall has suggested, however, this was part of a longer-term trend: Nuttall, 'Maternity Charities'.

91. 'Maternity and Child Welfare Scheme Memoranda', LHSA LHB 3/25/1–9.

92. R. Davidson, 'Venereal Disease, Sexual Morality and the State in Interwar Scotland',
     Journal of the History of Sexuality, 5:2 (1994), pp. 267–94.

3 Greenlees, '"The Peculiar and Complex Female Problem": The Church of Scotland and Health Care for Unwed Mothers, 1900–1948'

1.   Church of Scotland, 'Report of the Committee on Social Service to the General Assem-
     bly', *Report on the Schemes of the Church of Scotland with Legislative Acts passed by the
     General Assembly* (Edinburgh: William Blackwood & Sons, 1946), p. 199; hereafter,
     'Report of the Committee on Social Service'.
2.   *Life and Work*, November 1914, vol. 35, pp. 328–9; *Life and Work*, June 1912, vol.
     XXXIV, p. 215.
3.   Church of Scotland, 'Report of the Committee on Social Work to the General Assem-
     bly', *Report on the Schemes of the Church of Scotland with Legislative Acts passed by the
     General Assembly* (Edinburgh: William Blackwood & Sons, 1915), pp. 729–30, hereaf-
     ter, 'Report of the Committee on Social Work'.
4.   'Report of the Committee on Social Work', 1914, p. 753.
5.   G. R. Searle, *The Quest for National Efficiency: A Study in British Politics and Political
     Thought, 1899–1914* (Oxford: Blackwell, 1971); B. S. Rowntree, *Poverty: A Study of
     Town Life* (London: Macmillan, 1902); C. Booth, *Life and Labour of the People of Lon-
     don* (London, 1889).
6.   Between 1873 and 1875 there were 285 deaths of illegitimate births per 1,000 births
     compared with 152 infant deaths per 1,000 legitimate births. Glasgow Corporation,
     Report of the Medical Officer of Health (MOH) of the City of Glasgow, 1902 (Glasgow:
     Robert Anderson, 1903) (hereafter, *MOH Report*), p. 25 and A. K. Chalmers, *The Health
     of Glasgow, 1818–1925, An Outline* (Glasgow: Glasgow Corporation, 1930), p. 194.
7.   O. Checkland, 'Maternal and Child Welfare', in O. Checkland and M. Lamb (eds),
     Health Care as Social History: The Glasgow Case (Aberdeen: Aberdeen University Press,
     1982), p. 117.
8.   S. Koven and S. Michel (eds), *Mothers of a New World: Maternalist Politics and the
     Origins of Welfare States* (London: Routledge, 1993); L. Weiner, 'International Trends:
     Maternalism as a Paradigm', *Journal of Women's History*, 5:2 (1993), pp. 96–8; T.
     Skocpol, *Protecting Soldiers and Mothers: The Political Origins of Social Policy in the
     United States* (Cambridge, MA: Belknap, 1992); J. Lewis, *The Politics of Motherhood:
     Child and Maternal Welfare in England, 1900–1939* (London: Croom Helm, 1980),
     p. 35; M. Ladd-Taylor, *Mother-Work: Women, Child Welfare and the State, 1890–1930*
     (Urbana, IL: University of Illinois Press, 1994); and L. Bryder, *A Voice for Mothers: The
     Plunket Society and Infant Welfare 1907–2000* (Auckland: Auckland University Press,
     2003), pp. 1–2.
9.   For example, L. Marks, *Metropolitan Maternity: Maternal and Infant Welfare Services in
     Early Twentieth Century London* (Amsterdam: Rodopi, 1996); A. Digby and J. Stew-
     art (eds), *Gender, Health and Welfare* (London: Routledge, 1996); B. B. Gilbert, *The
     Evolution of National Insurance in Great Britain: Origins of the Welfare State* (London:
     Michael Joseph, 1973); P. Thane, *The Foundations of the Welfare State* (London and New
     York: Longman, 1982); E. Ross, *Love and Toil: Motherhood in Outcast London, 1870–
     1918* (New York: Oxford University Press, 1993), pp. 219–21.

10. S. Szreter, 'The Importance of Social Intervention in Britain's Mortality Decline *c.* 1850–1914: A Re-interpretation of the Role of Public Health', *Social History of Medicine*, 1:1 (1988), pp. 1–38.

11. Ross, *Love and Toil*, pp. 219–21; Thane, *Foundations*; G. McLachlan (ed.), *Improving the Common Weal: Aspects of Scottish Health Services, 1900–1984* (Edinburgh: Edinburgh University Press, 1984), pp. 413–40. A. Blaikie, 'Scottish Illegitimacy: Social Adjustment or Moral Economy?', *Journal of Interdisciplinary History*, 29:2 (1998), pp. 221–41; J. Jenkinson, *Scotland's Health, 1919–48* (London: Peter Lang, 2002), pp. 153–219. McCrae has shown that overall Scotland did enjoy long-term health improvements. M. McCrae, *The National Health Service in Scotland: Origins and Ideals, 1900–1950* (East Linton: Tuckwell Press, 2003).

12. Chalmers was Glasgow's MOH from 1898–1925. Chalmers, *Health of Glasgow*, p. 195.

13. 'The National Conference on Infant Mortality', *British Journal of Nursing*, 53:11 July (1914), p. 37.

14. For example, J. Welshman, *Municipal Medicine: Public Health in Twentieth-Century Britain* (Bern: Peter Lang, 2000), pp. 26–7; M. Tew, *Safer Childbirth? A Critical History of Maternity Care* (London and New York: Longman, 1990); A. Oakley, *The Captured Womb: A History of the Medical Care of Pregnant Women* (Oxford: Basil Blackwell, 1984); J. W. Leavitt, *Brought to Bed: Child-bearing in America 1750–1950* (New York: Oxford University Press, 1983); J. Murphy Lawless, *Reading Birth and Death: A History of Obstetric Thinking* (Bloomington, IN: Indiana University Press, 1998). More recently, the medicalization of childbirth has been defined as a process of increasing certainty and confidence, accepted by doctors and patients, and as what women wanted. W. Mitchinson, *Giving Birth in Canada 1900–1950* (Toronto: University of Toronto Press, 2002); L. M. Beier, 'Expertise and Control: Childbearing in Three Twentieth-Century Lancashire Communities', *Bulletin of the History of Medicine*, 78 (2004), pp. 379–409.

15. For example, S. J. Seligman, 'The Royal Maternity Charity: The First Hundred Years', *Medical History*, 24 (1980), pp. 403–18; Marks, *Metropolitan Maternity*; L. Marks, 'Mothers, Babies and Hospitals: "The London" and the Provision of Maternity Care in East London, 1870–1939', in V. Fildes, L. Marks and H. Marland (eds), *Women and Children First: International Maternal and Infant Welfare, 1870–1945* (London: Routledge, 1992), pp. 48–73. Notable exceptions for Scotland include: A. Nuttall, 'Maternity Charities, the Edinburgh Maternity Scheme and the Medicalisation of Childbirth, 1900–1925', *Social History of Medicine*, 24:2 (2011), pp. 370–88; L. Mahood, *The Magdalenes: Prostitution in the Nineteenth Century* (London: Routledge, 1990); O. Checkland, *Philanthropy in Victorian Scotland: Social Welfare and the Voluntary Principle* (Edinburgh: John Donald, 1980); S. Al-Gailani, 'Teratology and the Clinic: Monsters, Obstetrics and the Making of Antenatal Life in Edinburgh, *c.* 1900' (PhD dissertation, Cambridge University, 2010).

16. M. A. Crowther, 'Poverty, Health and Welfare', in W. Hamish Fraser and R. J. Morris (eds), *People and Society in Scotland, 1830–1914* (Edinburgh: John Donald, 1990), pp. 265–89, on p. 286.

17. M. M'Neill and A. Campbell, Draft for Board of Supervision Circular 1/7.1875, cited in T Ferguson, *Scottish Social Welfare, 1864–1914* (London, 1958), pp. 247–48; Crowther, 'Poverty, Health and Welfare', p. 275.

18. A. Higginbotham, 'Respectable Sinners: Salvation Army Rescue Work with Unmarried Mothers, 1884–1914', in G. Malmgreen (ed.), *Religion in the Lives of English Women* (Bloomington, IN: Indiana University Press, 1986); Mahood, *The Magdalenes*. A. Lev-

ine, T. Nutt and S. Williams (eds), *Illegitimacy in Britain, 1700–1920* (Basingstoke: Palgrave, 2005); I. Loudon, *Death in Childbirth: An International Study of Maternal Care and Maternal Mortality, 1800–1950* (Oxford: Clarendon Press, 1992).

19. For details about the rifts and unions in Scottish Presbyterianism, see C. Brown, *The Social History of Religion in Scotland since 1730* (London: Methuen, 1987), pp. 34–41.

20. G. P. Milne, 'The History of Midwifery in Aberdeen', in G. P. Milne (ed.), *Aberdeen Medico-Chirurgical Society, A Bi-Centennial History 1789–1989* (Aberdeen: Aberdeen University Press, 1989), p. 227, as cited in L. Reid, *Midwifery in Scotland: A History* (Erskine: Scottish History Press, 2011), p. 12.

21. Reid, *Midwifery in Scotland*, p. 14.

22. For example C. P. Williams, 'Healing and Evangelism: The Place of Medicine in Later Victorian Protestant Missionary Thinking', in W. J. Shiels (ed.), *The Church and Healing* (Oxford: Blackwell, 1982); S. J. Brown, 'Reform, Reconstruction, Reaction: The Social Vision of Scottish Presbyterianism, *c.* 1830–1930', *Scottish Journal of Theology*, 44 (1991), pp. 489–517. A. C. Ross, 'The Scottish Missionary Doctor', in D. A. Dow (ed.), *The Influence of Scottish Medicine: An Historical Assessment of its International Impact* (Carnforth: Parthenon Publishing, 1988).

23. Blaikie, 'Scottish Illegitimacy'; A. Blaikie, 'Accounting for Poverty: Conflicting Constructions of Family Survival in Scotland, 1855–1925', *Journal of Historical Sociology*, 18:3 (2005), pp. 202–26; A. Blaikie, *Illegitimacy, Sex and Society* (Oxford: Clarendon Press, 1993), p. 11.

24. L. Jamieson, 'Changing Intimacy: Seeking and Forming Couple Relationships', in L. Abrams and C. G. Brown (eds), *A History of Everyday Life in Twentieth-Century Scotland* (Edinburgh: Edinburgh University Press, 2010), ch. 3.

25. M. Hopkins, *Nobody wanted Sam: The Story of the Unwelcomed Child, 1530–1948* (London: John Murray, 1949); G. Clark, 'The Role of Mother and Baby Homes in the Adoption of Children Born outside Marriage in Twentieth-Century England and Wales', *Family and Community History*, 11:1 (2008), pp. 45–59; J. Nicholson, *Mother and Baby Homes: A Survey of Homes for Unmarried Mothers* (London: George Allen & Unwin, Ltd., 1968), esp. pp. 18–19; *MOH Report*, 1911, p. 19; *MOH Report*, 1914, pp. 24–5.

26. L. L. L. Cameron, *The Challenge of Need: A History of Social Service by the Church of Scotland, 1869–1969* (Edinburgh: Saint Andrews Press, 1971), p. 66.

27. Ibid., pp. 66–7.

28. D. Dow, *The Rottenrow: The History of the Glasgow Royal Maternity Hospital, 1834–1984* (Carnforth: Parthenon Press, 1984), pp. 31–2, 49.

29. W. L. Mackenzie, *Scottish Mothers and Children: Being a Report on the Physical Welfare of Mothers and Children, Scotland* (East Port, Dunfermline: The Carnegie United Kingdom Trust, 1917), p. 124.

30. Mahood, *The Magdalenes*, p. 115.

31. *MOH Report*, 1912, p. 19; *MOH Report*, 1913, pp. 24–5; *MOH Report*, 1911, p. 19 and *MOH Report*, 1913, pp. 24–5. See Nicholson, *Mother and Baby Homes*, esp. pp. 18–19. The move to hospital births came later. See *MOH Report, Glasgow*, 1934, p. 8; for an Edinburgh case study, see A. Nuttall, 'Taking "advantage of the facilities and comforts... offered": Women's Choice of Hospital Delivery in Interwar Edinburgh', this volume, ch. 4.

32. *MOH Report, Glasgow*, 1920, p. 29. See also Mackenzie, *Scottish Mothers and Children*, p. 122.

33. D. Watson, *Social Problems and the Church's Duty* (London, 1908). Stewart, 'Christ's Kingdom in Scotland', p. 2.

34. Watson's notes on the Maternity Home, as quoted in Mackenzie, *Scottish Mothers and Children*, p. 123.

35. Such as their Auldhousefield Rescue Home, Pollockshaws, 'Report of the Committee on Social Work', 1915, p. 729.

36. 'Report of the Committee on Social Work', 1915, p. 2 and 'Report of the Committee on Social Work', 1916, pp. 510–11.

37. 'Report of the Committee on Social Work', 1916, pp. 510–11.

38. Mackenzie, *Scottish Mothers and Children*, p. 123; Cameron, *Challenge of Need*, p. 64.

39. Mackenzie, *Scottish Mothers and Children*, p. 127; *MOH Report*, 1913, pp. 24–5.

40. Mackenzie, *Scottish Mothers and Children*, p. 123.

41. Ibid., pp. 123–4.

42. 'Report of the Committee on Social Work', various years, for example: 1921, p. 427; 1922, p. 475; 1925, p. 687.

43. It is unclear how many women gave birth at the home. 'Report of the Committee on Social Work', 1922, p. 475; 1923, p. 615.

44. Mackenzie, *Scottish Mothers and Children*, p. 124.

45. Mahood, *The Magdalenes*.

46. M. Foucault, *The History of Sexuality, Vol. 1: An Introduction,* trans. R. Hurly (New York: Random House, 1980). Discussed in relation to the Magdalene Homes in Mahood, *Magdalenes*, pp. 161–3.

47. Brown, 'Reform, Reconstruction, Reaction', p. 510; and S. J. Brown, '"A Solemn Purification by Fire". Responses to the Great War in the Scottish Presbyterian Churches, 1914–19', *Journal of Ecclesiastical History*, 45 (1994), pp. 82–104.

48. These were separate from orphanages. Babies stayed here until placed with relatives, boarded out or adopted. 'Report of the Committee on Social Work', 1919, pp. 700–2, 709; The Church acknowledged that this was 'perhaps *the most difficult and delicate work the Committee has ever undertaken*' [italics in original]. 'Report of the Committee on Social Work', 1920, p. 437.

49. Church of Scotland Commission on the War in *Reports on the Schemes of the Church of Scotland*, 1918, p. 629; C. M. Richardson, 'A Plea for the Industrial Drudges', *The Church and the War: Tracts for To-day*, no. 11 (Edinburgh, 1917), pp. 82–3, as cited in Brown, 'Solemn Purification by Fire', p. 99.

50. Local Government Board Scotland (LGBS), *Annual Report*, 1918 [Cmd 230] (Edinburgh: HMSO, 1919), p. xx; PRO, MH 55/218, LGBS, memorandum to all Scottish local authorities, 24 May 1918, 'Notification of Births (Extension) Act, 1915: Maternity Service and Child Welfare Schemes', as cited in Jenkinson, *Scotland's Health*, pp. 157–8.

51. Brown, *Social History of Religion*, pp. 217–18.

52. 'Report of the Committee on Social Work', 1921, p. 427.

53. 'Report of the Committee on Social Work', 1922, p. 475.

54. 'Report of the Committee on Social Work', 1923, pp. 607–8.

55. It is unclear how many, if any, births took place at the home. The hospital was preferred due to its more and better facilities and the limited space at Lansdowne House. 'Report of the Committee on Social Work', 1922, p. 475; 1923, p. 615; Cameron, *Challenge of Need*, p. 63.

56. 'Report of the Committee on Social Work', 1925, p. 687; 1926, p. 882; 1928, p. 1140 and 1935, p. 448.

57. Jenkinson, *Scotland's Health*, p. 166.

58. Nuttall, 'Taking 'advantage of the facilities and comforts... offered'.

59. S. Al-Gailani, 'Pregnancy, Pathology and Public Morals: Making Antenatal Care in Edinburgh around 1900', ch. 2 in this volume.

60. *MOH Report, Glasgow*, 1920, p. 29. A. K. Chalmers, 'Ante-Natal Hygiene and its Relation to Still and Premature Births and Mortality in the First Months of Life', in the *Proceedings of the National Conference on Infant Mortality Held at St. George's Hall Liverpool, 1914*, pp. 27–35.

61. Reid, *Midwifery in Scotland*, pp. 61–2.

62. D. Baird, 'Maternal Mortality in Hospital: A Review of 999 Fatal Cases in the Glasgow Royal Maternity and Women's Hospital during Ten Years, 1925–34', *Lancet*, 227:5867 (8 February 1936), pp. 295–299, on p. 298; PEP, *Report on the British Health Services*, p. 96. Both cited in Jenkinson, *Scotland's Health*, pp. 170–1. In 1937, Baird also took the position of chief obstetrician at Aberdeen Maternity Hospital and was Regius Professor of Midwifery (later Obstetrics and Gynaecology) at the University of Aberdeen.

63. Church of Scotland, 'Report of the Committee on Christian Life and Social Work', *Report on the Schemes of the Church of Scotland with Legislative Acts passed by the General Assembly* (Edinburgh: William Blackwood & Sons, 1938), p. 498.

64. *MOH Report, Glasgow*, 1929, p. 52; *MOH Report, Glasgow*, 1933, p. 68.

65. 'Report of the Committee on Social Work', 1931, p. 532; *Life and Work*, December 1935, pp. 476–81; it is unclear whether any births occurred at the home during the 1930s, but the better facilities at the hospital were preferred. 'Report of the Committee on Christian Life and Social Work', 1939, p. 488; 1941, p. 321; 1943, p. 225; Cameron, *Challenge of Need*, p. 63.

66. 'Report of the Committee on Social Work', 1931, p. 417.

67. 'Report of the Committee on Social Work', 1929, pp. 793, 799.

68. For example, 'Report of the Committee on Social Work', 1932, p. 484; 1933, p. 451; 1935, p. 455; 1938, p. 506.

69. Reid, *Midwifery in Scotland*, pp. 64–5.

70. My thanks to Muriel McEwan for the information on Cecile Henderson. M. McEwan, 'Ministering in Affliction: The 'Brown Deaconesses' of the Church of Scotland, 1888–c. 1948' (PhD Dissertation, Open University, 2008); 'Report of the Committee on Social Work', 1935, pp. 448, 455; 'Report of the Committee on Social Work', 1933, p. 451; 'Report of the Committee on Christian Life and Social Work', 1941, p. 301.

71. 'Report of the Committee on Christian Life and Social Work', 1939, p. 488. In 1940, just over 1/3 of the babies born went home with their mothers, 'Report of the Committee on Christian Life and Social Work', 1940, p. 364; in 1941, almost 1/4 went home with their mothers. 'Report of the Committee on Christian Life and Social Work', 1941, p. 321. In all years, mothers found situations with their babies. In contrast, in 1915, no babies were adopted. Mackenzie, *Scottish Mothers and Children*, p. 123. Figures not available for all years.

72. Clark, 'Role of Mother and Baby Homes', pp. 49, 51.

73. 'Report of the Committee on Christian Life and Social Work', 1938, p. 306; 1939, p. 488.

74. My emphasis. For example, 'Report of the Committee on Christian Life and Social Work', 1937, p. 484.

75. A. Reid, 'The Influences on the Health and Mortality of Illegitimate Children in Derbyshire, 1917–22', in Levine, et al., *Illegitimacy in Britain*, pp. 171–2.

76. Jenkinson, *Scotland's Health*, pp. 188–94; Reid, *Midwifery in Scotland*, p. 62.

77. 'Report of the Committee on Christian Life and Social Work', 1941, p. 321.

78. *Glasgow Herald*, 20 May 1944, p. 4.
79. 'Report of the Committee on Christian Life and Social Work', 1941, p. 302.
80. Ibid., p. 323 and 'Report of the Committee on Christian Life and Social Work', 1942, p. 259.
81. Cameron, *Challenge of Need*, pp. 65–6.
82. 'Report of the Committee on Christian Life and Social Work', 1944, p. 252. Cameron, *Challenge of Need*, p. 66.
83. Clark, 'Role of Mother and Baby Homes', pp. 51–2.
84. 'Report of the Committee on Christian Life and Social Work', 1944, p. 241; Cameron, *Challenge of Need*, pp. 64–6.
85. 'Report of the Committee on Social Service', 1949, p. 259.
86. A. Nuttall, '"Because of Poverty Brought into Hospital...": A Casenote-Based Analysis of the Changing Role of the Edinburgh Royal Maternity Hospital, 1850–1912', *Social History of Medicine*, 20:2 (2007), pp. 263–80.
87. 'Report of the Committee on Social Work', various years, for example: 1921, p. 427; 1922, p. 475; 1925, p. 687; 1927, p. 1050; 1933, p. 451;1935, p. 448.
88. When the National Council of Social Service initiated a Scottish Committee for the Unmarried Mother and Her Child, the Church of Scotland was well represented. This committee was designed to get voluntary and statutory bodies to invest and discuss illegitimacy and how to encourage more mothers to care for their child and more fathers to accept their responsibilities. 'Report of the Committee on Social Work', 1943, pp. 228–9. Cameron, *Challenge of Need*, pp. 61–2.

4 Nuttall, 'Taking "Advantage of the Facilities and Comforts ... Offered": Women's Choice of Hospital Delivery in Interwar Edinburgh'

1. Edinburgh Royal Maternity Hospital (ERMH) Annual Report, 1921, p. 4, Lothian Health Services Archive (hereafter LHSA) LHB 3/7/77.
2. M. Tew, *Safer Childbirth: A Critical History of Maternity Care* (London: Chapman and Hall, 1990), p. 65.
3. See, for example, S. Kitzinger, *Women's Experiences of Birth at Home* (Oxford: Oxford University Press, 1978); J. Lewis, *The Politics of Motherhood: Child and Maternal Welfare in England, 1900–1939* (London: Croom Helm 1980); R. Campbell and A. Macfarlane, *Where to be Born? The Debate and the Evidence* (Oxford: Oxford University Press for the National Perinatal Epidemiology Unit, 2nd edn, 1994); Tew, *Safer Childbirth*; R. Campbell and A. Macfarlane, 'Recent Debate on the Place of Birth', in J. Garcia, R. Kilpatrick and M. Richards (eds), *The Politics of Maternity Care: Services for Childbearing Women in Twentieth-Century Britain* (Oxford: Clarendon Press, 1990), pp. 217–37; H. Graham and A. Oakley, 'Competing Ideologies of Reproduction: Medical and Maternal Perspectives on Pregnancy', in H. Roberts (ed.), *Women, Health and Reproduction* (London: Routledge & Kegan Paul, 1981), pp. 50–74.
4. See, for example, E. Roberts, *A Woman's Place: An Oral History of Working-Class Women, 1890–1940*, paperback edn (Oxford: Basil Blackwell Ltd, 1985), pp. 108–9; J. W. Leavitt, *Brought to Bed: Child-bearing in America 1750–1950* (New York: Oxford University Press, 1986); P. Mein Smith, *Maternity in Dispute: New Zealand 1920–1939* (Wellington: Historical Publications Branch, Department of Internal Affairs, Govern-

ment Printer, 1986); L. Marks, *Metropolitan Maternity: Maternal and Infant Welfare Services in Early Twentieth Century London* (Amsterdam: Rodopi, 1996), pp. 200–14; W. Mitchinson , *Giving Birth in Canada 1900–1950* (Toronto: University of Toronto Press, 2002); L. M. Beier, 'Expertise and Control: Childbearing in Three Twentieth-Century Lancashire Communities', *Bulletin of the History of Medicine*, 78 (2004), pp. 379–409.

5. See, for example, E. R. van Teijlingen, 'A Social or Medical Model of Childbirth? Comparing the Arguments in Grampian (Scotland) and the Netherlands' (PhD thesis, University of Aberdeen, 1994); G. Chamberlain, A. Wraight and P. Crowley (eds), *Home Births, the Report of the 1994 Confidential Enquiry by the National Birthday Trust Fund* (Carnforth: Parthenon Publishing Group Ltd, 1996); L. Longworth, J. Ratcliffe and M. Boulton, 'Investigating Women's Preferences for Intrapartum Care: Home versus Hospital Births', *Health and Social Care in the Community*, 9:6 (2001), pp. 404–13; B. C. Madi and R. Crow, 'A Qualitative Study of Information about Available Options for Childbirth Venue and Pregnant Women's Preference for a Place of Delivery', *Midwifery*, 19 (2003), pp. 328–36.

6. E. F. Catford, *Edinburgh: The Story of a City* (London: Hutchison & Co., 1975), pp. 237–40.

7. Royal College of Obstetricians and Gynaecologists (RCOG), *Maternity in Great Britain: A Survey of Social and Economic Aspects of Pregnancy and Childbirth undertaken by a Joint Committee of the Royal College of Obstetricians and Gynaecologists and the Population Investigation Committee* (London: Oxford University Press, 1948), p. 55.

8. F. Whittaker, 'Edinburgh's Maternity Hospital', *Midwives Chronicle and Nursing Notes*, 62:740 (August 1949), p. 238; RCOG, *Maternity in Great Britain*, p. 68.

9. Alternate cases were taken from ERMH casebooks (1,500 cases in 1924, 1,671 in 1935); all the deliveries for 1924 were collected from Hospice and ELII casebooks (475 and 198 cases respectively), and from the Deaconess registers from February 1925 to February 1926 (130 cases). Cases from EIMMH in 1935 are only available for September to October (198); 202 cases were collected from the Western General casebook.

10. A. Nuttall, '"Because of Poverty Brought into Hospital ..." A Casenote-Based Analysis of the Changing Role of the Edinburgh Royal Maternity Hospital, 1850–1912', *Social History of Medicine*, 20:2 (2007), pp. 263–80.

11. In 1933 the MOH recorded 39 per cent of city births taking place under ERMH care, and none at the Western; in 1934, 2 per cent of such births occurred at the Western, and only 37 per cent in the care of the ERMH. J. Guy, *Reports of the Public Health Department of the City of Edinburgh 1933, 1934* (Leith: Mackenzie & Storrie Ltd).

12. A. M. Williamson, *Report of the Public Health Department of the City of Edinburgh 1912* (Edinburgh: Turnbull and Spears); W. G. Clark, *Report of the Public Health Department of the City of Edinburgh 1938* (Leith: George C. Mackay Ltd); Registers of Notifications of Births, LHSA LHB 16/47/6–7, 16–17, 1924 and 1935.

13. Clark, *Report of the Public Health Department ... 1938*, p. 73.

14. In 1925, the first year recorded, approximately 30 per cent of Edinburgh births took place within institutions, 25 per cent were under institutional care but in the patient's home, and 45 per cent in the care of privately engaged doctors or midwives. W. Robertson, *Report of the Public Health Department of the City of Edinburgh 1926* (Leith: Mackenzie & Storrie Ltd).

15. See, for example, ERMH Directors' Minutes, 7 October 1884, LHSA LHB 3/1/4.

16. ERMH Annual Reports, 1918, p. 5, 1920, pp. 7–8, LHSA LHB 3/7/74, 76.

17. ERMH Annual Reports, 1916–35, LHSA LHB 3/7/72–91.

18. Edinburgh Hospital and Dispensary for Women and Children and the Hospice (EHDWC&H) Annual Report, 1924, p. 3, LHB 8/7/45.

19. EHDWC&H Annual Report, 1920–35, LHSA LHB 8/7/41–57.

20. In 1933, the year of its closure, only twenty-three births took place under Lying-in Institution care, and ninety-four under that of the Deaconess. In 1934 Deaconess staff only delivered eighty-seven babies. Guy, *Reports of the Public Health Department, 1933, 1934*.

21. A. Oakley, *The Captured Womb: A History of the Medical Care of Pregnant Women* (Oxford: Basil Blackwell, 1986).

22. A. Nuttall, 'Maternity Charities, the Edinburgh Maternity Scheme and the Medicalisation of Childbirth, 1900–1925', *Social History of Medicine*, 24:2 (2011), pp. 370–88.

23. EHDWC&H Annual Report, 1923, p. 8, LHSA LHB 8/7/44.

24. Printed pamphlet on the Notification of Births Act 1918, sections 9 and 10, p. 5, Edinburgh City Archives, L26/4/1262.

25. J. Campbell, *Maternal Mortality*, HMSO, Reports on Public Health and Medical Subjects, no. 25, 1924, p. 39.

26. EHDWC&H Annual Report, 1926, pp. 4, 8; 1925, p. 10, LHSA LHB 8/7/47, 46.

27. See, for example, Oakley, *The Captured Womb*, p. 52.

28. Nuttall, 'Maternity Charities'.

29. In 1924, fifteen such patients had positive Wassermann results; three had gonorrhoeal symptoms; forty-one returned negative results for venereal disease.

30. In 1912, the ERMH admitted thirty antenatal eclamptics, twenty-six of whom fitted. Seven mothers and eighteen babies died. Nuttall, 'Maternity Charities'.

31. Case 88 (Dr Haultain's quarter), ERMH Indoor Casebook, 1912, LHSA LHB 3/16/3; ERMH Special and Ordinary Casebook, 1912, p. 60–2, LHSA LHB 3/17/13. All patients' names have been anonymized.

32. Case 827, ERMH Indoor Casebook, 1924, LHSA LHB 3/16/5.

33. Case 29 (Dr Halliday Croom's quarter), ERMH Indoor Casebook, 1912, LHSA LHB 3/16/3; ERMH Special and Ordinary Casebook, 1912, p. 210, LHSA LHB 3/17/13.

34. Case 1111, ERMH Indoor Casebook, 1924, LHSA LHB 3/16/5.

35. 'Here all mothers will be welcome, and will be able to obtain medical treatment, and learn the value of fresh air and sunshine, and proper food and clothing in the prevention of disease. Thus one more step will be taken to make their households healthy and happy, and to banish rickets and preventable diseases from their homes'. EHDWC&H Annual Report, 1923, p. 3, LHSA LHB 8/7/44.

36. A. M. Williamson, *Report of the Public Health Department of the City of Edinburgh 1919* (Edinburgh: H. & J. Pillans & Wilson), p. 86; W. Robertson, *Report of the Public Health Department of the City of Edinburgh 1924* (Edinburgh: H. & J. Pillans & Wilson), p. v.

37. Williamson, *Report of the Public Health Department ... 1919*, p. 83.

38. W. Robertson, *Report of the Public Health Department of the City of Edinburgh 1925* (Edinburgh: H. & J. Pillans & Wilson), p. 77.

39. H. Clark and E. Carnegie, *She was Aye Workin' – Memories of Tenement Women in Edinburgh and Glasgow* (Oxford, White Cockade Publishing, 2003), p. 23.

40. Tollcross Local History Project, *Waters under the Bridge* (Aberdeen: Aberdeen University Press, 1990), p. 2.

41. Ibid., p. 111.

42. J. Guy, *Report of the Public Health Department of the City of Edinburgh 1930* (Edinburgh: H. & J. Pillans & Wilson), p. v.

43. Case 379, ERMH Outdoor Casebook, 1924, LHSA LHB 3/18/21.
44. Robertson, *Report of the Public Health Department ... 1924*, p. v.
45. W. Robertson, *Report of the Public Health Department of the City of Edinburgh 1929* (Edinburgh: H. & J. Pillans & Wilson), p. 89.
46. In 1935 only sixteen women of the eighty-five resident in Craigmillar, Stenhouse, Longstone, Slateford, Meadowbank, Northfield and Willowbrae chose home delivery under ERMH care.
47. For example, from 1894 until 1931 the Cowgate dispensary regularly delivered approximately 350 midwifery cases a year, numbers only falling with the resettlement of many Cowgate residents. J. Wilkinson, *The Coogate Doctors: The History of the Edinburgh Medical Missionary Society, 1841–1991* (Edinburgh: Edinburgh Medical Missionary Society, 1991).
48. In 1912 only 12 per cent of Leith-resident ERMH patients were inpatients. By 1924 this had risen, but only to 31 per cent. By contrast, 31 per cent of central Edinburgh-resident ERMH patients were treated indoors in 1912, and 60 per cent in 1924. In 1935 half of Leith-resident ERMH patients still delivered at home. Nuttall, 'Maternity Charities'.
49. *Pelican*, 1929–35, LHSA LHB 1/109a/4–9. One of the two 'non-Edinburgh nursing home' births took place in one in London.
50. Registers of Notifications of Births, LHSA LHB 16/47/6–7, 16–17, 1924 and 1935.
51. Health and Hygiene Exhibition Official Catalogue and Guide, 1930, foreword, unpaginated, Edinburgh City Libraries (ECL), YRA438.
52. Health and Hygiene Exhibition Official Catalogue and Guide, 1928, p. 113, ECL, YRA438.
53. Health and Hygiene Exhibition Official Catalogue and Guide, 1930, foreword, unpaginated, ECL, YRA438.
54. 'Onward Edinburgh', Third Health and Hygiene Exhibition Official Catalogue and Guide, 1936, ECL, YRA438, p. 113.
55. ERMH Directors Minutes, 16 November, 21 December 1926, LHSA LHB 3/1/6.
56. ERMH Directors Minutes, 18 January, 19 April, 21 June 1927, LHSA LHB 3/1/6; EHDWC&H Annual Report, 1927, LHSA LHB 8/7/48.
57. ERMH Annual Report, 1927–38, LHSA LHB 3/7/83–94.
58. ERMH Directors' Minutes, 18 October 1927, LHSA LHB 3/1/6.
59. EHDWC&H Annual Report 1931, p. 13, LHSA LHB 8/7/52.
60. Ibid. 1936, p. 8, LHSA LHB 8/7/57.
61. 'EIMMH Inquiry into Maternal Morbidity, Bulletin no. 4, February, 1932' (no publisher given) 'Bulletin no. 6, February 1935', LHSA LHB 8/14/5, 7.
62. See, for example, 'Doctors, Nurse, Operating Theatre, Royal Edinburgh Maternity and Simpson Memorial Hospital', 79 Lauriston Place, Edinburgh, Scan ID: 000–000–093–065–C, LHSA.
63. ERMH Casefolder 693, 1935, LHSA LHB 3 CC/1, quoting from the 'Admission card and Directions for Patients' it contains.
64. Applying these criteria to the 1,114 inpatients from the 1935 sample (every second case) yielded 274 women. Age distribution between the indoor and outdoor groups was similar, with approximately 35 per cent in each group being aged between 20 and 25, suggesting such comparison is valid. However, parity did differ: 39 per cent of indoor patients were primgravid, compared with 15–16 per cent outdoors; 32 per cent of inpatients had had one previous pregnancy, whereas 22 per cent of dispensary patients had. In contrast, 61–3 per cent of domiciliary births were to women having their third or later

child; only 29 per cent of hospital births were. There were similar maternal outcomes, but perinatal mortality was appreciably higher among outdoor cases (6.7 per cent in Leith, 7.4 per cent in the main dispensary, compared with 4.3 per cent within the Hospital). The ninety-five EIMMH patients selected by the same criteria were noticeably healthier: no mother required treatment for anything other than minor consequences of childbirth; only one baby was stillborn.

65. V. Devlin (ed.), *Motherhood from 1920 to the Present Day* (Edinburgh: Polygon, 1995), p. 104. The Western General did not record any treatments other than delivery in its casebook.

66. Ten of the thirty-three primigravidae who had chloroform had also had morphine.

67. ERMH Casefolder 825, 1935, LHSA LHB 3 CC/1.

68. See, for example, ERMH Casefolders 467 (retention), 1001, 1935, LHSA LHB 3 CC/1.

69. ERMH Casefolder 579, 1935, LHSA LHB 3 CC/1.

70. ERMH Casefolder 1448, 1935, LHSA LHB 3 CC/1.

71. J. Beinart, 'Obstetric Analgesia and the Control of Childbirth in Twentieth-Century Britain', in J. Garcia, R. Kilpatrick and M. Richards (eds), *The Politics of Maternity Care* (Oxford: Clarendon Press, 1990), pp. 116–32, on p. 120; A. Susan Williams, *Women and Childbirth in the Twentieth Century* (Stroud: Sutton, 1997), pp. 128–9.

72. ERMH Casefolder 1609, 1935, LHSA LHB 3 CC/1.

73. ERMH Casefolder 527, 1935, LHSA LHB 3 CC/1.

74. ERMH Casefolder 307, 1935, LHSA LHB 3 CC/1.

75. There were 377 women in this category, of whom 198 (52 per cent) laboured for less than 12 hours, 63 for more than 24 hours and 8 for more than 48 hours.

76. Although this rate appears low compared with modern-day practice, the equivalent rate in the two dispensaries was 1.7 per cent (eight cases). However, it should be noted that Loudon claims 'forceps rates of 50 per cent or more' in private practice at this period. I. Loudon, *Death in Childbirth: An International Study of Maternal Care and Maternal Mortality, 1800–1950* (Oxford: Clarendon Press, 1992), p. 221.

77. The condition of 189 women (17 per cent) was not recorded.

78. ERMH Casefolder 29, 1935, LHSA LHB 3 CC/1.

79. ERMH Casefolder 215, 1935, LHSA LHB 3 CC/1.

80. ERMH Casefolder 1341, 1935, LHSA LHB 3 CC/1.

81. See, for example, A. Macdonald, 'Hints to Women Regarding their Health', in *Edinburgh Health Society, Health Lectures for the People, 1880–1* (Edinburgh: Edinburgh Health Society, 1881), pp. 130–1, while lack of such rest was the most common complaint of the Women's Co-operative Guild correspondents in 1915. Women's Co-operative Guild, *Maternity: Letters from Working-Women* (London: G. Bell and Sons Ltd., 1915).

82. First mobilization was recorded for 402 out of 977 delivered inpatients.

83. See, for example, L. Reid, *Scottish Midwives: Twentieth Century Voices* (Dunfermline, Black Devon Books, 2nd edn, 2008), p. 37.

84. Case 7, ERMH Leith Casebook, 1935, LHSA LHB 3/18/37; ERMH Casefolder 53, 1935, LHSA LHB 3 CC/1.

5 Bryder, '"What Women Want": Childbirth Services and Women's Activism in New Zealand, 1900–1960'

1. P. Mein Smith, *Maternity in Dispute, New Zealand 1920–1939* (Wellington: Historical Publications Branch, Department of Internal Affairs, Government Printer, 1986), p.147; UNICEF League table of Maternity Death; Progress of Nations 1996, http://www.unicef.org/pon96/leag1wom.htm [accessed 1 June 2012].

2. I. Loudon, 'Childbirth', in I. Loudon (ed.), *Western Medicine: An Illustrated History* (Oxford: Oxford University Press, 1997), pp. 206–20, on p. 219; see also I. Loudon, *Death in Childbirth: An International Study of Maternal Care and Maternal Mortality, 1800–1950* (Oxford: Clarendon Press, 1992).

3. T. McKeown, *The Role of Medicine: Dream, Mirage or Nemesis?* (London: Nuffield Provincial Hospitals Trust, 1976); T. McKeown, *The Modern Rise of Population* (London: Edward Arnold, 1976).

4. A. Oakley, *The Captured Womb: A History of the Medical Care of Pregnant Women* (Oxford and New York: B. Blackwell, 1984).

5. S. B. Ruzek, *The Women's Health Movement: Feminist Alternatives to Medical Control* (New York: Praeger, 1978), p. 117. Other classic feminist studies include B. Ehrenreich and D. English, *For Her Own Good* (New York: Anchor Press, 1979); B. Katz Rothman, *In Labour: Women and Power in the Birthplace* (New York: W. W. Norton, 1982). See also B. Duden; *Disembodying Women: Perspectives on Pregnancy and the Unborn*, trans. L. Hoinacki, (Cambridge, MA: Harvard University Press, 1993); R. E. Davis-Floyd, *Birth as an American Rite of Passage* (Berkeley, CA: University of California Press, 2003).

6. S. Coney, 'Alienated Labour – Foetal Monitoring', *Broadsheet*, May 1979, pp. 16–17, 38–9. See also A. Rich, *Of Woman Born: Motherhood as Experience and Institution* (New York: Norton, 1976).

7. J. Murphy-Lawless, *Reading Birth and Death: A History of Obstetric Thinking* (Cork: Cork University Press, 1998).

8. See for example M. Tew, *Safer Childbirth?: A Critical History of Maternity Care*, 2nd edn (London and New York: Free Association Books, 1998); for New Zealand, E. Papps and M. Olssen, *Doctoring Childbirth and Regulating Midwifery in New Zealand: A Foucauldian Perspective* (Palmerston North: Dunmore Press, 1997); J. Donley, *Save the Midwife* (Auckland: New Women's Press, 1986).

9. For this changing historiography which suggests women of the past had more 'agency', see also W. Mitchinson, 'Agency, Diversity, and Constraints: Women and the Physicians, Canada, 1850–1950' in which she cautions that women of the past should not be regarded as victims in the medical encounter, and argues that they participated in building their relationship with physicians through various demands, negotiation and renegotiation; 'that the patient–physician dynamic was composed of both sites of resistance and sites of compliance, that women as individual patients did have some agency'. pp. 122, 127, in S. Sherwin (coordinator), *The Politics of Women's Health: Exploring Agency and Autonomy* (Philadelphia, PA: Temple University Press, 1998).

10. See K. Sinclair, *A History of New Zealand*, rev. edn (Auckland: Penguin, 2000), p. 195.

11. *New Zealand Parliamentary Debates* (*NZPD*), 131, 1904, p. 481.

12. L. Bryder, *A Voice for Mothers: The Plunket Society and Infant Welfare 1907–2000* (Auckland: Auckland University Press, 2002), p. 2. See also A. Klaus, *Every Child a Lion: The Origins of Maternal and Infant Health Policy in the United States and France, 1890–1920* (Ithaca, NY: Cornell University Press, 1993) and D. Dwork, *War is Good for Babies and*

Other Young Children: A History of the Infant and Child Welfare Movement in England 1898–1918 (London: Tavistock, 1987).

13. *NZPD*, 131, 1904, p. 110. For similar trends in Britain, see B. Abel-Smith, *History of the Nursing Profession* (London: Heinemann, 1960), p. 77.
14. Report of the Inspector-General of Hospitals and Charitable Institutions, *Appendices to the Journals of the House of Representatives* (AJHR), H-22 (1906), p. 3.
15. G. Bourke, 'Illuminating the Dark Hour: Auckland's St Helens Hospital, 1906–1990' (MA Thesis, The University of Auckland, 2006), p. 97.
16. Department of Health, *The Expectant Mother and Baby's First Month* (Wellington: Government Printer, 1935), p. 2; Bourke, 'Illuminating the Dark Hour', pp. 60, 84.
17. On maternity services in the Netherlands, see H. Marland, 'Questions of Competence: The Midwife Debate in the Netherlands in the Early Twentieth Century', *Medical History*, 39 (1995), pp. 317–37; on Scandinavia see S. Vallgarda, 'Hospitalization of Deliveries: The Change of Place of Birth in Denmark and Sweden from the Late Nineteenth Century to 1970', *Medical History*, 40 (1996), pp. 173–96.
18. Report of the Inquiry into Maternity Services, *AJHR*, H-31a (1938), pp. 68–101.
19. Cited by M. A. Tennant, 'Grace Neill in the Department of Asylums and Hospitals', *New Zealand Journal of History*, 12:1 (1978), pp. 3–16, on p. 13.
20. Bourke, 'Illuminating the Dark Hour', p. 45.
21. Minutes of the New Zealand Obstetrical Society, 13 September 1929 (held by Professor Ron Jones, Auckland).
22. Minutes of the New Zealand Obstetrical Society, 16 March 1933; 'NZ Obstetrical Society Section: Doctor and Midwife, Colleagues or Rivals', *New Zealand Medical Journal* (*NZMJ*), 32 (1933), pp. 20–3, on p. 23.
23. Minutes of the New Zealand Obstetrical Society, 20 March 1934.
24. 'NZ Obstetrical Society Section: Doctor and Midwife, Colleagues or Rivals', pp. 20–3, 22.
25. T. F. Corkill: 'The Trend of Obstetric Practice in New Zealand', *NZMJ*, 32 (1933), pp. 42–52.
26. Mrs McGuire, Onehunga Labour Party, evidence before Inquiry into Maternity Services, 7 September 1937, MS 78, AMA.
27. Dr Lowe, evidence before Inquiry into Maternity Services, 8 September 1937, MS 78, AMA.
28. Mein Smith, *Maternity in Dispute*, p. 1.
29. H. Maclean, 'Report Nurses Registration Act, Midwives Act, Maternity Hospitals and Private Hospitals', *AJHR*, H-31 (1918), p. 9; (1919), p. 11.
30. Minutes of the Auckland Branch of the New Zealand Society for the Protection of Women and Children, 19 August 1936, p. 73, AMA.
31. In 1937, see also Corkill, 'The Trend of Obstetric Practice in New Zealand'.
32. Vallgarda, 'Hospitalization of Deliveries'.
33. P. Mein Smith, 'Midwifery Re-Innovation in New Zealand', in J. Stanton (ed.), *Innovations in Health and Medicine: Diffusion and Resistance in the Twentieth Century* (London and New York: Routledge, 2002), pp. 169–87.
34. Minutes of the Auckland Branch of the National Council of Women, 22 June 1936, NCW MS 879, 32, AMA, my emphasis.
35. V. Crowther, 'Maternity', *Woman To-day* (October 1937), pp. 150–1; 'Correspondence', *Woman To-day* (January 1938), p. 240.

36. Minutes of the Executive Committee of the Auckland Branch of the Society for the Protection of Women and Children, 19 August 1936, p. 73; Minutes of a Special Sub committee meeting 1 April 1936 To consider State Maternity Services, 23 July 1936, MS 1144/7, AMA.

37. Society for the Protection of Women and Children, 'Minutes of Executive', 9 November 1936, visit paid to St Helens Hospital, 22 October 1936 by Mrs Moore, Mrs Bates, Mrs Agnes Preston Chambers and Mrs Amy Hutchinson.

38. R. Dalziel, *Focus on the Family: The Auckland Home and Family Society 1893–1993* (Auckland: Home and Family Society, 1993), pp. 39–40.

39. Mrs Molesworth, representing the Society for the Protection of Women and Children, Evidence before 1937 Committee of Inquiry into Maternity Services, 6 September 1937, MS 78, AMA.

40. Dr Siedeberg McKinnon, Evidence before 1937 Committee of Inquiry into Maternity Services, 21 June 1937, MS 78, AMA.

41. D. Caton, *What a Blessing She had Chloroform: The Medical and Social Response to the Pain of Childbirth from 1800 to the Present* (New Haven, CT, and London: Yale University Press, 1999), p. 152.

42. Oakley, *The Captured Womb*, pp. 130–1.

43. J. W. Leavitt, *Brought to Bed: Child-bearing in America, 1750–1950* (New York: Oxford University Press, 1986), p. 173.

44. J. Lewis, 'Mothers and Maternity Policies in the Twentieth Century', in J. Garcia, R. Kilpatrick and M. Richards (eds), *The Politics of Maternity Care: Services for Childbearing Women in Twentieth-Century Britain* (Oxford: Clarendon Press; New York: Oxford University Press, 1990), p. 20; J. Lewis, '"Motherhood Issues" in the Late Nineteenth and Twentieth Centuries', in K. Arnup, A. Lévesque and R. Roach Pierson with the assistance of M. Brennan (eds), *Delivering Motherhood: Maternal Ideologies and Practices in the 19th and 20th centuries* (London: Routledge, 1990), p. 12.

45. Health Department Annual Report, *AJHR*, H-31B (1921), p. 4.

46. A. G. Kent-Johnson, Evidence before 1937 Committee of Inquiry into Maternity Services, Professor Dawson, 22 May 1937, MS 78, AMA. M. Lovell-Smith, 'Kent-Johnson, Agnes Gilmour', *Dictionary of New Zealand Biography. Te Ara – The Encyclopedia of New Zealand*, updated 30 October 2012, http://www.TeAra.govt.nz/en/biographies/5k8/kent-johnston-agnes-gilmour [accessed 1 June 2012].

47. Society for the Protection of Women and Children (SPWC), 'Minutes of Executive', 9 November 1936, visit paid to St Helens Hospital, 22 October 1936 by Mrs Moore, Mrs Bates, Mrs Agnes Preston Chambers and Mrs Amy Hutchinson, AMA.

48. Miss Every/Miss Paterson, representatives of the Obstetrical Branch of the NZ Registered Nurses' Association, 'Evidence to 1937 Committee of Inquiry', 22 June 1937, MS 78, AMA.

49. Minutes Auckland Branch, SPWC, 19 August 1936, p. 73, AMA.

50. D. Page, *The National Council of Women: A Centennial History* (Auckland: Auckland University Press with Bridget Williams Books, Wellington, National Council of Women, 1996), p. 73.

51. Donley, *Save the Midwife*.

52. H. Marland, 'Childbirth and Maternity', in R. Cooter and J. Pickstone, *Companion to Medicine in the Twentieth Century* (London and New York: Routledge, 2000), pp. 559–74, on p. 566.

53. Gordon, Evidence to Committee of Inquiry into Maternity Services, 13 September 1937, MS 78, AMA.

54. D. Gordon, *Backblocks Baby-Doctor: An Autobiography* (London: Faber & Faber; New Zealand: Whitcombe & Tombs, 1955), p. 207.

55. Doris Gordon to Nina Barrer, 29 November 1944, Doris Clifton Gordon Papers, MS 115, AMA.

56. Gordon, *Backblocks Baby-Doctor*, p. 224.

57. Evidence to Committee of Inquiry into Maternity Services, Mrs Cassey, Women's Auxiliary, Unemployed Workers Union, Mrs Stewart, Devonport Housewives' Union, 7 September 1937, MS 78, AMA.

58. Grace Marshall to Secretary, Commission of Inquiry, Public Health Department, 19 August 1937, Complaints, YCBH/4372/6b, Archives New Zealand, Auckland branch.

59. Vallgarda, 'Hospitalization of Deliveries'.

60. SPWC minutes, 13 November 1939, AMA.

61. Bourke, 'Illuminating the Dark Hour', p. 100.

62. Mein Smith, *Maternity in Dispute*.

63. Maternity Services in New Zealand: Report by a Sub-Committee of the Wellington Branch of the National Council of Women, 5 February 1960, p. 22, Federation of New Zealand Parents Centres (FNZPC) Archives, Wellington, box 1.1: Early federation files, executive minutes 1957–64–75.

64. H. Brew to J. R. Marshall, 22 September 1960, FNZPC Archives Wellington, box 2.1: FNZPC early correspondence 1958–63 miscellaneous.

65. J. Donnison, *Midwives and Medical Men: A History of the Struggle for the Control of Childbirth* (London: Historical Publications, 1988), p. 201, cites S. Arms, *Immaculate Deception: A New Look at Women and Childbirth in America* (Boston, MA: Houghton Mifflin, 1975), p. 61.

66. The Auckland Hospital Board, Obstetrical and Gynaecological Unit, Cornwall Hospital, Auckland, New Zealand, *Second Clinical Report for the Year ended 31 March 1950*, prepared by G. H. Green, 1951, pp. 106, 122.

67. T. Plunkett, lectures on paediatrics, Royal New Zealand Plunket Society archives, Hocken Library, AG 7 4–275.

68. Evidence before 1937 Committee of Inquiry into Maternity Services, Professor Bernard Dawson, 22 June 1937, MS 78, AMA.

69. K. M. Reiger, *Our Bodies, Our Babies: The Forgotten Women's Movement* (Carlton South: Melbourne University Press, 2001), p. v.

70. *Auckland Star*, 24 February 1956.

71. 'Taking Fear of the Unknown out of Childbirth', *New Zealand Herald*, 1 August 1956.

72. M. Dobbie, *The Trouble with Women: The Story of Parents Centre New Zealand* (Whatamongo Bay: Cape Catley, 1990), p. 43.

73. 'Taking Fear of the Unknown out of Childbirth'.

74. G. D. Read, *Natural Childbirth* (London, Heinemann Medical Books, 1933); G. D. Read, *Revelation of Childbirth: The Principles and Practice of Natural Childbirth* (London, Heinemann Medical Books, 1942); from 1944 in America and 1951 in Britain, published as *Childbirth without Fear: The Principles and Practice of Natural Childbirth*.

75. 'Maternity and the Working Woman', *Woman To-day* (October 1937), pp. 150–1. Vera Crowther (later Vera Ellis) later embraced the natural childbirth movement: 'Vera Ellis Crowther 1897–1983 Farewell to a Friend', *Parents Centre Bulletin* (Summer 1983), on p. 14.

76. H. Brew to W. Nash, 24 October 1960, FNZPC Archives, box 2.1: FNZPC early correspondence 1958–63 miscellaneous; 'Viewpoints in Antenatal Education. The Parents' Viewpoint', Helen Brew's speech at the National Women's Hospital, 1958. p. 3, FNZPC Archives, box 1.0: Early Wellington branch.

77. Dobbie, *The Trouble with Women*, p. 51.

78. Ibid., p. 48.

79. E. J. Campbell, honorary secretary, 22 August 1962, FNZPC Archives, Wellington, box 123: Branch news, 1959–91.

80. Dobbie, *The Trouble with Women*, p. 56.

81. National Council of Women, Records, 1924–1990, MS 91/47, AM. See also Dobbie, *The Trouble with Women*, F. Hercock, *Alice: The Making of a Woman Doctor, 1914–1974* (Auckland: Auckland University Press, 1999).

82. Maternity Services in New Zealand: Report by a Sub-Committee of the Wellington Branch of the National Council of Women, 5 February 1960, p. 22, FNZPC Archives, Wellington, box 1.1: Early federation files, executive minutes 1957–64–75.

83. Letter to the editor from the Senior Medical Staff at National Women's Hospital (twenty-two names), 'New Nursing Curriculum', *NZMJ*, 1960, p. 59.

84. Ibid.; see also Minutes of Hospital Medical Committee, National Women's Hospital, 5 September 1960, BAGC A638 38b, Archives New Zealand, Auckland branch.

85. *New Zealand Herald*, 6 December 1959.

86. Professor H. Green to Mrs H. Brew, 16 June 1960, FNZPC Archives, Wellington, box 2.1: NZPC early correspondence 1958–63 miscellaneous.

87. Minutes of the Auckland Branch of the National Council of Women, 24 August 1959, NCW MS 879, 39, AMA.

88. Maternity Services in New Zealand: Report by a Sub-Committee of the Wellington Branch of the National Council of Women, 5 February 1960, pp. 24, 26, FNZPC Archives, Wellington, box 1.1: Early federation files, executive minutes 1957–64–75; see also Dobbie, *The Trouble with Women*, pp. 65–6.

89. 'Are New Zealand's Maternity Services Perfect? Report by a Committee', *Women's Viewpoint* (Organ of the NCW Auckland Branch), 1:1 (January 1960), p. 35; Minutes of the Auckland Branch of the National Council of Women, 22 February 1960, NCW MS 879, 40, AMA.

90. Minutes of the Auckland Branch of the National Council of Women, 19 September 1960, NCW MS 879, 40, AMA.

91. Donley, *Save the Midwife*.

6 Earner-Byrne, "Twixt God and Geography: The Development of Maternity Services in Twentieth-Century Ireland'

1. This chapter is focused on what is now the Irish Republic; the Northern Irish state will only be referred to when relevant to that experience.

2. C. Cameron, *Report upon the State of Public Health in the City of Dublin for the Year 1916* (Dublin, 1917), p. 94.

3. R. Barrington, *Health, Medicine and Politics in Ireland 1900–1970* (Dublin: Institute of Public Administration, 1987), pp. 1–24; L. Earner-Byrne, *Mother and Child: Maternity and Child Welfare in Dublin, 1922–1960* (Manchester: Manchester University Press, 2007), pp. 8–23.

4. M. Ó hÓgartaigh, *Quiet Revolutionaries: Irish Women in Education, Medicine and Sport, 1861–1964* (Dublin: The History Press Ireland, 2011), pp. 153–6.

5. C. Cameron, *Report upon the State of Public Health in the City of Dublin for the Year 1919* (Dublin, 1920), p. 77.

6. J. Lewis, *The Politics of Motherhood: Child and Maternal Welfare in England, 1900–1939* (London: Croom Helm, 1980), pp. 19, 35.

7. 'Report of the Lady Sanitary Sub-Officers of Dublin', in C. Cameron, *Report upon the State of Public Health in the City of Dublin for the Year 1915* (Dublin, 1916), p. 206.

8. Lewis identifies the same motivations in England. Lewis, *The Politics of Motherhood*, p. 117.

9. W. Lawson, 'Infant Mortality and the Notification of Births Act, 1907, 1915', *Journal of the Statistical and Social Inquiry Society of Ireland*, 13 (October 1919), p. 479; J. Dunwoody, 'Child Welfare', in D. Fitzpatrick (ed.), *Ireland, the First World War* (Mulingar: Lilliput, 1988), pp. 69–75.

10. Cameron, *Report upon the State of Public Health in the City of Dublin for the Year 1915*, p. 195.

11. It was still cited as the first step in the chain of services provided to mothers and children in 1987. See *Health Care for Mothers and Infants: A Review of the Maternity and Infant Care Scheme* (Dublin: Department of Health, 1987), p. 79.

12. See Ellen Ross's description of their function in Britain. E. Ross, 'Mothers and the State in Britain, 1904–1914', in J. R. Gillis, L. A. Tilly and D. Levine (eds), *The European Experience of Declining Fertility: A Quiet Revolution 1850–1970* (Cambridge: Cambridge University Press, 1992), pp. 48–60, on p. 56.

13. Cameron, *Report upon the State of Public Health in the City of Dublin for the Year 1915*, p. 198.

14. 'Report of the Lady Sanitary Sub-Officers of Dublin', in Cameron, *Report upon the State of Public Health in the City of Dublin for the Year 1915*, pp. 207–8.

15. Ibid., p. 208.

16. Ibid., p. 199.

17. These developments were similar to England. P. Thane, 'Visions of Gender in the Making of the British Welfare State: The Case of Women in the British Labour Party and Social Policy, 1906–1946', in G. Bock and P. Thane (eds), *Maternity and Gender Policies: Women and the Rise of the European Welfare State, 1880s–1950s* (London: Routledge, 1991), pp. 93–114, on p. 103.

18. Ibid., p. 105.

19. Barrington, *Health, Medicine and Politics*, pp. 76–7.

20. See Ó hÓgartaigh, *Quiet Revolutionaries*, pp. 73–87.

21. *Dáil Debates*, vol. 7, col. 1986 (5 June 1924).

22. *Report of the Commission on the Relief of the Sick and Destitute Poor, including the Insane Poor* (Dublin, 1927), pp. 10–11.

23. The Local Government Act 1925 allowed for the appointment of county medical officers.

24. For example, in 1929 the department claimed that the high maternal mortality rate in Kerry was due to the lack of a medical officer of health. *Annual Report of the Department of Local Government and Public Health, 1928–9* (Dublin, 1929), p. 46.

25. *Annual Report of the Department of Local Government and Public Health, 1934–5* (Dublin, 1935), p. 87.

26. *Annual Report of the Department of Local Government and Public Health, 1933–4* (Dublin, 1934), p. 61.
27. 'The Health of Dublin', *Journal of the Irish Free State Medical Union* [hereafter *JIFSMU*], 111:17 (November 1938), pp. 56–8.
28. P. McCarvill, 'Presidential Address: Delivered to the Irish Free State Medical Union on 8 June 1939', *JIFSMU*, 5:25 (July 1939), pp. 4–8, on p. 7.
29. The Irish sweep was a lottery legalized in 1930 to help fund Irish hospitals. M. Coleman, *The Irish Sweep: A History of the Irish Hospitals Sweepstake, 1930–87* (Dublin: University College Dublin Press, 2009), p. 15.
30. Coleman, *The Irish Sweep*, p. 54.
31. M. E. Daly, 'The Curse of the Hospital Sweep Stakes?: A Hospital Service not a Health System', presented to the Centre for the Social History of Medicine of Ireland, 24 March 2011.
32. Lewis argues that there was a similar drive to medicalize and hospitalize childbirth in England after World War I. Lewis, *The Politics of Motherhood*, pp. 117–34.
33. *Annual Report of the Department of Local Government and Public Health, 1927–1928* (Dublin, 1928), p. 41.
34. *Annual Report of the Department of Local Government and Public Health, 1930–1931* (Dublin, 1931), p. 60.
35. *Annual Report of the Department of Local Government and Public Health, 1937–1938* (Dublin, 1938), p. 53.
36. Of course, many women did not avail themselves of a hospital birth because they could not afford to leave their family for so long, but for others this rest was a lifeline.
37. Mrs M. Q., Upper Dorest St., Dublin to Archbishop Byrne, 1926, Dublin Diocesan Archives [DDA], Byrne papers, AB 7, Charity Cases, box 2: 1926–9. Note the errors are too numerous in these citations to enter [*sic*] on each occasion.
38. Mrs C. W., Wellington St., Dublin to Archbishop Byrne, [n.d.], DDA, Byrne papers, AB 7, Charity Cases, box 5: 1931–5.
39. A. Browne (ed.), *Masters, Midwives and Ladies-in Waiting: The Rotunda Hospital 1745–1995* (1995); J. K. Feeney, *The Coombe Lying-in Hospital* (Dublin, [n.d.]); T. Farmar, *Holles Street 1894–1994: The National Maternity Hospital – A Centenary History* (Dublin: A. and A. Farmar, 1994).
40. The Rotunda tended to serve north Dublin, the Coombe the south-west of the city and Holles Street the south-east of the city.
41. See *Annual Report of the Department of Local Government and Public Health, 1927–8* (Dublin, 1928), p. 41.
42. Earner-Byrne, *Mother and Child*, pp. 172–226.
43. In Cork the Erinville Hospital, in Limerick the Bedford Row Hospital and in Drogheda the Lourdes Hospital.
44. A. Spain, 'Maternity Services in Éire', *Irish Journal of Medical Science* [hereafter *IJMSc.*], 229 (January 1945), pp. 1–11.
45. Ibid., p. 7.
46. Ibid., p. 8.
47. I. Loudon, *Death in Childbirth: An International Study of Maternal Care and Maternal Mortality, 1800–1950* (Oxford: Oxford University Press, 1992), p. 227.
48. Department of Health, *White Paper on Health Services: Outline of the Improvement of the Health Services* (Dublin, 1947), p. 15.

49. The Irish Medical Association wished to see the establishment of a Ministry of Health. 'A Ministry of Health?', *JMAÉ*, 14:81 (March 1944), pp. 28–9.

50. The NHS was introduced in Northern Ireland in July 1948. See T. Farmar, *Patients, Potions and Physicians: A Social History of Medicine in Ireland* (Dublin: A. and A. Farmar, 2004), p. 155. Porter noted that in England the battle between the medical profession and the state became the 'main threat to the implementation of the new health care system'. D. Porter, *Health, Civilization and the State: A History of Public Health from Ancient to Modern Times* (London: Routledge, 1999), p. 215.

51. 'The Beveridge Plan', *JMAÉ*, 12:67 (January 1943), pp. 5–6.

52. 'Events of the Month: Beveridge Report', *JMAÉ*, 11:98 (February 1943), p. 14.

53. See, for example, 'Editorial: The Voluntary Hospitals and the State', *JMAÉ*, 12:69 (March 1943), p. 25; 'Editorial: What is a State Medical Service', *JMAÉ*, 12:70 (April 1943), p. 37.

54. *Annual Report of the Registrar-General, 1938* (Dublin, 1939), p. viii.

55. The increase in urban infant mortality rates was even more dramatic: in 1938 the rate was 84 in urban areas and 110 in 1943. *Annual Report of the Registrar-General, 1943* (Dublin, 1944), p. viii.

56. W. R. F. Collis, 'Infant Mortality in Éire and the Proposed Mother and Child Service', *JMAÉ*, 23:138 (December 1948), pp. 82–5, on p. 83.

57. Prof. F. O Briain, OFM of University College Galway, 'State Medicine and Morality', *JIMA*, 31:182 (August 1952), pp. 224–8, on p. 228.

58. The Irish Medical Association claimed it had increased its representation of registered doctors from 60 to 90 per cent over the ten-year period from 1948 to 1958. 'Editorial: Ten Fruitful Years', *JIMA*, 42:250 (April 1958), pp. 128–9, on p. 129.

59. Thane argues that the introduction of the NHS in England was of the 'greatest benefit' to hard-pressed working-class mothers. Thane, 'Visions of Gender in the Making of the British Welfare State', p. 107.

60. 'Presidential Address by Dr Andrew Ryan to the AGM, 19 June 1947', *JMAÉ*, 21:121 (July 1947), pp. 1–2, on p. 2.

61. Most Rev. Dr Lucey of Limerick, 'The State and its Citizens', *JIMA*, 29:174 (December 1951), pp. 136–8.

62. 'Editorial: Mother and Child Health Services', *JIMA*, 27:162 (December 1950), pp. 93–5, on p. 94.

63. 'Editorial: Present Status of Irish Medicine', *JIMA*, 30:177 (March 1952), pp. 55–7, on p. 55.

64. Anon., 'Some Social Aspects of an Improved Medical Service', *JMAE*, 13:74 (August 1943), pp. 19–20.

65. *Report of the Maternity and Infant Care Scheme Review Group* (Dublin: Department of Health, 1994), p. 9.

66. For example, in 1979, although 85 per cent of women were eligible, only 40 per cent used the service. Department of Health, *Health Care for Mothers & Infants: A Review of the Maternity and Infant Care Scheme* (Dublin: Department of Health, 1987), p. 8. In 1992 only 54 per cent of births occurred under the scheme, although all births were eligible. *Report of the Maternity and Infant Care Scheme Review Group*, p. 11.

67. Barrington, *Health, Medicine and Politics*, p. 250.

68. M. E. Daly, *The Slow Failure: Population Decline and Independent Ireland, 1920–1973* (Wisconsin, WI: University Press Wisconsin, 2006), p. 4.

69. Ibid., p. 84.

70. Cited in E. Mahon, 'The Development of a Health Policy for Women', in J. Robins (ed.), *Reflections on Health: Commemorating Fifty Years of the Department of Health, 1947–1997* (Dublin: The Department of Health, 1997), pp. 77–96, on p. 78.

71. Ibid., p. 78.

72. *Commission on Emigration and Other Population Problems, 1948–54, Report* (Dublin, 1956), p. 69. Cited in Daly, *The Slow Failure*, p. 80.

73. Daly notes that the average marriage age had dropped significantly in Ireland by 1965, when the mean age for men was 29.4 years and for women was 26.1 years, a drop of 2.3 and 1.6 years respectively since 1957. Daly, *The Slow Failure*, p. 137.

74. The Church of Ireland was the next largest denominational grouping at 164,215. There were 32,429 Presbyterians, 10,663 Methodists, 3,686 Jews and 11,913 others. CSO, *Census 2006, Vol. 13 – Religion* (Dublin: Stationary Office, November 2007), p. 9.

75. M. Curtis, *A Challenge to Democracy: Militant Catholicism in Modern Ireland* (Dublin: The History Press Ireland, 2010), pp. 78–102.

76. See, for example, the Irish government's campaign (prompted by Irish doctors of the Guild of SS Luke, Cosmas and Damian) to have the wording changed of the League of Nation's 1933 booklet, *Maternal Welfare and the Hygiene of Infants and Children.* The Irish secured a change to allow states to refuse to provide birth control advice, but instead states were required to make couples aware of the dangers of further conception. Secretary of the Department of External Affairs, 17 November 1932. Department of Health, B130/59, National Archives of Ireland.

77. Gillis, Tilly and Levine (eds), *The European Experience of Declining Fertility*, p. 5.

78. L. Earner-Byrne, 'Moral Prescription: The Irish Medical Profession, the Roman Catholic Church and the Prohibition of Birth Control in Twentieth-Century Ireland', in C. Cox and M. Luddy (eds), *Cultures of Care in Irish Medical History, 1750–1970* (Hampshire: Palgrave Macmillan, 2010), pp. 207–28.

79. Symphysiotomy is an operation that severs one of the main pelvic joints, which unhinges the pelvis. It was (and in some parts of the world still is) used in cases of severe disproportion.

80. Cited in J. Morrissey, 'An Examination of the Relationship between the Catholic Church and the Medical Profession in Ireland in the Period 1922–1992' (PhD dissertation, University College Dublin, 1999), p. 159.

81. See M. O'Connor, *Bodily Harm: Symphysiotomy and Pubiotomy in Ireland, 1944–92* (Dublin: Evertype, 2011).

82. H. McVey, 'The Treatment of Disproportion by combined Lower Segment Section with Symphysiotomy', *IJMSc*, 355 (July 1955), pp. 299–307.

83. A. Niedermeyer, 'Gender Questions on Demography', in *Sixth International Congress of Catholic Doctors: Transactions of the Congress in Dublin, June 30th to July 4th, 1954* (Dublin, 1955), p. 53.

84. A. P. Barry, 'Conservatism in Obstetrics', in *Sixth International Congress of Catholic Doctors*, p. 122.

85. Ibid., p. 126.

86. The Department of Health is currently investigating the issue. According to O'Connor 1,500 women underwent this procedure between 1944 and 1992. See O'Connor, *Bodily Harm*; F. Garland, 'Inquiry to be Carried out on Controversial Childbirth Surgery', *Irish Times*, 22 June 2011.

87. Daly, *The Slow Failure*, pp. 92–5; M. Solomons, *Pro Life? The Irish Question* (Dublin: Lilliput Press, 1992), p. 16.

88. Cited in Daly, *The Slow Failure*, p. 95.
89. B. Solomons, 'The Dangerous Multipara', *Lancet*, 2 (7 July 1934), pp. 8–11.
90. M. Heanue, 'Matters of Life and Death', in A. Redmond (ed.), *That Was Then, This is Now: Change in Ireland, 1949–1999* (Dublin: Central Statistics Office, 2000), pp. 29–39, on p. 32.
91. J. H. Young, 'The Grand Multipara', in *Journal of the College of General Practitioner*, 8 (1964), pp. 49–59.
92. Ibid., p. 51.
93. Ibid., p. 52.
94. A mother cited in *Rotunda Maternity Hospital Annual Report, 1957*, p. 32.
95. L. Earner-Byrne, 'Aphrodite Rising from the Waves?': Women's Voluntary Activism and the Women's Movement in Twentieth-Century Ireland', in P. Thane and E. Breitenbach (eds), *Women and Citizenship in Britain and Ireland: What Difference Did the Vote Make?* (London: Continuum Books, 2010), pp. 95–112.
96. Mahon, 'The Development of a Health Policy for Women', p. 81.
97. *Holles Street: Annual Report of the National Maternity Hospital, 1964*, p. 94.
98. C. Hug, *The Politics of Sexual Morality in Ireland* (Basingstoke: Macmillan, 1999), pp. 85–6.
99. Ibid., p. 105.
100. *Holles Street: National Maternity Hospital Annual Report, 1976*, p. 80.
101. Hug, *The Politics of Sexual Morality*, p. 114.
102. J. Murphy Lawless and J. McCarthy, 'Social Policy and Fertility Change in Ireland', *European Journal of Women's Studies*, 6:1 (1999), pp. 69–96.
103. H. Murphy, D. O'Driscoll, M. Brogan, L. Hickey and K. O'Gorman, 'Opinions of Post-Natal Mothers on Family Planning', *JIMA*, 72:2 (February 1979), pp. 49–52.
104. Ibid.
105. *Health Care for Mothers and Infants: A Review of the Maternity and Infant Care Scheme*, p. 30.
106. Mahon, 'The Development of a Health Policy for Women', p. 81.
107. Heanue, 'Matters of Life and Death', p. 29.

7 G. Davis, 'Test Tubes and Turpitude: Medical Responses to the Infertile Patient in Mid-Twentieth-Century Scotland'

1. See, for example, J. Weeks, *Sex, Politics and Society: The Regulation of Sexuality since 1800*, 2nd edn (London: Longman, 1989); L. A. Hall, *Sex, Gender and Social Change in Britain since 1880*, 2nd edn (Basingstoke: Palgrave Macmillan, 2012).
2. See J. Keown, *Abortion, Doctors and the Law: Some Aspects of the Legal Regulation of Abortion in England from 1803 to 1982* (Cambridge: Cambridge University Press, 1988); T. Newburn, *Permission and Regulation: Law and Morals in Post-War Britain* (London: Routledge, 1992), ch. 6; G. Davis, 'The Medical Community and Abortion Law Reform: Scotland in National Context, *c.* 1960–80', in I. Goold and C. Kelly (eds), *Lawyers' Medicine: The Legislature, The Courts and Medical Practice, 1760–2000* (Oxford: Hart, 2009), pp. 143–65.
3. See, for instance, S. Sheldon, *Beyond Control: Medical Power and Abortion Law* (London: Pluto Press, 1997); M. Latham, *Regulating Reproduction: A Century of Conflict in Britain and France* (Manchester and New York: Manchester University Press, 2002); L.

Hoggart, *Feminist Campaigns for Birth Control and Abortion Rights* (New York: Edwin Mellen Press, 2003).

4. Sheldon, *Beyond Control*, p. 168.

5. N. Pfeffer, *The Stork and the Syringe: A Political History of Reproductive Medicine* (Cambridge: Polity, 1993).

6. R. Snowden, *The Artificial Family: A Consideration of Artificial Insemination by Donor* (London and Boston, MA: Allen & Unwin, 1981); F. Cannell, 'Concepts of Parenthood: The Warnock Report, The Gillick Debate, and Modern Myths', *American Ethnologist*, 17:4 (1990), pp. 667–86; S. Franklin and H. Ragone (eds), *Reproducing Reproduction: Kinship, Power, and Technological Innovation* (Philadelphia, PA: University of Pennsylvania Press, 1998).

7. J. McMillan, 'The Return of the Inseminator: Eutelegenesis in Past and Contemporary Reproductive Ethics', *Studies in History and Philosophy of Biological and Biomedical Sciences*, 38:2 (2007), pp. 393–410; M. Richards, 'Artificial Insemination and Eugenics: Celibate Motherhood, Eutelegenesis and Germinal Choice', *Studies in History and Philosophy of Biological and Biomedical Sciences*, 39:2 (2008), pp. 211–21; A. McLaren, *Reproduction by Design: Sex, Robots, Trees and Test-Tube Babies in Interwar Britain* (Chicago, IL: University of Chicago Press, 2012).

8. See, for example, H. Marland, *Dangerous Motherhood: Insanity and Childbirth in Victorian Britain* (Basingstoke and New York: Palgrave Macmillan, 2004).

9. Sheldon, *Beyond Control*, pp. 24–6; see, also, S. J. Macintyre, 'The Medical Profession and the 1967 Abortion Act in Britain', *Social Science and Medicine*, 7 (1973), pp. 121–34, on p. 130.

10. See G. Davis, 'Sexual Snapshots: Departmental Committees and their Value to the Historian of Sexuality', *Scottish Archives* (forthcoming, 2013).

11. *Glasgow Herald*, 22 July 1960.

12. National Records of Scotland (hereafter NRS), GRO 5/1838, Notes for Representatives of Government Departments appearing before the Committee on 7 December 1959.

13. NRS, HH 101/1628, Memorandum of Evidence by the Department of Health for Scotland, [n.d.].

14. These doctors included the Manchester practitioner Bernard Sandler, who established his infertility clinic in Manchester Jewish Hospital in 1947, and the Exeter-based physician Margaret Jackson.

15. NRS, GRO 5/1838, Notes for Representatives of Government Departments appearing before the Committee on 7 December 1959.

16. NRS, HH 41/1459, AI (59) 4, Home Office, London, 8 April 1959.

17. For an examination of artificial insemination as a pressing medico-legal problem in mid-century America, see K. Swanson, 'Adultery by Doctor: Artificial Insemination, 1890–1945', *Chicago-Kent Law Review*, 87:2 (2012), pp. 591–633.

18. NRS, HH 41/1455, Verbatim Report of Oral Evidence by the Royal College of Surgeons of Edinburgh, 13 October 1959.

19. NRS, HH 41/1458, Verbatim Report of Oral Evidence by Dr Albert Sharman, Royal Samaritan Hospital for Women, Glasgow, 11 February 1959.

20. NRS, HH 101/1628, Memorandum of Evidence by the Department of Health for Scotland, [n.d.].

21. NRS, HH 41/1461, Verbatim Report of Oral Evidence by Professor T. B. Smith, University of Edinburgh, December 1959.

22. NRS, HH 41/1453, Memorandum of Evidence by Dr Albert Sharman, Royal Samaritan Hospital for Women, Glasgow, 6 November 1958. Sharman also co-authored the textbook *Sterility and Impaired Fertility: Pathogenesis, Investigation and Treatment*

(London: Hamish Hamilton, 1939) in conjunction with fellow authorities in the field such as Kenneth Walker and Mary Barton.

23. NRS, HH 41/1458, Verbatim Report of Oral Evidence by Dr Hector MacLennan, 10 February 1959.
24. NRS, HH 41/1455, Verbatim Report of Oral Evidence by the Royal College of Surgeons of Edinburgh, 13 October 1959.
25. NRS, HH 41/1453, Memorandum of Evidence by Dr Albert Sharman, Royal Samaritan Hospital for Women, Glasgow, 6 November 1958.
26. NRS, HH 41/1458, Verbatim Report of Oral Evidence by Dr Albert Sharman, Royal Samaritan Hospital for Women, Glasgow, 11 February 1959.
27. NRS, HH 41/1458, Verbatim Report of Oral Evidence by Dr Audrey Freeth, 10 March 1959.
28. NRS, HH 41/1453, Memorandum of Evidence by Dr Albert Sharman, Royal Samaritan Hospital for Women, Glasgow, 6 November 1958.
29. NRS, HH 41/1453, Memorandum of Evidence by Dr Albert Sharman, Royal Samaritan Hospital for Women, Glasgow, 6 November 1958.
30. NRS, HH 41/1458, Verbatim Report of Oral Evidence by Dr Audrey Freeth, 10 March 1959.
31. NRS, HH 41/1453, Memorandum of Evidence by Dr Albert Sharman, Royal Samaritan Hospital for Women, Glasgow, 6 November 1958.
32. *Glasgow Herald*, 1 March 1958.
33. NRS, HH 41/1455, Verbatim Report of Oral Evidence by the Royal College of Surgeons of Edinburgh, 13 October 1959.
34. NRS, HH 41/1453, Memorandum of Evidence by Dr Albert Sharman, Royal Samaritan Hospital for Women, Glasgow, 6 November 1958.
35. NRS, HH 41/1453, Memorandum of Evidence by Dr Albert Sharman, 6 November 1958.
36. NRS, HH 41/1453, Memorandum of Evidence by Dr Hector R. MacLennan, [n.d.].
37. NRS, HH 41/1453, Memorandum of Evidence by the Royal College of Surgeons of Edinburgh, [n.d.].
38. NRS, HH 41/1455, Verbatim Report of Oral Evidence by the Royal College of Surgeons of Edinburgh, 13 October 1959.
39. Ibid.
40. NRS, HH 41/1453, Memorandum of Evidence by the Royal College of Surgeons of Edinburgh, [n.d.].
41. NRS, HH 41/1458, Verbatim Report of Oral Evidence by Dr Audrey Freeth, 10 March 1959.
42. NRS, HH 41/1453, Memorandum of Evidence by Dr Hector R. MacLennan, [n.d.].
43. NRS, HH 41/1453, Memorandum of Evidence by the Royal College of Surgeons of Edinburgh, [n.d.].
44. NRS, HH 41/1455, Verbatim Report of Oral Evidence by the Royal College of Surgeons of Edinburgh, 13 October 1959.
45. I. M. Ingram, 'Abortion Games: An Inquiry into the Working of the Act', *Lancet*, 2 (1971), pp. 969–70; G. Davis and R. Davidson, '"Big White Chief", "Pontius Pilate", and the "Plumber": The Impact of the 1967 Abortion Act on the Scottish Medical Community, *c.* 1967–1980', *Social History of Medicine*, 18:2 (2005), pp. 283–306, on pp. 301–4.
46. NRS, HH 41/1453, Memorandum of Evidence by Dr John McDonald, Murray Royal Hospital, Perth, 28 January 1959.
47. NRS, HH 41/1453, Memorandum of Evidence by the Royal College of Surgeons of Edinburgh, [n.d.].

48. 'The Royal College of Psychiatrists' Memorandum on the Abortion Act in Practice', *British Journal of Psychiatry*, 120 (1972), pp. 449–51, on p. 449.
49. Richards, 'Artificial Insemination and Eugenics', p. 217.
50. NRS, HH 41/1459, Note by the Feversham Secretary, 8 April 1959.
51. S. Wilmot (ed.), 'Between the Farm and the Clinic: Agriculture and Reproductive Technology in the Twentieth Century' special issue, *Studies in History and Philosophy of Biological and Biomedical Sciences*, 38:2 (2007), pp. 303–529.
52. NRS, HH 41/1454, Memorandum by the Public Questions and Religion and Morals Committee of the Free Church of Scotland, [n.d.].
53. NRS, HH 41/1454, Memorandum of Evidence by the United Free Church of Scotland, Glasgow, [n.d.].
54. NRS, HH 41/1459, Note by R. F. D. Shuffrey, Secretary, 'Summary of Written Evidence', 7 December 1959.
55. NRS, HH 41/1454, Memorandum of Evidence by the Committee of the Free Presbyterian Church of Scotland, [n.d.].
56. See, for example, NRS, HH 41/1453, Memorandum of Evidence by Dr John McDonald, Murray Royal Hospital, Perth, 28 January 1959.
57. NRS, HH 41/1458, Verbatim Report of Oral Evidence by Dr Audrey Freeth, 10 March 1959.
58. G. Davis and R. Davidson, '"The Fifth Freedom" or "Hideous Atheistic Expediency": The Medical Community and Abortion Law Reform in Scotland, *c.* 1960–75', *Medical History*, 50:1 (2006), pp. 29–48.
59. Ibid.
60. NRS, HH 101/1628, Free Presbyterian Church of Scotland to Ministry of Health, Edinburgh, 1 June 1959.
61. NRS, HH 41/1454, Report of the Committee on Church and Nation of the Church of Scotland, adopted by the General Assembly in May 1959.
62. NRS, HH 41/1454, Memorandum by the Public Questions and Religion and Morals Committee of the Free Church of Scotland, [n.d.].
63. NRS, HH 41/1458, Verbatim Report of Oral Evidence by Dr Hector MacLennan, 10 February 1959.
64. R. Davidson and G. Davis, *The Sexual State: Sexuality and Scottish Governance, 1950–80* (Edinburgh: Edinburgh University Press, 2012).
65. NRS, HH 41/1455, Verbatim Reports, 1959.
66. NRS, HH 41/1455, Verbatim Report of Oral Evidence by the Royal College of Surgeons of Edinburgh, 13 October 1959.
67. NRS, HH 41/1453, Memorandum of Evidence by Dr Hector R. MacLennan, [n.d.].
68. NRS, HH 41/1458, Verbatim Report of Oral Evidence by Dr Hector MacLennan, 10 February 1959.
69. NRS, HH 41/1458, Verbatim Report of Oral Evidence by Dr Audrey Freeth, 10 March 1959.
70. NRS, HH 41/1455, Verbatim Report of Oral Evidence by the Royal College of Surgeons of Edinburgh, 13 October 1959.
71. Lothian Health Services Archive (hereafter LHSA), LHB 1 C/C GOPD, Infertility Case Notes, 1946–1994, box 2425–71. Only initials are provided here, so as to protect patient confidentiality.
72. Ibid.
73. LHSA, LHB 1 C/C GOPD, Infertility Case Notes, 1946–1994, box 409–76.

74. See G. Risse and J. Warner, 'Reconstructing Clinical Activities: Patient Records in Medical History', *Social History of Medicine*, 5:2 (1992), pp. 183–205; G. Davis, *'The Cruel Madness of Love': Sex, Syphilis and Psychiatry in Scotland, 1880–1930* (Amsterdam and New York: Rodopi, 2008), pp. 22–30.

75. LHSA, LHB 1 C/C GOPD, Infertility Case Notes, 1946–1994, box 2425–71.

76. See, for example, J. Monach, *Childless: No Choice – The Experience of Involuntary Childlessness* (London and New York: Routledge, 1993); M. Marsh and W. Ronner, *The Empty Cradle: Infertility in America from Colonial Times to the Present* (Baltimore, MD: Johns Hopkins University Press, 1996).

77. Ibid.

78. NRS, HH 41/1458, Verbatim Report of Oral Evidence by Dr Albert Sharman, Royal Samaritan Hospital for Women, Glasgow, 11 February 1959.

79. Ibid.

80. NRS, HH 41/1453, Memorandum of Evidence by Dr Albert Sharman, Royal Samaritan Hospital for Women, Glasgow, 6 November 1958.

81. NRS, HH 41/1453, Memorandum of Evidence by the Royal Medico-Psychological Association, [n.d.].

82. NRS, HH 41/1453, Memorandum of Evidence by Dr John McDonald, Murray Royal Hospital, Perth, 28 January 1959.

83. NRS, HH 41/1458, Verbatim Report of Oral Evidence by Dr Albert Sharman, Royal Samaritan Hospital for Women, Glasgow, 11 February 1959.

84. NRS, HH 41/1461, Minutes of Meeting held in London, 14–15 April 1959; NRS, HH 41/1453, Memorandum of Evidence by Dr Albert Sharman, 6 November 1958.

85. NRS, HH 41/1453, Memorandum of Evidence by Faculty of Medicine, University of Edinburgh, February 1959.

86. See, for example, A. Oakley, 'Normal Motherhood: An Exercise in Self-Control', in B. Hutter and G. Williams (eds), *Controlling Women: The Normal and the Deviant* (London: Croom Helm, 1981), pp. 79–184; Sheldon, *Beyond Control*.

87. NRS, ED 11/511, Note by W. S. Kerr, 'Feversham Committee on Artificial Insemination', 13 October 1958.

88. A recent study of male sterility in the German context finds a similar pathologization of the male patient. See C. Benninghaus, 'Beyond Constructivism? Gender, Medicine and the Early History of Sperm Analysis, Germany, 1870–1900', *Gender and History*, 24:3 (2012), pp. 647–76.

8 A. Davis, 'Women's Experiences of the Maternity Services in Berkshire and Oxfordshire, *c.* 1970–1990'

1. S. McIntyre, 'The Sociology of Reproduction', *Sociology of Health and Illness*, 2 (1980), pp. 215–22, on p. 217.

2. A. Oakley, *Women Confined: Towards a Sociology of Childbirth* (Oxford: Martin Robertson, 1980), p. 20.

3. P. L. Brodsky, *The Control of Childbirth: Women versus Medicine through the Ages* (London: McFarland & Co., 2008); J. Donnison, *Midwives and Medical Men: A History of the Struggle for the Control of Childbirth* (London: Historical Publications, 1988); C. Hanson, *A Cultural History of Pregnancy: Pregnancy, Medicine, and Culture* (Basingstoke: Palgrave Macmillan, 2004); H. Marland and A. M. Rafferty (eds), *Midwives, Society and*

Childbirth: Debates and Controversies in the Modern Period (London: Routledge, 1997); O. Moscucci, *The Science of Woman: Gynaecology and Gender in England, 1800–1929* (Cambridge: Cambridge University Press, 1990); A. Oakley, *The Captured Womb: A History of the Medical Care of Pregnant Women* (Oxford: Basil Blackwell, 1984); P. Rhodes, *A Short History of Clinical Midwifery: Development of Ideas in the Professional Management of Childbirth* (Hale: Books for Midwives Press, 1995); E. Teijlingen, G. W. Lowis, P. McCaffery and M. Porter (eds), *Midwifery and the Medicalization of Childbirth: Comparative Perspectives* (New York: Nova Science, 1999); M. Tew, *Safer Childbirth? A Critical History of Maternity Care* (London and New York: Free Association Books, 1998).

4.   The interviews were conducted by the author between 2008 and 2010 for a Leverhulme Early Career Fellowship project entitled 'Motherhood *c.* 1970–1990: An Oral History'. Interviewees were principally found through women's and community groups and local media. The sample was self-selecting as the women volunteered to be interviewed, however the aim was to construct a sample that ranged in age, class and educational background. Although respondents did not require that their contributions be used confidentially, pseudonyms have been employed in the chapter. Interviewees are referenced by identifying codes. The recordings and transcripts are held by the author.

5.   Responding to an appeal from the Natural Childbirth Association for volunteers to show pregnant women how to breathe and relax for labour, she ran the first couples' classes in the country from the late 1950s. S. Kitzinger, *The Politics of Birth* (London: Elsevier, 2005), p. 46.

6.   The Agricultural Economics Research Institute Oxford, *Country Planning: A Study of Rural Problems* (London: Oxford University Press, 1944).

7.   M. B. McNay and J. E. E. Fleming, 'Forty Years of Obstetric Ultrasound 1957–1997: From A-Scope to Three Dimensions', *Ultrasound in Medicine and Biology*, 25 (1999), pp. 3–56, on p. 6. For a fuller account of the development and use of ultrasound imaging, see M. Nicolson and J. E. E. Fleming, *Imaging and Imagining the Fetus: The Development of Obstetric Ultrasound* (Baltimore, MD: Johns Hopkins University Press, 2013).

8.   A. Stewart, J. Webb, D. Giles and D. Hewett, 'Malignant Disease in Childhood and Diagnostic Irradiation in Utero', *Lancet*, 2 (1956), p. 447.

9.   I. Donald, J. MacVicar and T. G. Brown, 'Investigation of Abdominal Masses by Pulsed Ultrasound', *Lancet*, 1 (1958), pp. 1188–95.

10. M. H. Hall and R. A. Carr-Hill, 'The Significance of Uncertain Gestation for Obstetric Outcome', *British Journal of Obstetrics and Gynaecology*, 92 (1985), pp. 452–60.

11. McNay and Fleming, 'Forty Years of Obstetric Ultrasound', p. 28.

12. Andrea, SA9, p. 3.

13. Tara, SO15, p. 1416.

14. Hermione, NO15, p. 10.

15. Sandra, EW13, p. 5.

16. Pippa, CO13, p. 13.

17. Marilyn, BE13; Bet, CO1; Pippa, CO13; Harriet, CR8; Dawn, CR13; Bonnie, CR14; Sandra, EW13; Hermione, NO15; Liz, SA5; Andrea, SA9; Tara, SO15; April, SO16; Cynthia, WY12. Other interviewees may also have had scans but did not report this.

18. G. Lewando Hundt, J. Sandall, K. Spencer, B. Heyman, C. Williams, R. Grellier, L. Pitson and M. Tsouroufli, 'Experiences of First Trimester Antenatal Screening in a One-Stop Clinic', *British Journal of Midwifery*, 16 (2008), pp. 156–9, on p. 159.

19. Cynthia, WY12, p. 7.

20. J. G. Thornton, J. Hewison, R. J. Lilford and A. Vail, 'A Randomised Trial of Three Methods of Giving Information about Prenatal Testing', *British Medical Journal* (hereafter *BMJ*), 311 (1995), pp. 1127–30.

21. Thornton, et al., 'A Randomised Trial', p. 1127. This popularity has also been seen since the late 1990s in clinics offering scans to expectant parents for non-diagnostic purposes. J. Palmer, 'The Placental Body in 4D: Everyday Practices of Non-Diagnostic Sonography', *Feminist Review*, 93 (2009), pp. 64–80, on p. 66.

22. S. Kitzinger with R. Walters, *Some Women's Experiences of Episiotomy* (London: National Childbirth Trust, 1981), p. 1.

23. J. L. Reynolds and P. L. Yudkin, 'Changes in the Management of Labour: 2. Perineal Management', *CMAJ*, 136 (1987), pp. 1041–9, on p. 1048.

24. D. Banta and S. B. Thacker, 'The Risks and Benefits of Episiotomy: A Review', *Birth*, 9 (1982), pp. 25–30, on p. 27.

25. Reynolds and Yudkin, 'Perineal Management', p. 1048.

26. Kitzinger with Walters, *Episiotomy*, p. 2.

27. Ibid.

28. J. Kitzinger, 'Strategies of the Early Childbirth Movement: A Case-Study of the National Childbirth Trust', in J. Garcia, R. Kilpatrick and M. Richards (eds), *The Politics of Maternity Care* (Oxford: Clarendon Press, 1990), pp. 92–115, on p. 111.

29. Bet, CO1; Pippa, CO13; Harriet, CR8; Dawn, CR13; Sandra, EW13; Katherine, SA12; Jemma, SA13; Faith, SO12; Carol, TH14. There may have been other interviewees who also had episiotomies but did not remember, or did not consider it to be an important part of their birth stories, because they did not find it painful or traumatic.

30. Sandra, EW13, p. 6.

31. Dawn, CR13, p. 23.

32. Carol, TH14, pp. 10–11.

33. M. B. McNay, G. M. McIlwaine, P. W. Howie and M. C. MacNaughton, 'Perinatal Deaths: Analysis by Clinical Cause to Assess Value of Induction of Labour', *BMJ*, 1 (5 February 1977), pp. 347–50.

34. I. Chalmers, J. G. Lawson and A. C. Turnbull, 'Evaluation of Different Approaches to Obstetric Care: Part II', *British Journal of Obstetrics and Gynaecology*, 83 (1976), pp. 930–3.

35. The sample was not entirely random in that she excluded illegitimate births.

36. A. Cartwright, *The Dignity of Labour: A Study of Childbearing and Induction* (London: Tavistock Publications, 1979), pp. 69–70.

37. Ibid., p. 91.

38. Patsy, BA15; Marilyn, BE13; Pippa, CO13; Harriet, CR8; Bev, CR10; Viv, EW12; Anna, NO13; Megan, OX11; Liz, SA5; Andrea, SA9; Katherine, SA12; Jemma, SA13; Karen, SO4; Tasha, SO14; April, SO16; Josie, TH6; Mildred, TH11; Carol, TH14; Susan, WY11.

39. Patsy, BA15; Viv, EW12; Marilyn, BE13; Bev, CR10; April, SO16.

40. Patsy, BA15, pp. 11–12.

41. Liz, SA5, pp. 13–14.

42. Josie, TH6, p. 8.

43. Megan, OX11; Liz, SA5; Karen, SO4; Tasha, SO14; Josie, TH6; Mildred, TH11.

44. Pippa, CO13; April, SO16; Harriet, CR8; Bev, CR10; Anna, NO13; Andrea, SA9; Katherine, SA12; Jemma, SA13.

45. Anna, NO13, p. 8.

46. T. Lavender, S. A. Walkinshaw and I. Walton, 'A Prospective Study of Women's Views of Factors Contributing to a Positive Birth Experience', *Midwifery*, 15 (1999), pp. 40–6, on p. 42.
47. Viv, EW12, pp. 8–9.
48. Bev, CR10, p. 22.
49. I. Z. MacKenzie and J. Boland, 'Current Therapeutic Uses of Prostaglandins in Obstetrics in the United Kingdom', *Contemporary Reviews in Obstetrics and Gynaecology*, 5 (1992), pp. 9–14.
50. Kaye, WY14, p. 2.
51. Ibid., p. 7.
52. Ibid., p. 2.
53. V. A. Hundley, F. M. Cruickshank, G. D. Lang, C. M. A. Glazener, J. M. Milne, M. Turner, D. Blyth, J. Mollison and C. Donaldson, 'Midwife Managed Delivery Unit: A Randomised Controlled Comparison with Consultant Led Care', *BMJ*, 309 (1994), pp. 1400–4.
54. Mildred, TH11, p. 5.
55. Tasha, SO14, p. 7.
56. Geraldine, CR9, p. 6.
57. Georgie, OX2, p. 17.
58. Patsy, BA15; Bet, CO1; Pippa, CO13; Harriet, CR8; Geraldine, CR9; Dawn, CR13; Ellen, EW3; Hermione, NO15; Carmel, NO16; Katherine, SA12; Cynthia, WY12.
59. Bet, CO1; Dawn, CR13; Katherine, SA12; Cynthia, WY12.
60. Dawn, CR13, p. 21.
61. Patsy, BA15; Pippa, CO13; Harriet, CR8; Geraldine, CR9; Hermione, NO15.
62. Harriet, CR8, p. 5.
63. Carmel, NO16, p. 8.
64. Ellen, EW3, p. 9.
65. Jean, EW14, p. 4.
66. Bonnie, CR14, p. 22.
67. Pippa, CO13, p. 9.
68. Patsy, BA15, pp. 11–12.
69. While there was speculation at the time, and subsequently, that a difficult birth could affect bonding between mother and child, it seems that there is no clear correlation. S. Ayers and E. Ford, 'Birth Trauma: Widening Our Knowledge of Postnatal Mental Health', *European Health Psychologist*, 11 (2009), pp. 16–19.
70. Siobhan, BE1; Marilyn, BE13; Geraldine, CR9; Bev, CR10; Bonnie, CR14; Hermione, NO15; Carmel, NO16; Lynne, OX14; Pam, SA7; Katherine, SA12; Tara, SO15; Nina, TH3; Barbie, TH4; Mary, TH5; Alma, TH7; Mildred, TH11.
71. Carmel, NO16; Lynne, OX14; Pam, SA7.
72. Pam, SA7, p. 4.
73. Katherine, SA12, pp. 5–6.
74. Siobhan, BE1; Marilyn, BE13; Geraldine, CR9; Bev, CR10; Bonnie, CR14; Hermione, NO15; Lynne, OX14; Tara, SO15; Nina, TH3; Barbie, TH4; Mary, TH5; Alma, TH7; Mildred, TH11.
75. Tara, SO15, pp. 14–16.
76. An *elective caesarean* is performed before labour has begun and an *emergency caesarean* is carried out as a result of some complication arising during labour. By the 1980s, epidural anaesthesia was preferred over general anaesthesia in elective caesareans because it was

deemed safer for the mother and allowed the mother to be awake and immediately interact with her baby. General anaesthetic was still used in an emergency caesarean because it could be given very quickly when there was an immediate threat to life. Since the 1990s, spinal anaesthesia has become the technique of choice for elective and some *emergency caesareans* due to its more rapid onset and lower incidence of failed block than pure epidural techniques.

77. E. M. Hillan, 'Research and Audit: Women's Views of Caesarean Section', in H. Roberts (ed.), *Women's Health Matters* (London: Routledge, 1992), pp. 157–75, on p. 161.
78. Ibid., p. 169.
79. Bonnie, CR14, p. 24.
80. Bev, CR10, p. 18.
81. Ibid., pp. 10–11.
82. National Childbirth Trust, *Rupture of the Membranes in Labour: A Survey Conducted by the National Childbirth Trust, 1989* (London: National Childbirth Trust, 1989), p. 35.
83. Ibid., p. 36.
84. Ibid., p. 38.
85. S. Kitzinger, *Some Mothers' Experiences of Induced Labour* (London: National Childbirth Trust, 1975), p. 1.
86. Ibid.
87. Ibid.
88. Lynne, OX14, p. 6.
89. Carmel, NO16, p. 8.
90. Sandra, EW13, p. 5; Liz, SA5, pp. 13–14.
91. Katherine, SA12, p. 7. Consultants were also explicitly criticized by Katherine, SA12, pp. 6–7; Tasha, SO14, p. 7; Bonnie, CR14, p. 23.
92. Josie, TH6, p. 8.
93. Carol, TH14, pp. 10–11.
94. Pippa, CO13, pp. 13–14.
95. A. Davis, 'Motherhood in Oxfordshire *c.* 1945–1970: A Study of Attitudes, Experiences and Ideals' (DPhil Thesis, Oxford University, 2007), pp. 161–6.
96. Dawn, CR13, p. 23.
97. Katherine, SA12, pp. 5–6.
98. J. Robinson, 'Active Management of Childbirth "Reduces Hazards and Anxiety"', in *The Times*, 12 August 1974, p. 6.
99. S. Kitzinger, 'Women's Experiences of Birth at Home', in S. Kitzinger and J. A. Davis (eds), *The Place of Birth* (Oxford: Oxford University Press, 1978), pp. 135–56, on p. 136.
100. Ibid., p. 146.
101. Ibid., p. 143.
102. Margaret, EW15, p. 4.
103. Kaye, WY14, p. 4.
104. Bet, CO1, second child born at home in 1975; Stella, CR5, third child born at home in 1975; Margaret, EW15, first and second children born at home in 1969 and 1970; Martha, NO14, second child born at home in 1971; Kim, OX15, second child born at home in 1978.
105. R. Campbell and A. Macfarlane, *Where to Be Born? The Debate and the Evidence* (Oxford: Oxford University Press for the National Perinatal Epidemiology Unit, 1994), p. 117.
106. Davis, 'Motherhood in Oxfordshire', pp. 161–2, 167.
107. Jean, EW14, p. 4.

108. April, SO16, p. 11.
109. Amelia, CO15, p. 37.
110. Bev, CR10, p. 10.
111. Geraldine, CR9, p. 6.
112. Sheilagh, CO17, p. 37.
113. Tara, SO15, pp. 14–16.
114. Harriet, CR8, p. 5.

9 Hepler, 'From *Muller* to *Johnson Controls*: Mothers and Workplace Health in the US, from Protective Labour Legislation to Fetal Protection Policies'

1. A. Hamilton, 'Possibilities and Limitations of Employment of Women in Industry', *Monthly Bulletin of the Pennsylvania Department of Labor and Industry*, 5 (1918), pp. 37, 39.
2. *Muller* v. *Oregon*, 208 U.S. 412 (1908); *UAW* v. *Johnson Controls*, 499 U.S. 187 (1991).
3. *Lochner* v. *New York*, 198 U.S. 45 (1905); L. D. Brandeis and J. Goldmark, *Women in Industry: Decision of the United States Supreme Court in Curt Muller v. State of Oregon* (reprint, New York: National Consumers' League, 1908).
4. J. Goldmark, *Fatigue and Efficiency, A Study in Efficiency* (New York: Survey Associates, 1913). The National Consumers' League and the various state Consumer's Leagues offer voluminous records of women's working conditions in the early twentieth century. See, for example: National Consumers' League Papers, Library of Congress, Washington, DC; Consumers' League of Connecticut Papers and Consumers' League of Massachusetts Papers, Schlesinger Library, Radcliffe College, Harvard University Libraries, Cambridge MA; Consumers' League of New Jersey Papers, Special Collections and Archives, Rutgers University Libraries, New Brunswick, NJ; *Adkins* v. *Children's Hospital*, 261 U.S. 525 (1923).
5. The amendment was never ratified, despite repeated attempts.
6. See, for example, J. Baer, *Chains of Protection: The Judicial Response to Women's Labor Legislation* (Westport, CT: Greenwood Press, 1978); N. F. Cott, *The Grounding of Modern Feminism* (New Haven, CT: Yale University Press, 1987); N. Cott, 'What's in a Name? The Limits of "Social Feminism"; or Expanding the Vocabulary of Women's History', *Journal of American History*, 76 (December 1989), pp. 809–29; R. Muncy, *Creating a Female Dominion in American Reform* (Oxford: Oxford University Press, 1991); and W. Sarvasy, 'Beyond the Difference versus Equality Debate: Postsuffrage Feminism, Citizenship, and the Quest for the Feminist Welfare State', *Signs*, 17 (Winter 1992), pp. 329–62.
7. C. Sellers, 'Public Health Service's Office of Industrial Hygiene and the Transformation of Industrial Medicine', *Bulletin of the History of Medicine*, 65 (Spring 1991), pp. 42–73; H. Stevens, 'The Practice of Medicine in Industry', *New England Journal of Medicine*, 203 (13 November 1930), pp. 974–5.
8. M. T. Mettert, 'The Occurrence and Prevention of Occupational Disease Among Women, 1935–1938', *Bulletin of the Women's Bureau*, no. 184 (1941); 'The Employment of Women in Hazardous Industries in the United States', *Bulletin of the Women's Bureau*, no. 6 (1921).

9. S. Berger Gluck, *Rosie the Riveter Revisited: Women, the War, and Social Change* (Boston, MA: Twayne, 1989); 'Women Can Do 80% of War Jobs', *New York Times*, 23 May 1942. 'New Women War Workers are Women, 4 to 1', *New York Times*, 30 August 1943, p. 12. See also A. L. Hepler, *Women in Labor: Mothers, Medicine, and Occupational Health in the U.S., 1895–1980* (Columbus, OH: Ohio State University Press, 2000), ch. 4.

10. N. Stanton Barney, 'Women as Human Beings' (published by Barney, 1946), pp. 8–9, folder 38, box 2, Alma Lutz Papers, Schlesinger Library, Radcliffe College, Harvard University Libraries, Cambridge, MA.

11. N. F. Gabin, *Feminism in the Labor Movement: Women and the United Auto Workers, 1935–1975* (Ithaca, NY: Cornell University Press, 1990).

12. D. S. Cobble, 'Recapturing Working-Class Feminism: Union Women in the Postwar Era', in J. Meyerowitz (ed.), *Not June Cleaver: Women and Gender in Postwar America, 1945–1960* (Philadelphia, PA: Temple University, 1994), pp. 57–83, on p. 73.

13. *Pat L. Grant v. General Motors Corporation, et al.*, 743 F.Supp. 1260 (N.D. Ohio, 1989).

14. T. Oliver, 'Industrial Lead Poisoning in Europe', *Bulletin of the Bureau of Labor*, no. 95 (1911).

15. J. M. Stellman and S. M. Daum, *Work is Dangerous to Your Health* (New York: Random House, 1973); A. Baetjer, 'The Relation of Industrial Work to Obstetrical and Gynecologic Conditions', *Journal of the American Medical Women's Association*, 2 (1947), pp. 276–80, on p. 277.

16. *Dietrich v. Northampton*, 138 Mass. (1884); *Bonbrest v. Kotz*, 65 F. Supp. 138 (1946); *Brennan v. Smith*, 157 A.2d 497 (1960). See also R. Blank, *Fetal Protection in the Workplace: Women's Rights, Business Interests, and the Unborn* (New York: Columbia University Press, 1993) and C. R. Daniels, *At Women's Expense: State Power and the Politics of Fetal Rights* (Cambridge, MA: Harvard University Press, 1993), pp. 10–13.

17. E. Boris, *Home to Work: Motherhood and the Politics of Industrial Homework in the United States* (Cambridge: Cambridge University Press, 1994); and A. Kessler-Harris, *Out to Work: A History of Wage-Earning Women in the United States* (Oxford: Oxford University Press, 1982).

18. For more information on the origins of the EEOC, see R. Rosen, *The World Split Open: How the Modern Women's Movement Changed America* (New York: Viking Penguin, 2000), pp. 70–4.

19. N. Pedriana, 'From Protective to Equal Treatment: Legal Framing Processes and Transformations of the Women's Movement in the 1960s', *American Journal of Sociology*, 111 (May 2006), pp. 1718–61, on pp. 1735–7.

20. Ibid., pp. 1745–7.

21. R. Roth, *Making Women Pay: The Hidden Costs of Fetal Rights* (Ithaca, NY: Cornell University Press, 2000), pp. 76–7. According to Roth, five states passed such laws between 1979 and 1989: California, Connecticut, Louisiana, Minnesota and Oregon.

22. L. Vogel, *Mothers on the Job: Maternity Rights in the U.S. Workplace* (New Brunswick, NJ: Rutgers University Press, 1993), pp. 91–113.

23. For a more thorough understanding of this period, see Rosen, *The World Split Open*; S. Evans, *Personal Politics: The Roots of Women's Liberation in the Civil Rights Movement and the New Left* (New York: Knopf, 1979); and S. Morgen, *Into our Own Hands: The Women's Health Movement in the United States, 1969–1990* (New Brunswick, NJ: Rutgers University Press, 2002).

24. *Roe v. Wade*, 410 U.S. 113 (1973). For more discussion of the history and politics of abortion rights, see R. Solinger, *Abortion Wars: A Half Century of Struggle, 1950–2000*

(Berkeley, CA: University of California Press, 1998); and L. J. Reagan, *Dangerous Pregnancies: Mothers, Disabilities, and Abortion in Modern America* (Berkeley, CA: University of California Press, 2010).

25. Roth, *Making Women Pay*, p. 146; C. R. Daniels, 'Between Fathers and Fetuses: The Social Construction of Male Reproduction and the Politics of Fetal Harm', *Signs*, 22:3 (Spring 1997), pp. 579–616, on pp. 584–7, 594. See also L. E. Gomez, *Misconceiving Mothers: Legislators, Prosecutors, and the Politics of Prenatal Drug Exposure* (Philadelphia, PA: Temple University Press, 1997).

26. A. M. Hricko and C. Baglet Marrett, 'Women's Occupational Health: The Rise and Fall of a Research Issue', p. 8, folder 126, box 7, Harriet L. Hardy Papers, Schlesinger Library, Radcliffe College, Radcliffe University Libraries, Cambridge, MA.

27. Daniels, 'Between Fathers and Fetuses', pp. 594–6.

28. Daniels, *At Women's Expense*, pp. 63–4; Office of Technology Assessment, *Reproductive Health Hazards in the Workplace* (Washington, DC: Government Printing Office, 1985), p. 264; S. Kenney, *For Whose Protection? Reproductive Hazards and Exclusionary Policies in the United States and Great Britain* (Ann Arbor, MI: University of Michigan, 1992).

29. W. Williams, 'Firing the Woman to Protect the Fetus: The Reconciliation of Fetal Protection with Employment Goals under Title VII', *Georgetown Law Journal*, 69 (1981), pp. 641–704; Roth, Making Women Pay, p. 77. Roth argues that this case was mostly likely the rationale for the previously mentioned two state laws prohibiting sterilization as a condition of employment.

30. Roth, *Making Women Pay*, pp. 49–51.

31. New York Committee on Occupational Safety and Health (NYCOSH) Records, box 1, folder 'NYCOSH Minutes 1979–1981', Tamiment Library/Robert F. Wagner Labor Archives, New York University, New York; Hepler, *Women in Labor*, ch. 7; G. Markowitz and D. Rosner, *Deceit and Denial: The Deadly Politics of Industrial Pollution* (California: Millbank Books, 2003), pp. 123–8.

32. E. Bingham (ed.), *Proceedings of the Conference on Women and the Workplace, June 17–19, 1976* (Washington, DC: Society for Occupational and Environmental Health, 1977), p. 271, found in Library of the American College of Obstetricians and Gynecologists, Washington, DC.

33. *Proceedings of the Conference on Women and the Workplace*, pp. 287, 164, 272, 165, 359–60, ACOG. DES is diethelstibestrol, a drug prescribed to pregnant women to prevent miscarriages, was, in 1971, linked to increased risks of vaginal and cervical cancer in daughters exposed *in utero*.

34. *Reflections on OSHA's History* (Washington, DC: US Department of Labor, 2009); Daniels, *At Women's Expense*, p. 92.

35. R. K. Robinson, D. E. Terpstra and B. G. Malcolm, 'International Union v. Johnson Controls: Resolving the Dilemma between Fetal Protection Policies and Equal Employment Opportunities', *Employee Responsibilities and Rights Journal*, 5 (1992), pp. 309–21, on p. 311.

36. Ibid. The authors note on p. 311 that 'none of these eight pregnancies resulted in an abnormal birth'.

37. Daniels, *At Women's Expense*, p. 68.

38. L. Greenhouse, 'Justices Listen to Arguments on Fetal-Protection Policy', *New York Times*, 11 October 1990, p. A20; Daniels, *At Women's Expense*, p. 70.

39. P. Lehman, 'Women Workers: Are They Special?' *Job Safety and Health*, 3 (April 1975), p. 12.

40. Cited in Daniels, *At Women's Expense*, p. 73.

41. P. Kilborn, 'Who Decides Who Works At Jobs Imperiling Fetuses?' *New York Times*, 2 September 1990, pp. A1, 28; Daniels, *At Women's Expense*, p. 88.

42. D. Stone, 'Fetal Risks, Women's Rights: Showdown at Johnson Controls' (Robert Wood Johnson Fund, September 1990); J. M. Stellman, *Women's Work, Women's Health: Myths and Realities* (New York: Pantheon Books, 1977), p. 179 (emphasis in original).

43. Kilborn, 'Who Decides Who Works At Jobs Imperiling Fetuses?', pp. A1, 28; Greenhouse, 'Justices Listen to Arguments On Fetal-Protection Policy', p. A20; UAW brief cited in Daniels, *At Women's Expense*, p. 84.

44. 'Court Backs Right of Women to Jobs with Health Risks', *New York Times*, 21 March 1991, p. A1; *International Union, United Automobile Workers* v. *Johnson Controls, Inc.*, 111 S.Ct. 1196 (1991).

45. Daniels, *At Women's Expense*, pp. 90, 94 (emphasis in original).

46. Roth, *Making Women Pay*, pp. 79, 87.

47. R. Rosen, 'What Feminist Victory in the Court?' *New York Times*, 1 April 1991, p. A32.

48. These are proposed by Robinson, et al., 'Resolving the Dilemma between Fetal Protection Policies and Equal Employment Opportunities', pp. 317–20; http://govpulse. us/entries/1994/05/20/94-12311/johnson-controls-inc-bennington-vt-negative-determination-on-reconsideration (United States Department of Labor, 20 May 1994) [accessed 15 April 2010].

49. Roth, *Making Women Pay*, p. 87.

50. S. U. Samuels, 'The Fetal Protection Debate Revisited: The Impact of UAW v. Johnson Controls on the Federal and State Courts', in *Women's Rights Law Reporter 17* (Spring 1996), pp. 1–20, on pp. 4–6, found in *Lexsee 17 Women's Rights L. Rep. 209*.

51. Roth, *Making Women Pay*, p. 49.

52. Hricko and Marrett, 'Women's Occupational Health: The Rise and Fall of a Research Issue'.

53. Roth, *Making Women Pay*, p. 196.

INDEX

abortion, 11, 16, 35, 109, 110, 113, 114, 119, 120, 121, 126, 154
   spontaneous, 152, 155, 162
Abortion Act 1967, 114
Addams, Jane, 147
adoption, 10, 39, 50, 51, 52, 54, 58–9, 60–1, 62, 121, 124, 126
Adoption Act 1926, 51, 59, 60
Adoption of Children (Regulations) Act 1943, 60
adultery, 120, 124, 125
alcohol, and pregnancy, 35, 43, 117, 154, 155
Alliance of Honour, 33
American Academy for the Advancement of Science, 156
American Civil Liberties Union, 159
American Cyanamid, 155, 158
antenatal care, 1, 2, 9, 28, 31–46, 48, 56–7, 59, 61, 62, 69–70, 71, 100, 104, 105, 112, 129, 132, 140
antenatal hygiene, 32–6, 40, 43, 44, 75
Arney, William R., 3
artificial insemination, 10, 112–27
   by donor (AID), 115
   by husband and donor (AIHD), 125
Association for Improvements in the Maternity Services, 143

Baetjer, Anna, 152
Baird, Sir Dugald, 2, 11, 12, 57
Balfour, Lady Frances, 38
Ballantyne, Dr John W., 9, 10, 31, 32–9, 40–1, 42, 43, 44, 45, 46, 56
Balls-Headley, Dr Walter, 33
Banta, Dr H. David, 132
Baptist Union of Scotland, 121

Barney, Nora S., 151
Barrer, Nina, 90
Barry, Dr Arthur P., 110
Bevan-Brown, Dr Maurice, 94
Beveridge Report, 61, 105–6
birth abnormalities *see* teratology
birth control, 107–9, 111, 113, 120
Booth, Charles, 47
Borst, Charlotte, 7
Boston Women's Health Collective, 2
Boyd, Dr Hugh, 23
Brew, Helen, 92, 94
British College of Obstetricians and Gynaecologists, 77, 84
British Medical Association, 44, 84
Burke, Seamus, 102

caesarean section, 6, 24, 28, 70, 71, 79, 92, 109–10, 130, 131, 137, 139–40, 141, 145, 146
Cameron, Sir Charles A., 100–1
Campbell, Dame Janet, 69
Campbell, Mary, 17, 21, 25
Carey, Dr Harvey, 93, 94–5, 96
Carnegie UK Trust, 44, 53, 54
Cartwright, Ann, 134, 135
Catholic Action, 109
Catholic Truth Society, 108
Censorship and Publication Act 1929 (Ireland), 109
Central Midwives Board for Scotland, 53
Chalmers, Dr Archibald K., 48, 51, 56–7
childbirth, hospitalization of, 1, 2, 3, 4, 6, 7, 8, 14, 29, 45, 57, 65–6, 67–9, 73, 74, 79–80, 81–2, 84, 85, 86–92, 96–7, 100, 101, 103–4, 112, 130
Children's Act 1908, 48

Church of England, 49, 109
Church of Ireland, 109
Church of Scotland, 10, 47–73, 121
    Committee for Christian Life and Social
        Work, 60
    Committee of Life and Work, 60
    Committee on Social Work, 47, 52, 58,
        60
    Moral Welfare Scheme, 60
Civil Rights Act 1964 (US), 153, 154, 157,
    159
Coalition for the Reproductive Rights of
    Workers (US), 156
Collis, Dr W. R. F., 106
Commission on the Relief of the Sick and
    Destitute Poor 1927, 102
Committee of Inquiry into Maternity Ser-
    vices 1937 (NZ), 85, 86, 87, 89, 90
Concerned Women of America, 158
Coney, Sandra, 82
contraception *see* birth control
Coombe Lying-In Hospital, Dublin, 104,
    109, 110
Corkill, Dr Thomas, 85
Coroners Act 1890 (Victoria), 15
Country Women's Association (Victoria),
    27
Coutts, Ann, 19, 26
Craig, Miss M., 60
Craiglockhart Poor Law Institution, Edin-
    burgh, 66, 73
craniotomy, 35, 71
Criminal Law Amendment Act 1935 (Ire-
    land), 109
Croom, Dr John H., 38
Crowther, Vera, 87, 93

Daly, Mary E., 103, 108
Daniels, Cynthia, 154–5, 160
Davidson, Flora L., 61
Davis-Floyd, E., 4
Dawson, Dr J. Bernard, 85, 86, 92
DBCP, 155, 157
Deaconess Hospital, Edinburgh, 66, 68, 77
Department of Health (Ireland), 105, 106
Department of Health for Scotland, 57, 115,
    116

Departmental Committee on Human
    Artificial Insemination *see* Feversham
    Committee
DES Action Network (US), 157
dibromochloropropane *see* DBCP
Dick Read, Dr Grantly, 93
Dobbie, Mary, 94
domiciliary birth *see* home birth
Donald, Dr Ian, 131
Donnison, Jean, 7, 92
Dougall, Miss, 60, 61
Douglas and McKinlay Report *see Report on
    Maternal Morbidity and Mortality in
    Scotland* 1935
Dublin Corporation, 100, 101
    Chief Health and Medical Officer, 100
    maternity and child welfare services, 104

Edinburgh City Council/Corporation, 45,
    71, 73
    Maternity and Child Welfare Depart-
        ment, 45
    Maternity and Child Welfare Scheme,
        32, 45
Edinburgh Lying-In Institution, 66, 77
Edinburgh Medical Missionary Society, 33
Edinburgh Obstetrical Society, 34
Edinburgh Royal Maternity Hospital, 31,
    65–80
    Ladies Committee, 67
    Married Women's Pavilion, 67
    pre-maternity ward, 31, 37, 39, 40–3, 46
    Stenhouse branch, 74
Edinburgh Women Citizens Association, 75
Ehrenreich, Barbara, 4, 7
Elliot, Eliza, 26
Elliot, Dr T. E., 77
Elsie Inglis Memorial Maternity Hospital,
    Edinburgh, 66, 67, 68, 69, 74, 75, 76,
    77, 80
English, Deirdre, 4, 7
epidural anaesthesia, 6, 130, 137–9, 142
    see also pain relief
episiotomy, 6, 92, 130, 132–3, 134, 136, 146
Equal Employment Opportunity Commis-
    sion (US), 153
Equal Rights Amendment 1923 (US), 150
eugenics, 36, 113, 117, 118
Exxon, 155, 158

fallen women *see* unmarried mothers
Faludi, Susan, 161
family planning, 110, 111–12
  see also birth control
Federation of Parents Centres (NZ) *see*
  Parents Centre (NZ)
Feeney, Dr J. K., 110
feminism, 1, 2–6, 10, 11–12, 81–2, 86, 87,
  89, 93, 113, 126, 129, 134, 147, 148,
  149–50, 152–4, 156–7
Fenwick, Dr Henry M., 24, 25
Ferguson, Dr James H., 31, 38, 42, 43, 56
fetal protection laws, 11, 152, 153, 154–6,
  162
  workplace policies, 157–9
fetal rights, 11, 152, 153, 154, 154–6, 160,
  161, 162
Feversham Committee, 114, 115–16, 117,
  118, 119, 120–1, 122, 123, 124, 125–6
Foucault, Michel, 3, 81
Free Church of Scotland, 121
Free Presbyterian Church of Scotland, 121
Freeland Barbour, Dr A. H., 37
Freeth, Dr Audrey, 117, 119
Frimley Park Hospital, Camberley, 130, 139,
  140, 141, 143

General Motors, 152
Glasgow Home for Deserted Mothers, 51,
  54
Glasgow Lock Hospital, 51, 53, 54
Glasgow Royal Maternity Hospital, 51, 57
Globe Union, 157
Goldstein, Hannah, 17, 19–20, 24, 25, 26
Gordon, Dr Doris, 89–90
Gordon, Mrs, 61
grand multiparae, 72, 110–11
Green, Dr Herbert, 95–6

Hamilton, Alice, 147–8, 152, 162
Hamilton, Dr James, 37
Hamilton Ward *see* Edinburgh Royal Mater-
  nity Hospital pre-maternity ward
Health Act 1953 (Ireland), 107
Health (Amendment) Act 1991 (Ireland),
  107
Health (Family Planning) Act 1979 (Ire-
  land), 109, 111
Health and Hygiene Exhibition 1928, 75

health visitors, 5, 6, 31, 45, 59, 102, 105
Henderson, Cecile, 58, 59, 60
Herbert Street Maternity Home, Glasgow,
  52–3
home birth, 6, 8, 13, 14, 43, 65, 66, 67–9,
  72, 73, 74, 77, 80, 84, 86, 88, 91, 104,
  129, 143–4
Hospice, The, Edinburgh *see* Elsie Inglis
  Memorial Maternity Hospital
Hricko, Andrea, 162
Humane Vitae 1968, 111

illegitimacy *see* unmarried mothers
induced birth, 6, 23, 40, 43, 70–1, 130, 132,
  134–7, 130, 140, 141, 146
industrial toxicology, 147, 148
Industrial Welfare and Efficiency Confer-
  ence, Pennsylvania, 147
Infant Aid Society, 101
infant mortality, 31, 35, 43, 47–8, 55, 56, 62,
  83, 90, 99–100, 101, 102, 106, 129
infertility, 1, 9–10, 90, 113–27
Institute of Epidemiology and Health Ser-
  vices Research, Leeds University, 132
Inter-Departmental Committee on Physical
  Deterioration, 48
Irish Free State, 99, 109
Irish Hospitals Sweepstake, 103
Irish Housewives Association, 111
Irish Medical Association, 105, 106–7

Jamieson, Dr James, 16, 21, 23, 27, 28
Jellett, Dr Henry, 84
John Radcliffe Hospital, Oxford, 130, 132,
  136
  GP Unit, 130
Johnson, Agnes K., 88–9
Johnson Controls v. *UAW* 1991, 148–9,
  159–61

Kennedy, Dr Alexander, 125
Kitzinger, Sheila, 93, 129, 133, 140–1, 143
Knight's Index, 15–16

Lady Dudley Nursing Scheme, 102
Lansdowne House, Glasgow, 56, 58–9,
  60–1, 62
Lauriston Pre-Maternity Home, Edinburgh,
  9, 31, 32, 37, 38–9, 40, 41, 42, 43, 46

Leavitt, Judith W., 2, 8
Lewis, Jane, 3, 88
Liston, Dr, 78
Local Government Board for England, 44, 54
Local Government Board for Scotland, 44, 54, 56, 69
Loudon, Irvine, 7–8, 8–9, 81, 88, 91, 105
Lowe, Dr Edward, 85

Macgregor, Dr Alexander S., 57
MacGregor, Dr Duncan, 83
Mackenzie, Sir William L., 44, 53
Maclean, Hester, 86
MacLennan, Hector, 116, 118, 119, 120, 121, 122
Magdalene Homes, 49, 51, 54
Mansie, Revd John, 52
Marks, Lara, 5, 6
Marland, Hilary, 5
maternal and child welfare movement, 31, 41, 44–5, 46, 48, 54, 55
maternal mortality, 1, 8, 9, 16, 18, 28, 48, 57, 58, 62, 69, 70, 76, 81, 83, 88, 90, 99, 100, 102, 103, 105, 108, 129
Maternity and Child Welfare Act 1918, 45, 55, 102
Maternity and Child Welfare Scheme (Edinburgh), 32, 45, 68, 69
Maternity Hospital, Wokingham, 130
Maternity Services (Scotland) Act 1937, 48, 58
Mazzochi, Anthony, 156–7
McDonald, Dr John, 125
McKeown, Thomas, 7
McVey, Dr Hugo, 109
Medical Defence Union, 116
Medical Research Council, 40, 44
Melbourne, General Hospital, 24
Midwives Act 1902, 7
Midwives Act 1936, 84
Midwives and Maternity Homes (Scotland) Act 1927, 57
Midwives Registration Act 1904 (NZ), 83, 86
Midwives (Scotland) Act 1915, 48, 53
midwives, training and regulation of, 8, 13, 17–18, 26, 29, 31, 37, 49, 53, 65, 66, 83, 84, 103

milk depots, 45, 48
Miller, Dr Douglas, 75–6
Ministry of Health, 44, 84
Minnitt 'gas and air' machine, 77
Mitchinson, Wendy, 4, 8, 9
Molesworth, Nellie, 87
More, Sister, 73
Muller, Curt, 149
Muller v. Oregon, 1908, 148, 149–50
Murphy-Lawless, Jo, 4, 82

National Birthday Trust Fund, 5, 88, 89
National Childbirth Trust, 6, 133, 140, 143, 144, 145–6
National Conference on Infant Mortality 1914, 43, 48
National Consumer Council (NZ), 96
National Council for Public Morals, 33
National Council of Women (NZ), 86, 90, 92, 95, 96
    Auckland branch, 89
    Christchurch branch, 89
national efficiency, 47, 48, 83, 90
National Health Service, 50, 116
National Institute for Occupational Safety and Health (US), 157
National Maternity Hospital, Dublin, 104, 105, 109, 110, 111
National Organization for Women (US), 153
National Woman's Party (US), 150
National Women's Hospital, Auckland, 91, 92, 94, 95
natural childbirth, 6, 8, 18, 22, 27, 29, 88, 93–4, 95, 133, 142, 143, 144, 145
Natural Childbirth Association (NZ) *see* Parents Centre (NZ)
Natural Childbirth Association (UK) *see* National Childbirth Trust
Neild, Dr James, 26
New Deal, 150
New Zealand Department of Health, 82, 85, 88, 89, 91–2
    Consultant Obstetrician, 84
    Director of the Division of Nursing, 86, 95
    General Principles of Maternity Nursing, 95
    Inspector of Maternity Hospitals, 85

New Zealand Nurses and Midwives Board, 95–6
New Zealand Obstetrical Society, 84, 89–90
New Zealand Registered Nurses' Association, Obstetrical Branch, 89
Newman, Sir George, 44
Newsholme, Sir Arthur, 44
Notification of Birth (Extension) Act 1915, 45, 101, 102
Notification of Births Act 1907, 48, 100–1
Nurses Registration Act 1901 (NZ), 82

Oakley, Ann, 2, 3, 4, 81, 129
obstetric anaesthesia *see* epidural anaesthesia; pain relief
Occupational Safety and Health Act 1970 (US), 157
Oil, Chemical and Atomic Workers Union (US), 156–7

Paget, Dr Tom, 85
pain relief, 19–20, 22, 76–8, 79, 80, 85, 86–7, 88, 89, 91, 92, 93–4, 97, 134, 138, 141, 142, 146
paraldehyde, rectal, 77–8
Parents Centre (NZ), 92–3, 94, 96
perinatal mortality, 1, 129, 131, 134
Pfeffer, Naomi, 113
Pleasant Sunday Afternoon Brotherhood, 33
Plunkett, Dr Tom, 92, 93
Pope Pius XII, 111
postnatal care, 53, 54, 56, 61, 62, 74, 76, 112, 141
post-partum haemorrhage, 2, 15, 16, 19, 20, 21–2, 23, 25, 28, 92
Pregnancy Discrimination Act 1978 (US), 154, 156, 159
Pre-maternity *see* antenatal
Protchownick, Dr Ludwig, 40
Public Health Department, Edinburgh, 45, 69, 74, 75
puerperal infection, 2, 3, 23, 57, 69, 76, 92, 95

Queen's Institute for District Nursing, 102

Ramsay, Mrs, 17–18, 19, 25
Reiger, Kerreen, 5, 93
religion, impact on maternity, 10, 11, 12, 32, 33, 36, 47–63, 99, 104, 105, 106–7,

108–10, 111, 112, 114, 117, 119, 120–1
Report of the Royal Commission on Physical Training (Scotland) 1903, 48
Report on Maternal Morbidity and Mortality in Scotland 1935, 57, 59
Report on the British Health Services (PEP), 57
Report on the Physical Welfare of Mothers and Children ... Scotland 1917, 53
rescue work *see* unmarried mothers
Roberts, Dr Norbert, 158
Robinson, Jean, 143
Roe v. *Wade*, 1973, 154
Roth, Rachel, 156, 160
Rotunda Hospital, Dublin, 84, 104, 106, 109, 110
Routh, Dr Amand, 44
Rowntree, B. S., 47
Royal Berkshire Hospital, Reading, 130, 135, 143
Royal Buckinghamshire Hospital, Aylesbury, 130, 136
Royal College of Surgeons of Edinburgh, 115, 118, 119, 122
Royal Infirmary of Edinburgh, 33, 74
    infertility and gynaecological outpatient clinic, 114, 122–3, 124
    out-patient infertility clinic, 10
    Royal Samaritan Hospital for Women, Glasgow, 116
Royal Society of Medicine, Obstetric and Gynaecological Section, 44
Russell, Dr Matthew J., 103
Ruzek, Sheryl, 3, 81
Ryan, Dr Andrew, 106–7
Ryan, Dr Charles S., 20

Salvation Army, 38, 49, 83
Sanitary Association, 43
Scalia, Antonin, 159
Scottish Committee of Catholic Union, 121
Scottish Episcopal Church, 121
Seddon, Richard J., 83
Sharman, Dr Albert, 116, 117, 118, 124
Siedeberg McKinnon, Dr Emily, 87–8
Simpson, Dr Alexander R., 33–4, 37, 38, 42, 56
Simpson, Sir James Y., 33

Sixth International Congress of Catholic Doctors, 110
Skene, Dr David, 49
Smith, Dr Elizabeth, 53
Smith, Professor T. B., 116
Social Security Act 1938 (NZ), 91
Society for Occupational and Environmental Health (US), 156
Society for the Protection of Women and Children (NZ), 86, 89, 91
    Auckland branch, 87
Society for the Study of Inebriety, 53
Solomons, Dr Bethel, 109, 110
Spain, Dr Alex, 105, 109, 110
sperm donors, 10, 114, 115–16, 117–18, 119, 120–1, 122, 124, 125, 126–7
St Helens hospitals (NZ), 83–4, 86, 87, 89, 97
    Auckland, 87, 91
    Christchurch, 89
    Dunedin, 88
    Wellington, 83
St Luke's Home, Edinburgh, 38
St Machar's Kirk Session, Aberdeen, 49
St Mary's Hospital, Manchester, 110–11
St Peter's Hospital, Chertsey, 140
St Thomas's Hospital, London, 136
Stanton, Elizabeth C., 151
Stellman, Jeanne, 159
stillbirth, 70, 71, 89, 91, 152, 154
Stopes, Marie, 120
Sweetnam, William F., 25
syphilis *see* venereal disease

temperance movement, 33, 35, 36, 46
teratology, 34–5, 36
termination of pregnancy *see* abortion
Tew, Marjorie, 4, 7
Thacker, Dr Stephen B., 132
Thompson, Susannah, 26
Thornton, Miss C., 101
Torrance, Miss, 53, 54, 56, 58, 62
Tracy, Dr Richard, 22
twilight sleep, 5, 78, 89

UAW v. *Johnson Controls* 1991, 148, 159–61
ultrasound scans, 6, 129, 130, 131–2, 141
United Auto Workers, 158, 159

United Free Church of Scotland, 33, 43, 49, 52, 57, 120
University of Melbourne, obstetrics course, 22
unmarried mothers, 38
    in Australia, 24
    in Ireland, 104, 105, 111
    in New Zealand, 83
    in Scotland, 9, 10, 11, 31, 37, 38, 39, 40, 42, 46, 47–63, 67
US Catholic Conference, 158
US Department of Labor, Women's Bureau, 150–1
US Supreme Court, 148, 149, 153, 159, 161, 162

Vallgarda, Signild, 86, 91
venereal disease, 33, 35, 45, 51, 70
Venereal Diseases (Scotland) Act 1917, 45
Voluntary Health Insurance Board (Ireland), 108

Wallingford Community Hospital, 130, 130
Walters, Rhiannon, 133
Watson, Revd David, 52
West London Hospital, 141
Western General Hospital, Edinburgh, 66, 67
Whitson, Thomas B., 75
Williams, Susan, 5
women, and agency, 2–6, 9, 11–12, 46, 50, 54, 79, 90, 91, 92, 96–7, 123, 124
Women's Cooperative Guild, 3, 44
women's health movement, 2, 3, 4
Women's Hospital, The, Melbourne, 14, 18, 19, 24, 25
women's movement, 11, 38, 81, 111, 153, 154
Women's Political Action-Occupational Health Caucus (US), 156
World War II, impact of, 50, 60–1, 106, 151
Wright, Nurse M. C., 78

Young, Dr J. H., 110–11
Young Women's Christian Association (YWCA), 51, 74